LIBRARY

College of Physicians and Surgeons
of British Columbia

Health Management for Older Adults

Health Management for Older Adults: Developing an Interdisciplinary Approach

Edited by

David G. Satin, MD

Division on Aging
Assistant Clinical Professor of Psychiatry
Harvard Medical School

OXFORD
UNIVERSITY PRESS

2009

OXFORD
UNIVERSITY PRESS

Oxford University Press, Inc., publishes works that further
Oxford University's objective of excellence
in research, scholarship, and education.

Oxford New York
Auckland Cape Town Dar es Salaam Hong Kong Karachi
Kuala Lumpur Madrid Melbourne Mexico City Nairobi
New Delhi Shanghai Taipei Toronto

With offices in
Argentina Austria Brazil Chile Czech Republic France Greece
Guatemala Hungary Italy Japan Poland Portugal Singapore
South Korea Switzerland Thailand Turkey Ukraine Vietnam

Published by Oxford University Press, Inc.
198 Madison Avenue, New York, New York 10016
www.oup.com

Oxford is a registered trademark of Oxford University Press

Library of Congress Cataloging-in-Publication Data
Health management for older adults : developing an interdisciplinary approach / edited by David G. Satin.
   p. ; cm.
Includes bibliographical references.
ISBN 978-0-19-533571-2
1. Geriatrics.   2. Health services administration.   3. Older people—Services for—Management.
4. Gerontology. I. Satin, David G.
[DNLM: 1. Health Services for the Aged—organization & administration.
   2. Aged.   3. Delivery of Health Care.   4. Long-Term Care.   5. Organizational Case Studies.
   6. Patient Care Team—organization & administration. WT 31 H4343 2008]
RA564.8.H4283 2008
618.97—dc22
2008021761

9 8 7 6 5 4 3 2 1

Printed in USA
on acid-free paper

This textbook on the health-care system as it affects the health of older adults is dedicated to four older adults who helped us, both in the textbook and in the education program on which it is based, to keep our theory and practice congruent with the real lives of older adults. They were part of the core faculty of the education program, participating in the questioning and discussion in all class sessions. They acted as resource people when the validity or applicability of concepts and practices was being tested. They acted as mentors to students individually and in teams, offering mature support, information on real-life experience, and second opinions on student projects. In core faculty meetings they provided the perspective of the world of the older adult in curriculum planning and student evaluation. We are grateful for their enrichment of the health team with the role of the recipient of health care and for their mature comradeship.

Fay Salmon participated in the course from 1984 to 1990, when she was 85–92 years old. She demonstrated the sharp intellect and indomitable courage of an older adult who was disabled and living in an assisted living facility but interested and eager to continue as part of the world at large.

Margaret Lafferty participated in the course from 1997 to 2003, when she was 75–81 years old. Her sharp observational and literary skills gave us a perspective on five generations of her family spanning three centuries. She taught us the "inside feel" of growing into older ages and family roles.

Jeanette Burack participated in the course from 2004 through 2007, when she was 80–83 years old. Her indomitable will carried her—and us—through physical and emotional struggles with practical wisdom, a wry wit, and grandmotherly love.

Joanne Prince contributed to the course from 2005 through 2008 and beyond, when she was 74–77 years old. As older adult, nurse, and African-American she called our attention especially to concerns about advance planning for old age, the needs of the disadvantaged, and the realization that all generations share this voyage.

We are charged by their contributions and support to help young professionals help real older adults in a real world. This textbook is one way of doing so.

Preface

This text was written by the faculty of the interdisciplinary gerontology program which shares its title and embodies the educational approaches and goals progressively developed in that program. There are three goals:

1. *Environmental factors*: We teach about the environmental factors that shape the health care that older adults get and the practices of the health professionals who provide that care. These include policy, economics, regulation, administration, and social philosophy. This does not directly address clinical issues of health, illness, and treatment. However, it is addressed to clinicians as well as planners and administrators since the clinicians are directly affected by these environmental factors: They have a major influence on the ways clinicians practice in terms of program goals, resource allocation, job availability, reimbursement, standards of practice, legal liability, etc. They also have a major impact on the health care that older adults get as affected by health-care goals, programs, resources, funding, allowed professional services, availability, access, and so on. Thus, these matters are relevant to the education of those who create the environmental influences, those who practice under them, and those whose health and welfare are affected by them. For these reasons, this text should be valuable to all three groups.

2. *The interdisciplinary working relationship*: Theory and practice of various models of collaboration among health-care professionals are rarely, if ever, taught in programs that educate the various health disciplines. They are usually either considered irrelevant to disciplinary expertise, assumed to be intuitive, or left to experience. Thus, this approach can be learned well, inadequately, or not at all.

   We consider working relationships important to both the quality of health care that results from this work and the quality of the professional lives of the workers. Effective collaboration among multiple disciplines adds depth and breadth to understanding and addressing problems—whether the problems are individuals, populations, planning, or research. Dealing with the above-mentioned environmental factors emphasizes the fact that effective collaboration is important not only among clinicians, planners, and administrators but also between these groups. Planners need to know the clinical issues that will be affected by their plans, administrators need to know the plans they implement and the effects of this implementation, and clinicians need to know why and how plans are made and implemented that enable or disable their practices.

   Details of the interdisciplinary working relationship are addressed in several chapters. In addition, it is a theme in all the chapters that focus on other issues. And, finally, it is demonstrated in Chapter 2: The Reality of Being an Older Adult and Getting Health Care; Chapter 14: Functioning Interdisciplinary Teams; and Chapter 16: An Interdisciplinary Case Conference.

3. *New professional roles and skills*: The interdisciplinary approach introduces professionals in health care for older adults to a broader range of disciplines than they are likely to experience in their own disciplinary educations. In addition to learning to work with them, they learn from them, enriching their own disciplinary knowledge, skills, and values with relevant expertise from other disciplines. This text includes the perspectives and skills of a broad range of disciplines.

   Planners, administrators, and clinicians have considerable flexibility in their foci of practice. In learning more about each other's practices they can prepare themselves for cross-practice. For instance, planners and administrators may learn to apply their professional skills clinically to individuals or small groups. Clinicians may also expand their professional skills in administrative and planning roles. This text gives some perspective on all these spheres of practice.

   Finally, critical analysis, education, advocacy, and change agency are roles that may not be familiar in many professional identities. All disciplines may add one or more of these as a matter of career choice or out of a sense of larger professional responsibility. This text addresses these roles not only in Chapters 15 and 17 but also as professional practice to consider in almost all topic areas.

The context in which the health needs of older adults are addressed is increasingly important. To ignore it leads to confusion, frustration, and ineffectiveness. To address it helps understanding, appropriate response, the health of older adults, and the enrichment of professional lives. Therefore, this text is intended for planners, administrators, clinicians, older adults, and interested citizens. Its perspectives should be a useful addition to the literature and education in gerontology, geriatrics, and public policy.

In structure, the text begins with a prologue: the rationale for this text, the reality of older adult lives and health that anchors this education, as well as a case study that is referred to in all substantive chapters as a way of linking their various perspectives. Then, the climate of health management for older adults is explored in three modules, giving a societal perspective (issues generally applicable), an institutional perspective (addressing the institutional contexts in which health and health management are dealt with), and a health team perspective (dealing with the health disciplines and their working relationships). A bibliography for further reading is offered in each chapter. Finally, an epilogue applies this education in both a case conference by health professionals and reflections on the relation of this education to other professional education and professional practice. Thus, the text takes the issues of older adult health, health care, and professional practice from current realties through theory and context (from macro to micro) and finally to practical application. Build on this core education with other study, experience, and enrichment from colleagues from the widest possible range of disciplinary and life backgrounds.

David G. Satin

Contents

Contributors   *xiii*

1   Introduction: Health Management for Older
Adults and Disciplinary Working Relationships   3
Terry R. Bard, Nancy A. Lowenstein, and David G. Satin

2   The Reality of Being an Older Adult and Getting
Health Care   18
*Jeanette Burack, Janet Coté, Kay McGuire, Joanne Prince,
Renée Summers, Albert Taylor, and Charlotte Yacker*

3   The Older Adult Care, Training, Research, and
Planning Program   35
David G. Satin

4   The Structure and Financing of the Health-Care System:
Reality and Consequences   38
Laurence G. Branch and Kathryn H. Petrossi

5   Elder Autonomy and Consumer-Directed Care   67
Mark Sciegaj

6   Prevention   79
Sarita Bhalotra and John Orwat

7   Justice in Community Care   *106*
     John A. Capitman

8   Health Law for Older Adults   *130*
     Ellen A. Bruce

9   Acute Care: Access to Health Care   *149*
     Martin P. Solomon; David G. Satin, Editor

10   Long-Term Care   *163*
     Len Fishman with David G. Satin

11   Community-Based Care for the Elderly   *189*
     Seymour J. Friedland

12   Models of Disciplinary Practice   *207*
     Clare E. Safran-Norton and Susan Neary

13   Knowing the Individual Disciplines and Introduction to Team
     Development, Function, and Maintenance   *223*
     Jennifer L. Kirwin and Teresa T. Fung
     with Myrna D. Bocage, Nancy A. Lowenstein, Susan Neary, Clare
     E. Safran-Norton, David G. Satin, Ann Stahlheber

14   Functioning Interdisciplinary Teams
     A. The Mt. Auburn Hospital Multiple Sclerosis Comprehensive Care Center:
     Linda Y. Buchwald and Nancy A. Lowenstein
     with Kathleen Leahy, Donald Meyer, Steven Moskowitz, Susan Nutile, and
     Ann Pisani   240
     B. Sawtelle Hospice House:
     David G. Satin
     with Jane Duggan, Terry Fallon, Joan Key, Pat Kumph,
     Deborah Moore, and Sue Berger   258

15   Policy Making and Policy Changing   *272*
     Theodore Chelmow

16   An Interdisciplinary Case Conference   *301*
     Terry R. Bard, Sarita Bhalotra, Myrna D. Bocage, Laurence G. Branch,
     Ellen A. Bruce, John A. Capitman, Teresa T. Fung, Jennifer L. Kirwin,
     Nancy A. Lowenstein, Ralph Ranald, Clare E. Safran-Norton,
     David G. Satin, and Mark Sciegaj

17   Interdisciplinary Health Management for Older Adults:
     Professional Education and Practice   *318*
     Kimberly Armstrong, Terry R. Bard, Kathleen Boyle, Shannon Broverman,
     Peggy Brown, Jeanette Burack, Joan R. Drevins, Peter Maramaldi, Jennifer
     Pritchard, Erica Raine, Julie Salinger, David G. Satin, Kimberly Sauder,
     and Melanie Vaughn

Index   339

Contributors

TERRY R. BARD, DD, PhD   Clinical Instructor, Harvard Medical School, Boston, MA

SARITA BHALOTRA, MD, PhD   Associate Professor, Schneider Institute for Health Policy, Florence Heller Graduate School for Social Policy and Management, Brandeis University, Waltham, MA

LAURENCE G. BRANCH, PhD   Distinguished University Professor, College of Public Health, University of South Florida, Tampa, FL

ELLEN A. BRUCE, JD   Associate Professor, Gerontology Institute, University of Massachusetts Boston, Boston, MA

LYNDA Y. BUCHWALD, MD   Medical Director, Multiple Sclerosis Clinical Care Center; Chief of Neurology, Mt. Auburn Hospital, Cambridge, MA

JOHN A. CAPITMAN, PhD   Executive Director, Central Valley Health Policy Institute, California State University Fresno, Fresno, CA

THEODORE CHELMOW, MEd, MA, LMHC   Formerly Executive Office of Elder Affairs, Commonwealth of Massachusetts, Northampton, MA

LEN FISHMAN   President, Hebrew SeniorLife, Jamaica Plain, MA

SEYMOUR J. FRIEDLAND, PhD   Executive Director, Jewish Family and Children's Service, Waltham, MA

TERESA T. FUNG, ScD, RD   Assistant Professor, Department of Nutrition, Graduate School for Health Sciences, Simmons College, Boston, MA

JENNIFER L. KIRWIN, PharmD, BCPS   Associate Clinical Professor, Bouve College of Health Sciences, School of Pharmacy, Department of Pharmacy Practice, Northeastern University, Boston, MA

NANCY A. LOWENSTEIN, MS, OTR/L, BCPR   Associate Clinical Professor, Department of Occupational Therapy, Boston University College of Health & Rehabilitation Sciences: Sargent College, Boston, MA

SUSAN NEARY, PhD, RN, CS   Associate Clinical Professor, Department of Nursing, Graduate School for Health Sciences, Simmons College, Boston, MA

JOHN ORWAT, PhD   Assistant Professor, Loyola University Chicago, School of Social Work, Chicago, IL

KATHRYN H. PETROSSI, PhD   Tampa, FL

CLARE E. SAFRAN-NORTON, PhD, MS, PT, OCS   Assistant Professor, Physical Therapy Program, Graduate School for Health Sciences, Simmons College, Boston, MA

DAVID G. SATIN, MD   Assistant Clinical Professor, Division on Aging, Harvard Medical School, Newton, MA

MARK SCIEGAJ, PhD, MPH   Associate Professor of Health Policy and Administration, and Associate Director, Smart Spaces Center, Pennsylvania State University, State College, PA

MARTIN P. SOLOMON, MD   Medical Director, Brigham and Women's Primary Care Associates of Brookline, Brookline, MA

ANN STAHLHEBER, MS, RD, LD   Public Health Coordinator, Cardiovascular Health Program, Cuyahoga County Board of Health, Parma, OH

Health Management for Older Adults

1

Introduction

Health Management for Older Adults and Disciplinary Working Relationships

TERRY R. BARD, NANCY A. LOWENSTEIN, AND DAVID G. SATIN

The Need for This Text and Its Evolutions
TERRY R. BARD

Why Another Textbook on Geriatric Care?

As the core faculty for the only Harvard Medical School elective course on interdisciplinary care of aged persons gathered to prepare for the spring 2003 semester, discussion arose about how our students could benefit from a text that would include the scope of the course they were about to experience. This was not the first time that this faculty had raised this concern. About 15 years before, the same question emerged from the core faculty teaching an earlier iteration of the course. The textbook that the faculty wrote to meet this need, Satin, Blakeney, Bottomley, Howe, and Smith (editors), *The Clinical Care of the Aged Person: An Interdisciplinary Perspective* (NY: Oxford University Press, 1994), marked the first effort to explore the concept of truly interdisciplinary care, particularly from the clinical perspective. At that time, the field of geriatrics had achieved formal status as a clinical specialty in medicine and psychiatry; other clinical disciplines, too, began to offer specialized education. In addition, nonclinical professions were developing a special interest focus on aging. Interdisciplinary Care of the Aged Person remained a unique course offering within the Division of Aging at the Harvard Medical School. Its two-fold focus was on helping its students learn about and experience interdisciplinary care as well as providing specific clinical information about aging as understood from experts in a variety of disciplines. Class composition then and now includes students in medicine, nursing, social work, occupational and physical therapy, law, divinity school, public health, business and community administration, as well as a number of other academic arenas. Students gather from a number of universities and professional schools in addition to the Harvard University schools in an effort to achieve a broader-based and focused perspective on the care of the aged.

Many shifts have taken place since the formation of this class and the appearance of its first textbook. Social shifts; shifts in the provision and reimbursement of health care; changes in housing, rehabilitation, and acute care; and legal changes in estates, wills, and indemnification are but a few of the dimensions that suggested a shift as well in the focus of this ongoing course. Students were now receiving much more detail about clinical concerns for the elderly within their disciplines of study. New focus on time management and a variety of models for clinical reimbursement coupled with reduced resources and institutions for continuing care and rehabilitation began to threaten the application of the interdisciplinary construct offered in this course. The core faculty recognized these new challenges by shifting the focus of the course to reflect the realities faced by its students.

The course's evolution was not new, but the new focus constituted a dramatic shift in content. The faculty determined that the organizing feature of professional interdisciplinary care and/or management should remain central. Similarly, the aging person remained focal. Recognizing that students were now learning about particularities about the aging process within their own disciplinary education, the faculty decided that it would be helpful to consider three primary nexus arenas wherein aging and society interact. The first focus would be the community at large, in the provision of health care to the aged person, methods of medical coverage and reimbursement, access to care and support, and the social, ethical, political, and legal challenges these pose. The second focus would be on those institutions entrusted to the care of the aged including hospitals, long-term care and rehabilitation facilities, and community organizations. The third focus would be on the aged individual as he or she engages the world during this later stage in life.

After teaching this new curriculum over the past 3 years, it is not surprising that the faculty, once again, would reflect on the dearth of a common text to assist future students. Hence, this book provides the answer to the questions why another textbook and why another textbook now.

History and Theory of the Interdisciplinary Working Relationship
DAVID G. SATIN

> ... the social process of a ward is likely to involve typical patterns of stress. These patterns are derived from a number of factors—such as, the emotional impact of illness and death, typical ambivalences about nurturance and dependence so prevalent in human affairs, shifts in role functions emanating from within a profession or from somewhere up the hierarchy, and conflicting value orientations and expectations within a complex organization. Hospital staff groups, having to live in such continuous proximity and to function at a generally high level of task efficiency, appear prone to develop protective devices against disruption by ever-present stresses. Numbered among such protective reactions are: barriers to communication; carefully guarded lines of hierarchy and the rights of initiation of activities; and well defended functional domains. Because they serve a defensive function, these arrangements are not easily altered even though they seem, at times, to react adversely upon the emotional well-being of patients ... many staff members themselves are troubled by some of the inappropriate protective arrangements....[1]

The interdisciplinary approach is one of the main foci of this text and, thus, will be a constant motif. We present here one schema of the range of disciplinary working relationships, not because it is the only one but to provide a concept of "interdisciplinary" for perspective on the discussions that follow. Chapter 12 models of disciplinary practice will explore more deeply variations in definitions and applications of this approach.

We will start with the concept of "disciplines." We are referring to professions that have knowledge, skill, and value bases sufficiently different from one another that it requires some new learning to understand, much less join, them. Examples are psychiatry, nursing, public health, and law. Professions that may be said to be variants of one another, and thus share knowledge, skill, and value bases, we are not considering different disciplines. Examples are psychiatry, pediatrics, and gynecology. Thus, it is the working relationship among these significantly different disciplines that interests us.

Next, let us get a sense of bases of these disciplinary differences. Perhaps social need and the development of special expertise resulted in the development of early disciplines such as the priesthood, medicine, and the military. As needs multiplied and societal resources became available for division of labor, new disciplines developed, such as seamanship and engineering.

Of importance is the subdivision of existing disciplines, such as medicine elaborating surgery, internal medicine, and dentistry or the priesthood elaborating denominational clergy, politics, law, and policing. Also, additional disciplines may have developed as adjuncts and extenders of previous ones, such as medicine stimulating the development of nursing, occupational therapy, and physical therapy. And disciplines may have moved together as they subscribed to contemporary ideologies or opportunities to maintain or extend their practices. Examples are medicine, psychology, and social work. Finally, disciplines have moved apart, defining their own knowledge, skill, and value bases, such as medicine and nursing; or psychiatry, psychology, social work, and a variety of counseling specialties.

An understanding of this creation, subdivision, seeding, amalgamation, and segregation of disciplines is important in addressing their singularity or overlap with others. Since there is so much interrelation in their lineage, much overlap would be expected and is found. This leads to a tension between collaboration and integration among disciplines vs. autonomy and self-definition. Collaboration is motivated by an interest in collegiality, responding to the complexity of problems and professional growth. Autonomy is motivated by reaffirmation of identity, competition for recognition and status, and the search for and expansion of job security. Of course, disciplines have some special expertise that supports their separate identities. Beyond this, society has assigned them roles and statuses that maintain these identities. Beyond these, there is testing and adjusting of roles, scopes of practice, control of disciplinary membership and credentialing, and disciplinary relationships. These often justify disciplinary identities, but there are also motivations for disciplinary power, security, and income.

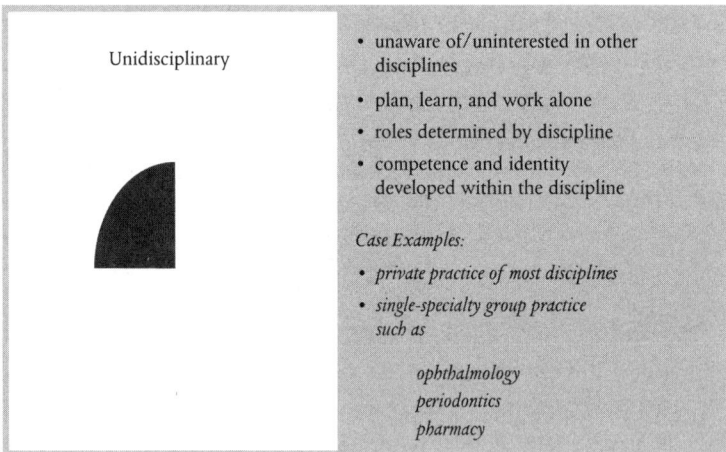

Unidisciplinary

- unaware of/uninterested in other disciplines
- plan, learn, and work alone
- roles determined by discipline
- competence and identity developed within the discipline

Case Examples:
- *private practice of most disciplines*
- *single-specialty group practice such as*

    ophthalmology
    periodontics
    pharmacy

Figure 1.1 Unidisciplinary.

We offer the following conceptual schema of disciplinary working relationships to provide a vocabulary with which to address the interdisciplinary aspect of the topics that follow in this text. This model can be tested and revised as it is applied and, in Chapter 13, will be placed in the perspective of other alternatives and experience.

First, let us organize the concept of uniqueness and overlap of disciplinary expertise as "spheres of competence" (see Tables. 1.1–1.3):

It can be asserted that all disciplines have primary, secondary, and tertiary spheres of competence, the specific domains constituting the real differences among the disciplines. Bear these distinctions and overlaps in mind when considering models of collaboration.

Now, we will apply these concepts of disciplinary expertise and overlap to a suggested range of disciplinary working relationships (see Figs. 1.1–1.5):

In the unidisciplinary model, disciplines exist without reference to any other. In the paradisciplinary model, disciplines are aware of other disciplines but not of their nature and do not interact. In the multidisciplinary model, disciplines understand one another but act autonomously; areas of

TABLE 1–1. Primary Competence

—unique or superior expertise
—function as sole or one of few consultants and trainers

TABLE 1–2. Secondary Competence

—useful expertise equaled by other disciplines
—problems referred to and training obtained from discipline with primary competence

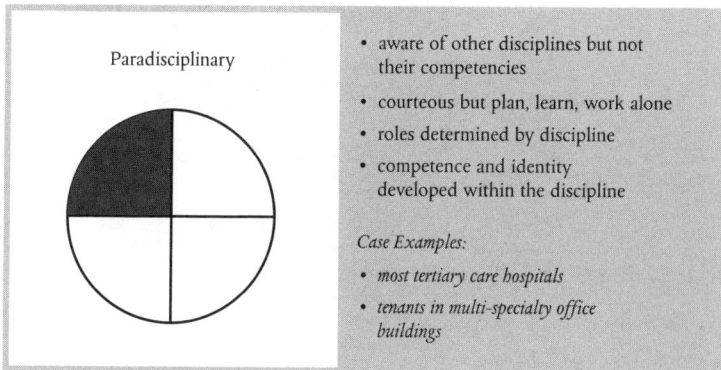

Paradisciplinary

- aware of other disciplines but not their competencies
- courteous but plan, learn, work alone
- roles determined by discipline
- competence and identity developed within the discipline

Case Examples:

- *most tertiary care hospitals*
- *tenants in multi-specialty office buildings*

FIGURE 1.2 Paradisciplinary.

- know other disciplines and their competences
- plan together
- learn and work alone; avoid intrusion on territories of other disciplines
- roles and determined by discipline
- competence and identity developed within the discipline

Case Examples:

- *geriatric "interdisciplinary" training with social work and nursing students working together and medicine fellows participating when they have time*

- *child psychiatry team—psychiatrist treats the child, psychologist tests the child, social worker gets history and supports the family, nurse supervises activities and medications*

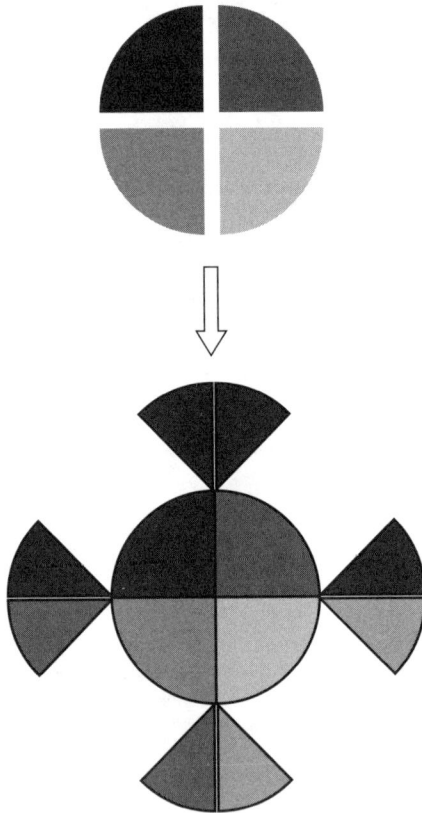

FIGURE 1.3 Multidisciplinary.

- know other disciplines and their competences
- learn and work together according to tasks
- assign roles by competence—disciplinary, personal, situational
- overlapping and flexible disciplinary roles
- competence and identity modified by experience, interests, and learning from other disciplines

Case Examples:

- *Mt. Auburn Hospital Multiple Sclerosis Team., with neurologist, nurse, occupational therapist, physical therapist, social worker getting information, deciding treatment, and assigning roles in appropriate task groups*

- *rural group practice – physicians, public health officers, nurses, clergy pooling information, determining treatment approach, assigning staff members' roles, and implementing treatment in appropriate task groups*

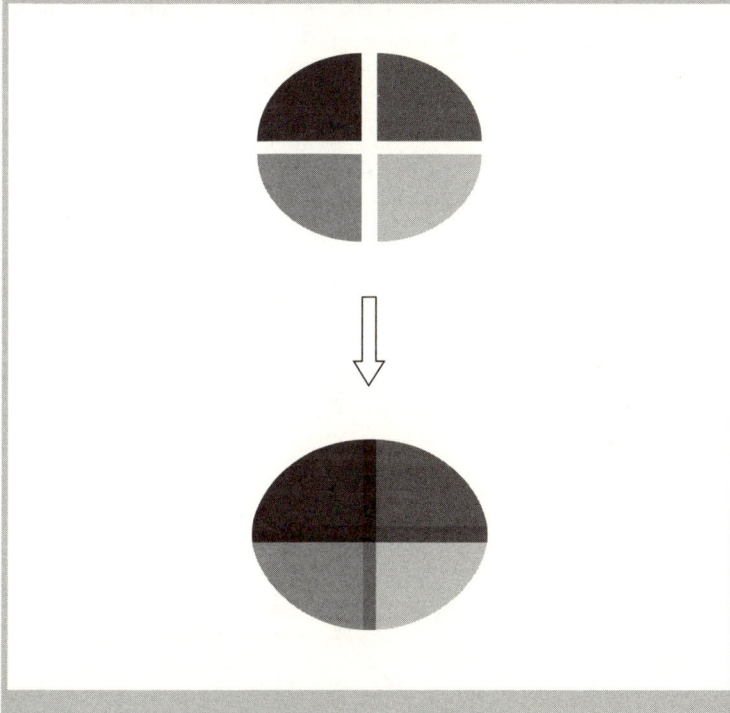

FIGURE 1.4 Interdisciplinary.

TABLE 1–3. Tertiary Competence

—little expertise
—refer all cases to disciplines with secondary or primary competence except give basic emergency help
—may or may not want training from discipline with secondary or primary competence

overlapping competence are excluded as conflicting and, thus, lost to use. In the interdisciplinary model, disciplines understand one another and areas of overlapping competence are integrated into (and enrich) team functioning. In the pandisciplinary model, the discipline again functions without reference to others.

Note that certain factors define and distinguish the working relationships:

1. The degree to which the disciplines know and care about one another
2. The degree to which they learn and work together
3. The flexibility of their roles and tasks in response to the needs of the project
4. The influence of factors other than discipline in determining roles and tasks
5. The degree to which professional identity and development are influenced by factors outside the parent discipline, including interaction with other disciplines

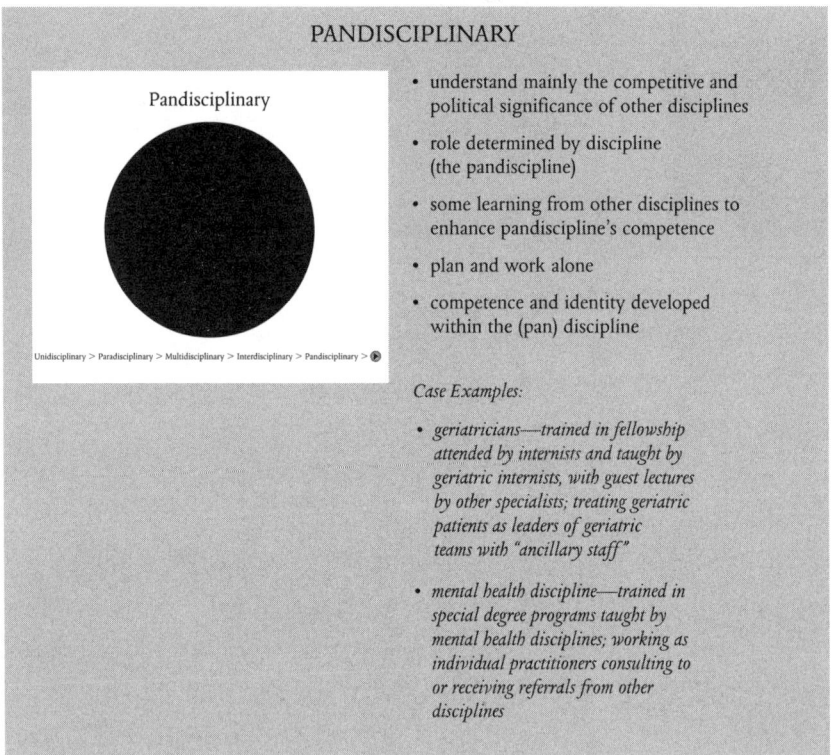

PANDISCIPLINARY

Pandisciplinary

Unidisciplinary > Paradisciplinary > Multidisciplinary > Interdisciplinary > Pandisciplinary > ▶

- understand mainly the competitive and political significance of other disciplines
- role determined by discipline (the pandiscipline)
- some learning from other disciplines to enhance pandiscipline's competence
- plan and work alone
- competence and identity developed within the (pan) discipline

Case Examples:

- *geriatricians—trained in fellowship attended by internists and taught by geriatric internists, with guest lectures by other specialists; treating geriatric patients as leaders of geriatric teams with "ancillary staff"*

- *mental health discipline—trained in special degree programs taught by mental health disciplines; working as individual practitioners consulting to or receiving referrals from other disciplines*

FIGURE 1.5 Pandisciplinary.

Note that the interdisciplinary model embodies the greatest interaction with other disciplines and the greatest flexibility and adaptability of role, task, and professional identity. It is also interesting that the pandisciplinary model, far from embodying the greatest disciplinary flexibility, returns to the disciplinary isolation of the unidisciplinary model.

Bibliography

Satin, D.G. A conceptual framework for working relationships among disciplines and the place of interdisciplinary education and practice: clarifying muddy waters. Gerontology and Geriatrics Education 1994;14(3):3–24.

Satin, D.G. The difficulties of interdisciplinary education: lessons from three failures and a success. Educational Gerontology 1987;13:53.

Satin, D.G. The interdisciplinary, integrated approach to professional practice with the aged. In: Satin, D.G. (ed.) The Clinical Care of the Aged Person: An Interdisciplinary Approach. New York: Oxford University Press, 1994, pp. 391–403.

References

1. Lindemann, E. The Role of Psychiatry at the M.G.H., 1965. Boston: Erich Lindemann Collection, Center for the History of Medicine, Francis A. Countway Library of Medicine, Harvard Medical School, 1965.

Teaching Interdisciplinary Teamwork
NANCY A. LOWENSTEIN

There are many different elements to consider in developing a curriculum on interdisciplinary teamwork, such as the content of the curriculum, barriers to implementing the curriculum, institutional support, and faculty training. This section will take a look at these and other issues that may arise when developing a curriculum to teach about interdisciplinary teamwork.

Each individual program needs to determine the content of the curriculum depending on its resources, but at least three distinct areas should be included. These are the basics of gerontology, how teams work, and an understanding of the current health-care delivery system related to elder care. Work by Reuben et al.[1] and Hall and Weaver[2] found that three other elements to consider when planning a curriculum are (1) faculty/students, (2) academic institutions, and (3) clinical sites. All three of these elements must buy into and be supportive of the concept of the interdisciplinary team. Students and faculty must understand how working on an interdisciplinary team is different from working on a multidisciplinary team; they must be instructed in the definitions and workings of the different types of teams and on group dynamics and teamwork. The institution must support the concept and logistics necessary for teaching about interdisciplinary teams, which might include multiple faculty members involved in one class in order to model teamwork; and any clinical sites used must agree to let students function as an interdisciplinary team and not a multidisciplinary team. Additionally, the curriculum should be a combination of didactic and clinical training.

There can also be barriers to implementing this type of curriculum. Hall and Weaver[2] looked at the literature on interdisciplinary education and found that issues or barriers emerged in two main areas: (1) the content of the curriculum and (2) the training of the professionals who are to be providing the care. Since the curriculum needs to involve didactic and clinical training and modeling of team roles by faculty, it is necessary for representatives from the different professions to be included in determining and creating the curriculum. All parties must come to a consensus on what needs to be included and the best ways to teach the content. Additionally, it is not clear when in the curriculum is the best time to include this content. It is important to consider the timing of this education in a professional's life. Since the underlying hallmark of interdisciplinary teams is a blurring of professional roles, the question arises as to whether these skills should be taught before students have a good understanding of the profession or later, after they have had time to understand their own professional philosophy, roles, etc. No clear consensus has been found in the literature on this issue, so it needs to be discussed before the content of the curriculum can be clearly laid out. In terms of methods employed to teach the skills for interdisciplinary care, Hall and Weaver[2] found that there is a large variety of methods employed, from problem-based learning and service learning formats to classroom instruction with use of role plays, videos, and case studies.

The role of faculty is key in developing a good program. Skinnar,[3] Fulmer et al.,[4] Reuben et al.,[1] and Hall and Weaver[2] all noted that most faculty currently in health-care disciplines are not trained in or are not comfortable teaching the concepts of interdisciplinary teamwork. Many have not worked as part of a team and must themselves learn new "knowledge, attitude and skills when facilitating interdisciplinary education."[2] Skinnar[3] also found another barrier to be that faculty does not have the necessary skills to advise and mentor students in this type of teamwork. This is important as one of the hallmarks of interdisciplinary education is good role modeling of interdisciplinary team work.[5]

One last systems issue described by Reuben et al.[1] and Hall and Weaver[2] is that of institutional support. Both note that without strong institutional support, interdisciplinary training is difficult to accomplish. This support must come in the way of financial support; time allowance for faculty to develop programs to coteach courses, mentor students, and process team issues; space support so that team members can have offices near each other; and finally, recognizing and valuing the work of interdisciplinary teams.

In regard to the curriculum itself, Hall and Weaver[2] found that skills in group development, communication, leadership, and conflict resolution were important to include in the curriculum. Others have found that the content of the curriculum needs to include information on the health-care system, geriatrics, and gerontology.[6] Additionally, it is expected that the different health-care disciplines will learn about their disciplines from each other, which returns to the earlier point of when to teach about interdisciplinary teams. If students are learning about other disciplines from each other, then shouldn't students have a good understanding of their own disciplines? On the flip side is the argument that students may be better able to understand and appreciate interdisciplinary care when they are more open to exploring what other disciplines have to offer and how their discipline can support or overlap with other members of the team.

There can be several professional or disciplinary barriers to developing interdisciplinary education. These may be put into a few general categories: the different level of knowledge and skills brought by students, differing jargon among disciplines, different philosophies of practice, different academic schedules among programs/schools, funding of programs, and faculty development.[3,6] Additionally, establishing partnerships with clinical settings that utilize interdisciplinary teams and are willing to develop a student-training program may be an obstacle. None of these barriers is insurmountable, but they should all be addressed when developing a curriculum.

The development of clinical training sites where students can see the interdisciplinary team in action is a consideration as well. These sites need to have faculty who are familiar with working as part of a team and willing to take time to involve students in a training program. Most academic settings are geared for this, but many community settings, where care of the elderly is given, are not set up as interdisciplinary teams or do not have the time to devote to student education. Some of the other challenges in these settings can be the differing academic schedules and required length of clinical rotations for students. Rotations may vary in length, time, and starting dates, as well as students' schedules of classes and other programmatic commitments. All of these issues need to be resolved before a clinical facility can commit to taking students.[5]

Perhaps the most comprehensive guide for developing training programs for interdisciplinary teams is the book *Geriatric Interdisciplinary Team Training*, edited by Siegler, Hyer, Fulmer, and Mezey.[5] This excellent book came about as a project funded by the John A. Hartford Foundation to implement training programs in geriatric interdisciplinary team training, or GITT. Eight sites around the country were funded to establish this curriculum, and this book describes the process fully.

In conclusion, there is no one way to implement a training program for interdisciplinary teams. A multitude of factors must be taken into account, and each institution involved must look at the resources, in terms of both financial and personnel resources that they are willing to give in developing, implementing, and maintaining the program. Without good support on the administrative level, the barriers to implementing a team training program may be too large to overcome. However, those institutions which have developed such programs have found them to be valuable and beneficial to all parties.

Bibliography

Fulmer, T., Flaherty, E., Hyer, K. The Geriatric Interdisciplinary Team Training (GITT) program. Gerontology and Geriatrics Education 2003;24(2):3–12.

Hall, P., Weaver, L. Interdisciplinary education and teamwork: a long and winding road. Medical Education 2001;35:867–875.

Howe, J.L., Mellor, M.J., Cassel, C.K. Cross-disciplinary approaches to teaching interdisciplinary teamwork and geriatrics. Gerontology and Geriatrics Education 1999;19(4):3–17.

Mellor, M.J., Hyer, K., Howe, J.L. The geriatric interdisciplinary team approach: challenges and opportunities in educating trainees together from a variety of disciplines. Educational Gerontology 2002;28:867–880.

Parham, I.A., Coogle, C.L., Welleford, E.A., Netting, F.E. Institutionalizing a multifaceted approach to geriatric interdisciplinary team training. Gerontology and Geriatrics Education 2003;23(4):41–56.

Reuben, D.B., Yee, M.N., Cole, K.D., Waite, M.S., Nichols, L.O. Benjamin, B.A., Zellman, G., Frank, J.C. Organizational issues in establishing geriatrics interdisciplinary team training. Gerontology and Geriatrics Education 2003;24(2):13–34.

Siegler, E.L., Hyer, K., Fulmer, T., Mezey, M. (eds.) Geriatric Interdisciplinary Team Training. New York: Springer, 1998.

Skinnar, J.H. Transitioning from multidisciplinary to interdisciplinary education in gerontology and geriatrics. Gerontology and Geriatrics Education 2001;21(3):73–85.

References

1. Reuben, D.B., Yee, M.N., Cole, K.D., Waite, M.S., Nichols, L.O. Benjamin, B.A., Zellman, G., Frank, J.C. Organizational issues in establishing geriatrics interdisciplinary team training. Gerontology and Geriatrics Education 2003;24(2):13–34.

2. Hall, P., Weaver, L. Interdisciplinary education and teamwork: a long and winding road. Medical Education 2001;35:867–875.

3. Skinnar, J.H. Transitioning from multidisciplinary to interdisciplinary education in gerontology and geriatrics. Gerontology and Geriatrics Education 2001;21(3): 73–85.
4. Fulmer, T., Flaherty, E., Hyer, K. The Geriatric Interdisciplinary Team Training (GITT) program. Gerontology and Geriatrics Education 2003;24(2):3–12.
5. Siegler, E.L., Hyer, K., Fulmer, T., Mezey, M. (eds.) Geriatric Interdisciplinary Team Training. New York: Springer, 1998.
6. Mellor, M.J., Hyer, K., Howe, J.L. The geriatric interdisciplinary team approach: challenges and opportunities in educating trainees together from a variety of disciplines. Educational Gerontology 2002;28:867–880.

Interdisciplinary Implications for Policy and Administrative Aspects of Health Management for Older Adults

DAVID G. SATIN

The interdisciplinary approach has implication in three areas for policy and administration of health management for older adults:

1. Attitude affected by the interdisciplinary perspective
2. Resources tailored by the interdisciplinary approach
3. Effect of the interdisciplinary approach on health-management policy and practice

Attitude Affected by the Interdisciplinary Perspective

The interdisciplinary approach is not the conventional one in education, professional practice, or the planning of health management; instead, these are based on the unidisciplinary approach (see earlier, "History and Theory of the Interdisciplinary Working Relationship"). Concepts of the identities of individual professionals, of the various professions, and of their training and practice are described in terms of autonomous disciplines. Health-care systems and health-management policies are built around these identities and practices.

The introduction of the interdisciplinary perspective challenges these personal and organizational disciplinary identities, suggesting their overlap in expertise, enrichment from exchange, and shared contributions to professional practice. While this cross-fertilization is intended to clarify, enrich, and empower the individual disciplines, it can be feared as questioning them or demeaning their value. It may be seen as adulterating the preparation and practice of these disciplines. It may be feared as converting professionals from their initial disciplines to others. New perspectives that require self-examination and change can also cause anxiety. These concerns may be overcome by the stimulation and opportunity that this new perspective offers. However, in the absence of supportive leadership and institutions, the new perspective often leads to skepticism, resentment, and resistance.

The contributions of the interdisciplinary approach to professional thinking are the enrichment of knowledge, skills, and values that comes from openness to other disciplines; the energizing that comes from self-reevaluation and opening of new pathways; the strength that comes from a mutually respectful and supportive work group; and the excitement of experiencing even repetitive tasks in new ways and with new approaches. The satisfaction of better outcomes of professional efforts goes without saying.

Resources Tailored by the Interdisciplinary Approach

As mentioned previously, educational institutions, professional organizations, and health-care agencies are organized around discrete disciplines, each with its own organizational hierarchy, location, schedule, membership, etc. Each discipline has acquired authority over these instruments of group function.

The interdisciplinary approach requires an interrelationship among disciplines. This applies not only to understanding, practice, and identity but also to the infrastructure in which disciplines function. Creative renovation is called for so that disciplines are physically accessible to one another, have common schedules, have units of function that accommodate multiple disciplines, and have time allocated for interaction. It also calls for supportive attitudes: a system of authority that will respect all disciplines, professional rewards for interdisciplinary effort (promotion, tenure, awards), and a general atmosphere of appreciation.

These require considerable thought and effort—and perhaps money. This renovation can be an exciting interdisciplinary exercise in itself, creating skills and comradeship through a common project. It can also represent public evidence of institutional affirmation of the interdisciplinary approach. On the other hand, this may represent a daunting task in reconfiguring institutional structure and thinking.

The benefits of these institutional reorganizations are more effective teaching, health care, planning, research, or whatever the program goals may be; reenergized staff, which is communicated to the recipients of their efforts; and more efficient functioning by reconsideration and improvement of structure and function, utilizing the widest range of disciplinary contributions.

Effect of the Interdisciplinary Approach
on Health-Management Policy and Practice

In terms of atmosphere, the attitudes and resource configuration encouraged by the interdisciplinary approach themselves influence the ways in which the host institutions function. Understanding of and involvement with a wide range of disciplines and access to a wide range of resources orient the institutions toward a broader and more inclusive approach to their tasks. An interdisciplinary perspective facilitates this approach, while a unidisciplinary perspective presents barriers to this approach.

In terms of task performance, the interdisciplinary approach presents health management with a broad, integrated perspective, whether it is regarding policy making, teaching, health care, or research. This encourages a comprehensive and integrated program. In contrast, the unidisciplinary approach presents a segmented perspective of special problems and solutions. This encourages a fragmented program, which may overlook or electively exclude some issues and areas of expertise.

Finally, these approaches may have implications for the level of prevention addressed in the programs in which they are applied. Some disciplines may be more oriented toward primary or postevent prevention (see Chapter 6 for a discussion of levels of prevention)—such as preventive medicine and public health. Some may be more oriented toward secondary prevention—such as medicine, nursing, and pharmacy. Some may be more oriented toward tertiary prevention—such as occupational and physical therapy and physiatry. And the prevention orientation of some disciplines (such as nursing, pastoral counseling, and social work) and some individuals in the above-mentioned disciplines may be broad and flexible, determined by the interests and experiences of individual practitioners or by the requirements of the problem at hand. The interdisciplinary approach is more likely to include all these levels of prevention among their varied participating disciplines and, thus, to offer all options. A unidisciplinary approach includes only those disciplines filling preplanned approaches to the program and the prevention levels they are used to. It risks missing the opportunity to build into the program other levels of prevention that had not been considered by the planners.

In summary, the disciplinary approach implicitly or explicitly influences the attitudes, structures, and products of programs. In addition, it brings a special openness, comprehensiveness, and creativity.

2

The Reality of Being an Older Adult and Getting Health Care

MODERATOR DAVID G. SATIN

PARTICIPANTS JEANETTE BURACK, JANET COTÉ, KAY McGUIRE, JOANNE PRINCE, RENÉE SUMMERS, ALBERT TAYLOR, AND CHARLOTTE YACKER

Introductions

RENÉE SUMMERS: *Shall we introduce ourselves? I'm Renée Summers. I've been told I should give my age: I'm 71. I'm married. My husband's still alive. He still works part-time. I work part-time as a counselor in the Pension Assistance Project at University of Massachusetts in Boston 2 days a week. And I was recently the editor of a newsletter from the alumni association.*

ALBERT TAYLOR: *I'm Al Taylor. I'm 77 years old. I'm retired and I love it. I'm a widower. My wife passed away in 2001 after a long bout with Alzheimer's. And I got involved with the University of Massachusetts in their educational programs and also a few doors opened up for me with the legislature, and now I am a Public Policy intern for the Legislative Caucus on Older Citizens Concerns. It's created a tremendous interest in me. Essentially, I feel great about my life right now. When my wife passed away I felt I had no obligations to anybody anymore except to myself, so I have to keep my mind active. And I decided I better go and get some more information about life, so I took a couple of courses here in the Gerontology Institute at the University of Massachusetts Boston, and I have a certificate from the Gerontology course that was offered by the institute called the Manning Certificate Course, and I went on to their Advanced Certificate Course, so I have two certificates, for which I'm lucky. I work with the elderly in many other ventures and I volunteer for many positions. I also read for the blind and in the Talking Information Center in Marshfield, Massachusetts, which broadcasts over the radio to blind people. We carry the frequency of the WATD radio station in Marshfield, and I just got into that last June and I'm loving it. I've never talked so much in my whole life. With that, I'll pass it on.*

KAY MCGUIRE: *My name is Kay McGuire, and I live in South Weymouth, Massachusetts. I'm 74 years old; I'll be 75 in September. My husband and I will be married for 55 years in August, and we have five grown children, eight grandchildren, and three great-grandchildren. Our newest great-granddaughter was just born January first. My husband worked till he was 74 and I had stayed at home with my five children most of their growing up years. But then when my youngest son was in the third grade—I was about 38 at that time—I started working as a kindergarten teaching assistant in the public schools, and I did that for 16 years and I really enjoyed it. Then my dad became too ill to live alone and my husband and I took him to live with us. So I quit my job, and my dad only lived a year but it was a very wonderful year for us and the family to help him and be able to have him at home with us. After that I saw an article about gerontology in the Boston Globe newspaper and I said, "Well, here's my opportunity! I don't have a job and my kids are grown up." And I went back to school at age 61 and I've been there ever since. I got a BA in gerontology, and I'm the legislative liaison for the Gerontology Institute, and Al and I work together up at the State House with the Elder Caucus. And I work with many other elderly groups as well. So, that's what I've been doing.*

SUMMERS: *I thought you were president of the Alumni Association.*

JANET COTÉ: *Good girls and fella! I'm Janet Coté, 74. I do volunteer work 2 days a week, Monday and Tuesday, at the New England Pensions Project, finding pensions for people. I'm in my sixth year doing that. And I recently took on 2 more days of volunteer work, Thursday and Friday, at the Massachusetts Association of Older Americans— here's our newspaper. So that leaves Wednesday for appointments, Sunday for daughter and grandchildren, and Saturday for shopping. It's a really good schedule! Well, that's basically it.*

JOANNE PRINCE: *I'm Joanne Prince and I'm 74 years old. I've been widowed since the age of 50. My husband was diagnosed with prostate cancer, and the first 3 years weren't too difficult but the last 2 years of his illness was quite trying. I'm a retired licensed practical nurse, and I would say I spent the last 20 years of my 39 years of nursing in geriatric nursing practice. I did 6 years in the community and 14 years as evening charge nurse in a long-term care facility. And I observed when I first went into long-term care that much of our hands-on staff, the CNAs [certified nursing assistants], were American-born and English-speaking for the most part. Then I suddenly seen the change where there were people coming from third-world countries taking the jobs. And some had accents. And I also observed that many of our residents, especially our European elder residents who had never been exposed to any other but their own kind, come into long-term facility and they had a very difficult time dealing with someone who looked different than they taking care of them. I'm sure some of you have experience and know exactly what I'm talking about. I thought that this needed to be addressed. A lot of people discouraged me until I met this wonderful woman, Roberta Rosenberg, who is now at the Jewish Community for Housing, and together we sat down and talked about forming the Multicultural Coalition on Aging. And it's been running for 10 years. It's the most wonderful organization. We meet once a month at the Hebrew Rehabilitation Center, the first Wednesday, 8:30 in the morning, and you all are welcome to come.*

JEANETTE BURACK: *My name is Jeanette Burack and I am 81 years old. Being 81 gives me license to better understand what old age might be like. It occurs to me that I might have a few qualifications for being on this panel, namely, I have had a variety of mishaps, accidents, poor health. And many blessings as well—don't misunderstand. I have been a victim of a terrible elevator plummet, and I'm a survivor of breast cancer, and I have various and sundry serious illnesses. But I try to forget them as much as possible because I cannot bear to be a sick person. And I'm delighted to be in the company of people who can help me think about all these issues. Thank you so much.*

CHARLOTTE YACKER: *My name is Charlotte Yacker and I am the chair emerita of the board of directors of the Osher Lifelong Institute at the University of Massachusetts Boston Gerontology Institute.*

Although it is said that a woman who will tell her age will tell anything, I do not hesitate to tell my age because of the reaction of those inquiring, ranging from disbelief to admiration. I am 89 years old and have lived a long, busy life. I have been widowed for 4 years, and my only child died in 1998.

When I graduated from high school in 1934, college was not an option for me. The country was still in the throes of the Great Depression and I was fortunate to have a job. I worked as a legal secretary until 1939, when I took a civil service exam and went to work for the U.S. in Washington, D.C., first at the War Department—now the Department of Defense—and then at the National War Labor Board, transferring back to Boston in 1942, when my agency was decentralized. My position was assignment officer, one of 12 in the country and the only one held by a woman. While I was in Washington I took courses at George Washington University in the evenings on a variety of subjects. After my return to Boston, I continued to take evening courses at Harvard Extension School.

In 1945 I left the workforce to become a homemaker and mother until 1951, when I returned to work as administrative assistant to a justice of the Massachusetts Court of Appeals. That led to my involvement with Brandeis University as executive director of the National Women's Committee, a 75,000-member national organization whose mission was and still is the support of the libraries at Brandeis University.

After 7 years there were other irresistible opportunities that presented themselves, including appointment as a U.S. delegate to an international conference in Brussels, Belgium.

I retired from gainful employment in 1985, when I became a full-time volunteer for AARP [American Association of Retired Persons] as associate director of the New England region. After a period of training in Washington, I served as a national volunteer trainer. It was in that capacity that I became caught up with the need for national health-care reform when, in 1992, President Clinton presented his proposal for a national health-care program. It was inconceivable to me that the United States was one of just two industrialized nations in the world which did not have national health care, the other being South Africa. Under the sponsorship of AARP I traveled the country speaking to groups about the need for health-care reform.

It was through my AARP connection that I learned about the Gerontology Institute at the University of Massachusetts Boston, and I was "hooked." I enrolled in the Manning Certificate Program in Gerontological Social Policy and, in 1991, received my certificate, followed in 1993 by an Advanced Certificate. I then enrolled in the College of Public and Community Service as a degree candidate, and in 1997 I received my BA in Gerontology, replete with the Dean's Award and election to the National Honor Society. This was followed in 1998, when I was granted the university's Distinguished

Alumni Award. For all these years—1992 to 1997—I worked as a counselor in the U. Mass. Pension Assistance Project, a national program instituted and funded by the U.S. Administration on Aging. It was during that time, also, that I served as chair of the Citizen's Advisory Committee of the state Executive Office of Elder Affairs. That committee ceased to exist when it was decided to combine the EOEA with the state's Department of Health and Human Services.

In 1998 I was on the founding committee of the Lifelong Learning Institute at University of Massachusetts Boston, eventually serving first as a board member and then, for two terms, as chair of the board.

Health and Illness in Older Adults

DAVID G. SATIN: *We've really started off with the discussion of the first question we hope you will address. Would you talk further about what aging has been like for you, and what has it done to your health?*

YACKER: *Age has never been a factor that I thought about very much. My health was good and I just never thought of myself as aging. Of course, I have had my share of illnesses over the years, including breast cancer; but once the radiation was completed, I picked myself up, dusted myself off, and went back to doing what I enjoyed doing without looking back. I have always defied age limitations. As a matter of fact, when I was 67 years old I volunteered for service in the Israel Defense Force, even though the age limit was 65. I convinced the recruiting officer that I was of sound mind and body, produced the necessary medical records and other certifications, and served 1 month a year for 7 years in military bases there throughout the country. It is only in the past 2 years that I find I am not quite able to continue at the same pace as previously. I agree with a previous speaker that attitude is an important component of successful aging. I have gone through the healing process. As difficult as radiation and surgery are, nothing compares to the death of a child. And I feel that if I was able to learn to cope with that, I can take anything. My greatest salvation came from my years at the University of Massachusetts. I commuted for 5 years from my home on Cape Cod to the University of Massachusetts Boston, and sometimes it was not easy but I kept the destination in mind. I knew that when I got there I would be reborn, whether it was as a student, employee, or counselor. The people at University of Massachusetts at every level are exceptional, and they sustained me through everything.*

I can empathize with Joanne because my husband, too, suffered with cancer, first at home, where I alternated with professional caregivers, and finally in a long-term care facility. And I know how stressful that can be. It's amazing how we find the strength to survive all the painful things life hands us but also to learn from them.

MCGUIRE: *I always was very healthy as a child, except for having a bout of scarlet fever that I had to stay in bed for 4 months after I had it when I was 11. But most of my younger adult years I was always very healthy. Now, I have to admit I take several medicines and I do have arthritis. But for the most part I'm able to function very well and I don't think of myself as a sick person. I think of myself as a well person.*

PRINCE: *I think everything about aging is our attitude. I feel that our culture does not respect aging. Aging is hardly shown in a very positive way, but we can't let that disturb our attitude. It's a process; and if we slow down and things happen, I think it's really chronic illness or it's a disease. I don't know how the rest of you feel about that.*

SUMMERS: *You're right about that. Chronic illness or a bad disease is the one that will slow us down. But if we're not slowed down, we have all kinds of opportunities. We can do anything we want; we are given those opportunities now. But you're right, there's a feeling about the elderly that's not quite what we would prefer.*

COTÉ: *In my case I'm really pleasantly surprised that after 65 you don't have to just sit in the rocking chair. I fortunately don't have a chronic disease. I didn't expect to be so active and alert and enthusiastic at this age. But I find I'm relieved by not having the career and child-rearing responsibilities any longer. That frees up a lot of time for more interesting things. I won't say that they weren't important things but not always so interesting. I have time now to pay more attention to my diet, do a little exercising. All that has been good. Sometimes I think I do have a little drop in my energy level. And I say, "Maybe I am slowing down," but I have a cup of coffee and I'm ready to go. I just have—it's minor—a slight weakness in one knee, and I have to be careful that my pelvic floor doesn't drop.*

TAYLOR: *I'm pretty fortunate in my health except until the time that I was diagnosed with prostate cancer just a little bit after my wife passed away. And when I was told I was diagnosed with prostate cancer, it didn't seem to sink in because I was still going through the process of mourning for my wife, and it just didn't seem to hit me right. And, fortunately for me, it wasn't a cancer that had to be surgically attended to. They attended to it with outside radiation and hormone treatments. And I think that was one of the things about the hormone treatments—it really dragged down my energy. And as my energy dragged down I gained a lot of weight, and I weighed about 199 pounds eventually. And they took me off of the hormone treatments about a year and a half ago, and since then my energy has come back slightly. My doctor, who is a geriatrician, thank God, because he understood what I was going through, and he suggested a little bit of physical activity. So I joined a health club last July and I got into exercising, resistance training, and aerobics, and things like that. And I'm glad I did because I lost 22 pounds and I got my energy back—I can climb up stairs now without huffing and puffing. And it's something that I want to keep up. Since I have met with such great success in exercising I feel more energetic now. I don't feel like I'm getting old until I look in the mirror, and I don't recognize that person anymore. But I think part of the key in getting old gracefully is being able to laugh at yourself. I had an older brother who always laughed at himself. And he never laughed at anybody but always laughed with them. And I think I took his example. So I try to laugh at the things that happen to me and make fun of them, and I don't take myself that seriously.*

SUMMERS: *Don't you all think that laughter is really important?*

MCGUIRE: *Definitely. We were talking about that earlier.*

SUMMERS: *Laughing in itself is helpful to feel better.*

BURACK: *Making someone else laugh.*

SUMMERS: *If you have that opportunity.*

BURACK: *If you have an opportunity to bring a smile to someone's face. That's been my goal for practically my entire life. It's a pleasure to see people smile. So there! Now all of these people represent areas of my life that I won't repeat. But mine have been more traumatic, I think. I've been a victim of ill health. I've been a victim of an accident that*

*caused irreparable damage. I lost a husband after being married to him for 52 won-
derful years. Following almost in the wake of that was an episode of breast cancer that
required radiation, and to this day requires going to an "ist" You know what "ists" are?
Ists are psychiatrists, podiatrists, oncologists—all the ists.*

*Grieving is a very personal issue, right Al? No matter how wonderful the life has
been, you have to almost put it to a side, remember it with a smile, and go on. And
it takes a lot of doing. I've been very fortunate in facing the tribulations of grief and
ill health and absence of facilities that I used to take for granted by pursuing the care
of an ist who's specialty is geriatric psychiatry. And it is my pleasure, the one major
pleasure that has evolved among other small ones, in getting the help to help oneself.
And if one can go into the aging process—the adventure of aging—by having the privilege of learning to help oneself, then that is a gift beyond description. Now, I am a
senior member of this panel; I'm going to be 81 years old next month. So here, show me
respect! I'm a little kid!*

MCGUIRE: *We have to show her respect. But who will show us respect? That's what the
problem is, that there's not always the respect. It doesn't come from your various ists.
And sometimes the respect isn't there. And that's one of the things we miss—I miss.
I know I've run into it with social workers, with health-care workers. They're just not
always aware that we're people and not numbers and not just names on a piece of
paper. And if we could make young people realize that we are not just numbers, not
just people with gray hair, and not just somebody who doesn't have any place anymore,
and it's time to push us aside. And it's time for us to realize, also, that we're not going
to be pushed aside. And this is why we do these types of things. That's why I work at
the Gerontology Institute. That's why I was a volunteer at one time for Dr. Herbert
Benson at the Mind Body Institute. And that's why I worked for Joan Borysenko, PhD,
who also did that kind of work in the relaxation response. And that's why I go to work
2 days a week. And that's why I'm going to work again doing the same thing that Al
does—I'm going to be reading for the blind at the Information Center. And all of the
things that I've done in the past can't even make up for what I can do today. I had a
terrible period of 20 years when I was mentally ill. And I had to live through that.
And as soon as I reached an older age everything seemed to get better. In most cases it
doesn't, but in my case I was very fortunate. I went through 20 years of it. And after
the 20 years and I turned 65 or I went through menopause it ended. And everybody
who told me to pull myself up by my own bootstraps and I couldn't do it, something
clicked but we don't know what. Whether it was a combination of being able to do the
things that I wanted to do when I could. . . . Mental illness is not the same as physical
illness, but it's just as bad if not worse.*

PRINCE: *I'm so glad to hear you talk about Dr. Benson and Joan. I had the opportunity,
when I was going through that experience with my husband, when Joan had that circle
for cancer patients and they allowed me to join that circle. And I found that when we're
helping someone going through an illness like that that we have to help them to tap into
their inner self, their inner spirit. And it was a wonderful, wonderful experience.*

MCGUIRE: *I worked for Joan as her assistant.*

PRINCE: *I think we were 6 weeks in the program, and it did a lot for me at the time.
There was no caregiver support, and even as a nurse I can recall we always focused in
on the patient. We would send the patient home and tell the caregiver, "This is what
you have to do," not realizing what caregiving can do to the caregiver. But when my
husband reached a point where the cancer had metastasized through his entire body,*

he just looked at me one day and he said, "Jo, I can't stay with you any longer." And what he was saying was, "Let me go." Then I had to step in and be his advocate. But that was before we had hospice. And I sat down with the doctor and he said, "Oh, now, Mrs. Prince, we could do thus and such." I said, "No." You couldn't manage his pain. I said, "He has made this decision."

SUMMERS: *You were fortunate you were a nurse.*

PRINCE: *That's why I do the work that I'm doing now, because it just opened my eyes. I said, "What in the world do other people do?" So we worked through all of that. And of course in my early years of training it was just wonderful. We had an excellent nurse clinician that taught us about dying; no one should die alone, and to be there. Consequently, I am now part of the pastoral care at the Sherrill House, where we have a chaplain there. And we feel very strong because the nurses are busy, the CNAs are busy. And many of our residents are opting to stay in a facility and not be moved into hospitals for further intervention. But you need that spiritual care, that spiritual well-being. And you have to remember that. After my husband died—he died in '81—and in 1988 I went to work one day, and all of a sudden I was just so dizzy—I was acutely ill. And I really think it was from all the stress of caregiving. I could not function for 3 months. My immune system, I do believe, just shut down. And I still have residue of inner ear infection that triggered the vertigo that I suffer with off and on now. But having that attitude and saying, "Hey, you just go on and do and try to help others." That's why I'm very much supporting our family caregivers, supporting our caregivers in the profession who are there caring for people, and supporting hospice workers who are caring for the dying.*

TAYLOR: *At the time that my wife was diagnosed with Alzheimer's, it was in 1989. In those days Alzheimer's was a very feared word; it still is, but even more so then because less was known at the time. And the people who did the clinical diagnosis was University Hospital, and the help that they gave me was that I would be presented more with the task of caregiver. I come from a culture where the men were not caregivers; women were the caregivers of the family: The mother took care of the sick and the daughter took care of the sick, and that's the way it was in my family. When my father got ill, my sister and mother took care of him and my brother and I sort of stepped aside and watched. When my mother got ill, my sister took care of her and my brother and I sort of stepped aside and watched. When my wife got ill, I was totally unprepared for any caregiving duties. In those days, in 1989, there were not many help groups for Alzheimer's. I think there were three at the time. One was in Stoughton, one was in Hingham, and one was in Kingston, which were the ones that were recommended to me by the University Hospital. We settled on the one in Hingham, and I have to say that without their help I would have really been lost. They helped me a lot to understand caregiving, especially with an Alzheimer's person, and recommended a few pieces of literature to study. One of them was called The 36 Hour Day; it's probably a very popular book right now, and there's probably several of them out now. And even today, now, practically every town and city has a support group for Alzheimer's. But in those days there wasn't much help for me. I was devastated. I didn't know where to go or which way to turn. Fortunately, there were many, many people from church and from neighbors who knocked on my door and asked me if they could help out. I was grateful for them. In the early stages she could still take care of herself, but as the illness progressed, she got to the point where I was afraid to leave her alone. And then I had to determine for myself: What am I supposed to do? Should I continue to work, or should*

I stay home with her? And I was pretty close to retirement age, so I opted to retire just before my retirement age to stay home with her. After she passed away or the last year of her life I took this certificate course in gerontology. And that surely opened up the door for me in terms of understanding aging and caregiving, which I never knew before. And it really helped, a little too late, of course, but it helped for me to understand more about aging and caregiving.

MCGUIRE: *A lot of people who are fortunate enough to have their husband or wife with them as they age, they end up being the caregiver for that person. So while you're aging and maybe you're having certain problems, you have to take care of another aging person as well. And I think that's the situation you were in, Al.*

TAYLOR: *That's right. And I wish that I would have had training in it before. But I'm glad I had learned more about it even after the fact.*

SUMMERS: *The interesting thing about that is that you need to find resources. And the only places to find resources are from other people who have been in the same position or people who are outside, like a physician. But you need to find the resources. And you need the resources early on; you don't want to find the resources later on.*

MCGUIRE: *I was lucky: Taking care of my dad opened my eyes. I was 59 and 60 when I was taking care of him, and it made me realize that I needed to know a lot more about this subject and that my husband and I were going to be older and were getting older by the minute. It's been a big help to us in dealing with problems we have had with our health. I think it's helped us not to let our health problems overwhelm us. I've been a caregiver for him and he's been a care-giver for me. I had an automobile accident a year ago and I dislocated my right foot. I was out of commission for about 3 months and my husband had to be my home health aide. Right now he's going through a problem with his eye: He has a growth on the back of his eye, and we just went today for him to get an X-ray because the eye may not be the primary site. We don't even know if it's malignant or benign, but we have to go through the process of investigating the whole thing. So we're very supportive of each other. And I think it's wonderful. And I think we're very lucky people. We've made a lot of mistakes in our lives and a lot of things have gone wrong, and every family has its trauma and tragedies; but I think we've been able to learn something from them.*

PRINCE: *I think it's wonderful, Kay, that you went through all of this. But what I'm also saying (I don't know how the rest of you feel) is that now, with the move for us to age in our homes and in our communities rather than in a nursing home because of the cost, I'm beginning to wonder how many of us who have functional health and are well are looking down the road. My big concern is that many of our baby boomers, our adult children, should begin to learn how the elder network works.*

SUMMERS: *Absolutely.*

PRINCE: *Not wait until they're in the crisis. When I was working, I can't begin to tell you how many adult children stood in front of me when the resident, their parent, could not make any further choices. And we would say, "Now, here are your options." And they would say, "Oh, well, Joanne, tell us what to do." I said, "We can't do that." And then I would ask one question: "Have you ever had this conversation with your parent?" "No." It was amazing. It was an eye-opener. Some did not know who their parent's primary-care doctor was. They knew nothing about their financial affairs. I don't know about your family, but in my family, when you tried to bring up that discussion it was like "Don't be so fresh! Don't ask me. What kind of question is that?"*

It seems those issues were a big, dark secret. But I think we have to move forward today and be more open-minded. If we can't trust our children, we certainly need to have someone we can trust. I hate to see any elder go into the system without an advocate so that they will not get lost in the cracks. You could get lost in the hole, and that's a given.

YACKER: *I would like to mention lifestyle changes, which have a very direct bearing on health-care delivery. Lifestyle changes occur in many ways for the elderly. One is the development of communities that offer different forms of community living for older Americans. Some are called "retirement villages," "assisted living communities," and other identities. These have become extremely popular, and they all offer some form of health care to the residents, ranging from general oversight by health-care professionals, assisted care that has several levels of caregiving, and, finally, nursing homes. Lifestyle changes occur in several ways—becoming a single spouse, becoming caretakers for grandchildren or a spouse, and making changes in actual living arrangements.*

The need for proper health care is important on all levels and should be available for everyone.

Older Adults and the Health-Care System

SATIN: *Could you all say something more about the health-care system? What's been helpful and what's been unhelpful in the health-care system? Specifically, how much control have you had over your health and your health care? And finally, what suggestions do you have about improving the health-care system? Young professionals are coming into the health-care system or are in it and need some guidance about how they should be treating older adults.*

YACKER: *My personal experience with the health-care system has been fairly positive. I belong to an HMO [health maintenance organization] and all my needs are eventually met. I joined the HMO when I moved from Cape Cod to Boston because I did not have a regular physician here. Prior to enrolling in the HMO, I was living on the Cape and there we had our own physicians and other health-care workers, such as home health aides for my husband. My son died unexpectedly—running a road race—so he never had the need for professional care. However, I have always been concerned with the need for national health care and the lack of its availability for the population as a whole. Hopefully the new Medicare coverage for medications now before us will close some of the gaps in health-care availability, but the information we are given is so confusing it's difficult to determine which plan is best for which people. It's true that costs are enormous on almost every level, and that's why I believe more strongly than ever that the government has to step up to the plate and provide its citizens of every age with a national health-care program which will be all-inclusive. Insurance rates have gone through the roof, and there is no indication that that will change. The time to do something about it is right now, before the situation becomes really catastrophic. As a national trainer for AARP, I traveled the country talking about President Clinton's health-care proposal.*

We have a responsibility to become health-care advocates—be directly involved with groups or organizations that have taken this as their primary concern: Health Care for All, AARP, and Community Councils on Aging, for example. But it's important to bear in mind that what we do now is not just for our benefit. If the proper changes are put in place now, they will affect the generations that come after us. Think of what Social Security and Medicare—enacted in 1935 and 1965, respectively—have done for our generation. It truly is an intergenerational problem.

TAYLOR: *When I hear so many problems that people have today with their health care or those without any health care—you know they have to put up the money themselves—I am a little bit appalled. I'm pretty fortunate: I'm retired from MIT [Massachusetts Institute of Technology], and MIT takes care of many of their retirees. I've been retired for 11 years, and I still don't have to pay a premium for my HMO. I do have to pay a copayment for my prescription drugs and a copayment for my doctors' visits, but I almost cannot understand how people get along without this and I feel very fortunate. MIT sponsors many HMOs, and I'm happy with them so far. The first one was Tufts Health Care, and then there was a changeover for me of the area they were responsible for, and then I had to change over to Harvard Pilgrim Health Care. But I retained the same doctor, which was pretty fortunate because I have been with this man for 23 years; and it's hard to give up a doctor when you've had one for 23 years because he knows you personally and he knows your history and we can talk to one another. But the third time it was the same story: The HMO decided not to support this area where I live, so I had to give up my doctor even when I changed back to Tufts. I was fortunate enough to be assigned a geriatrician, and he understood much of my problems even more than my old doctor did. But as for paying for it, like I said, I'm pretty fortunate. I know there are a lot of people on the panel here who have had more problems paying for their medical care, HMOs, and premiums. I'm devastated when I hear some of the things that go on. I don't know how much longer MIT is going to support me. They have sent me letters saying that there's a possibility in the future that I might have to pay some of the premium, but I've been with MIT for so long now that anybody who was there before 1970 is under the grandfather clause and I wouldn't have to pay. But the people who come after that have to worry about it. These are some of the things that are happening in a lot of the health care. The cost is going to be transferred over to the employee or retiree—that's what's happening. I don't know how to correct that. There are a lot of health issues that are up to the legislature this year. It's going to be a big item this year, health issues and social security, so be prepared.*

BURACK: *I'm on the other end of the spectrum. I pay for my health insurance independently, and it has gone up now to a premium of $ 7,156 a year, $1789 a quarter just for me. True, they're losing money on me because I have had so many health-care expenses, but still that's an enormous amount of money for a premium for health insurance. I, too, consider myself lucky because I am able to pay that premium—with difficulty, but it is top priority. The kids today, I don't know how they manage. Look at these baby boomers who have no conception—really don't have any conception—of what is involved. And this is just me as an individual. When my husband was alive, there was no such thing as joint insurance; each of us had a premium to pay. It's astronomical, absolutely astronomical! Plus the prices of pharmaceuticals, even with copayments and saving a great deal of money under my coverage. It's mind-boggling, absolutely mind-boggling! So the health-care system has been fine for me because I've been very fortunate to have been on top of things. It is very important as one ages to be on top of your own affairs as long as you possibly can, but share the concerns with your children or a confidant or somebody else who understands the dilemma that you're in so that, should there be an emergency, you have an advocate.*

SUMMERS: *But you don't have advocates sometimes with managed-care programs. In a managed-care program you have to be your own advocate.*

PRINCE: *I think that's what she's talking about: having a confidant, another person.*

BURACK: *A confidant, a personal advocate like my daughter or son. I have been an advocate. I have had a talent over my lifetime, including as I've grown older, in that I have always had the ability to deal with the terminal illnesses of friends and family who had nobody who would recognize the reality of their illnesses and nobody with whom they could speak openly about the reality of what was happening to them. People are afraid. The word "cancer" causes trepidation. People turn off and close relationships; sometimes relationships become very distant because not everybody can handle the reality of it all. I have, fortunately or unfortunately, been able to do this. "Jeanette the Hospice" is the term my kids created. But I'm glad to have had the opportunity to do this because I don't know how things would have worked out had I not. It's important for everybody to have somebody or some group. But you know they say "Give your kids enough rope but hang on to the end of it." That's what you have to do when you grow old: You have to hang on to the end of that rope because when push comes to shove the final decisions are those that you have got to make for yourself. And when you can't there's your advocate. You've got to have an alternative.*

TAYLOR: *I want you on my side!*

PRINCE: *I think you've brought up a very good point about payment. It's not only elders, many of whom cannot even afford to pay the premiums of the HMOs now because it's gone way out of sight. I think it's across the country. How many uninsured people we have with jobs disappearing: Along with the jobs disappearing the insurance disappears. So we have many young people out here working who have no health care. Or they have low-paying jobs or part-time jobs, and they can't afford to pay the premiums. I think the cost of health care is a serious problem in this country across the board.*

MCGUIRE: *I agree totally. I'm in the same predicament as Jeanette because my husband has been a mechanical engineer for over 50 years, but one company after another was bought out; and after Raytheon bought out United Engineers, they created their own engineering and constructing company and they gave no retirement health benefits. My husband worked till he was 74, 2 and a half years ago, so that we could pay the premiums on our health care. We had Blue Cross Medex Gold [Medicare extension insurance via Blue Cross Blue Shield health insurance company] as a supplement; that went up to $523 a person a month this year; for two people it's over $1000 a month now. In December we said we just can't do this any longer. Either fortunately or unfortunately, we weren't getting our full money's worth of it as you were.*

BURACK: *I have. It's the biggest bargain in the world!*

MCGUIRE: *We found out that by getting the Medicare discount card and paying for our own prescriptions, we're saving money by just having Medex Bronze [the lowest-cost and -coverage Medicare extension plan from Blue Cross Blue Shield]. We get wonderful health care from a doctor we have had for over 25 years. And we come to Boston because there's no place like Boston for medical care. And we go to the Beth Israel Hospital and get wonderful care there when we've had a problem. We've been lucky we were able to have control over our care because we're not in an HMO, so we can choose our doctor. When my husband had this problem with his eye, we could go right to the ophthalmologist, right to Massachusetts Eye and Ear Infirmary, because we* could choose where we wanted to go. We had excellent doctors that were able to get us the appointments. Not everybody's that lucky.

PRINCE: That's right. There are too many people in managed care.

MCGUIRE: It's the money that's causing the problem. Right now we can pay for it, but I don't know how much longer we'll be able to. Another big thing is dental care: My husband had to have three implants in his teeth, and that was a tremendous expense because there's no dental care coverage for older people usually unless they have extremely low income.

PRINCE: And it's minimal at that.

MCGUIRE: There's something wrong with the way they figure poverty in this country and what people are supposed to be able to exist on.

SUMMERS: Especially when they have medicine to buy and premiums to pay, which we all do.

BURACK: A propos of what I just said, I remembered I picked my mail up and my health insurance premium is $1556.88 per quarter for me alone.

SUMMERS: If I got a bill like that, I'd have my hair snow white too!

Improving the Health-Care System

SATIN: Do you folks have any suggestions about how the health-care system could be improved?

MCGUIRE: I think we need to have universal health care. And I think the profit . . . I think doctors and health-care professionals and health-care givers should make excellent salaries; they deserve all the financial benefits they can accrue for themselves. But I don't think there should be shareholders; I don't think it should be a profit-making thing, which people profit from because of other people's illness.

CÔTÉ: A lot more should be done to help keeping people home—which would save money in the long run—instead of forcing them into nursing home situations.

PRINCE: That's where we have to be very vigilant and watch the home care budget because where's the care going to be coming from and the money to provide this care? We also have to remember that we have many elders who are raising their grandchildren and great-grandchildren, and they are taking some of their meager funds to help to support these children and to help their adult children going along. So it's a generational thing. I just don't want to see the old pitted against the young 'cause that's not workable. We are all in this together, generations together. And we all have to work together to find a way to provide a good-quality, healthy lifestyle for all of us: for the children, for the young adults, and for the elderly. And right now the bottom line is money.

BURACK: Not right now. It always has been, but it's become a crisis.

TAYLOR: Right. Especially for the professions. Doctors today face a tremendous malpractice insurance premium. Many doctors are even expressing the idea they want to get out of the practice because of that. It's getting to be a real problem. It doesn't look like it's ever going to cap.

SUMMERS: So we're not down to dollars, we're down to insurance companies. Insurance for the health care, insurance for the doctors, and insurance to pay for prescriptions!

Everything is insurance companies! There's an awful lot of big insurance companies out there. What can we do for that?

PRINCE: *I can remember one time a doctor had ordered some medications for one of his nursing home patients, and I called the pharmacist and he said, "Ah, you better tell the doctor MassHealth [Medicaid] is not gonna pay for that." So I had to call the doctor, and, oh, I had to hold the phone away from my ear because of what the doctor was saying! So he ended up saying, "Who's runnin' health care?" I said, "The insurance companies. Doctor, you better get in here. The house will pay for this medication 'cause I know the patient needs it. But you better get in here tonight and sign the papers." That's the way it is.*

BURACK: *So, how does one go about improving this? I mean, we sit here and talk about it. I would like to think that we can do more, but what? It's such a dilemma.*

SUMMERS: *There are organizations that are advocating. We should belong to those organizations. MAOA [Massachusetts Association of Older Americans] is one of them; OWL [Older Women's League] is another. Somebody has to advocate. We can't all be advocates by ourselves, but maybe the younger people could be advocates at some point and that will teach them what's going on. Students come to an interdisciplinary gerontology program studying to become health professionals. And you talk to people like them. Maybe they're learning enough, and maybe they'll help us advocate. We can't always do it on our own.*

BURACK: *I sure hope so. In an interdisciplinary gerontology program the varied students come primarily because they're concerned for the problems in the care of the elderly. I am so grateful for their interest. But they have got to spread the gospel; they have to get other people involved. They must not just say "I attend a class that is fascinating, interesting, marvelous, wonderful." "What do you do there?" "Well, we talk about things." But you've got to stimulate translating this talk into action.*

SUMMERS: *We have to talk to the young people to make them the advocates. A lot of us can't advocate for ourselves; we just don't have any more time. We're doing the things that we're doing. We can't do all the advocating for health.*

TAYLOR: *This is really an intergenerational problem. Anytime the elderly do anything to improve the situation is, in essence, paving the road for the people that come behind them—the younger people.*

BURACK: *Those are going to be the elderly.*

TAYLOR: *In order to convince the younger people to support our efforts we have to show them that we are doing something for them.*

MCGUIRE: *You talk about the legislative process, and that's a scary thing. You think, "Oh, how do I do this? How do I get the legislation?" It takes a lot of grassroots work, a lot of persistence. I started working with the Elder Caucus in 1992, and it took 9 years before we were able to get support for prescription medication through the state legislature. That is a wonderful achievement for a lot of people, but it takes a long time and it takes a lot of hard work. So you can't just write to your congressman and say, "Oh, please do this or that"; you have to get out there in the grassroots and work.*

SUMMERS: *We also have to think about the people who have no advocates at all: the younger people, the groups who have no insurance, who have no anything. And they're of all ages, not just old.*

PRINCE: *And then there is the property tax. We have many widows who have beautiful homes—best-kept secret, there are gorgeous homes in the minority community—and they have unbelievable prices on them now. But, you have a generation—my generation* of African Americans, prior to the civil rights movement—who did not retire from the corporate world.

SUMMERS: *They didn't retire from anything. They just kept working and working and working.*

PRINCE: *At service jobs and menial jobs. So, therefore, many of them just have a Social Security check as their main source of income, and they're concerned about how are they going to pay the property taxes in the homes that they have worked so hard for.*

MCGUIRE: *Property taxes and sewage taxes: That's the other one.*

PRINCE: *I'm not embittered. I always did say, "You know, it might not be your problem today, but trust me, it will be your problem tomorrow." So, just because your plate is full today doesn't mean your plate is going to be full tomorrow. We have to look at the least among us in our society. This is the season for it, this is Holy Week. It's been too much greed, too much corporate greed. And there have been honest, hard-working people that have worked hard all their lives to provide for their families. They paid their taxes. And look at them! You hear some of these seniors talk, "I can't afford to buy my medicine."*

MCGUIRE: *Never mind the seniors. There are young people who can't afford their medicine!*

PRINCE: *It's all of us together. We're in the same boat together now.*

MCGUIRE: *And all this uproar over Social Security and Medicare. Unfortunately, I remember the days during the Depression when older people didn't have jobs, and they had to go from one child to another to live a few months with each one because they couldn't afford to have their own homes. None of us want that situation to happen again, but who are we going to fall back on? Our children. If hard times hit us, we took care of the children and now the children have to take care of the parents. We want to be independent. And we want young people to be independent when they're retired, too. That's why these programs were set up, because there was a desperate need for them. We can't let them go by the wayside.*

BURACK: *Just as students are learning interdisciplinary gerontology, there's something about doing for somebody else and ultimately getting at the roots of a problem and hopefully making a contribution toward the solution thereof that brings us together.*

SUMMERS: *To make the transition from thinking about doing something for somebody else to doing it, you get up and you do it.*

PRINCE: *It was a lot of my own personal experience that motivated me into advocacy. When I went through the caregiving experience and my work experience in nursing, as we begin to see the shift in who is doing the direct, hands-on care and those issues were not being addressed, I said to myself, "It needs to be addressed."*

Intergenerational Relationships

SUMMERS: *It's nice to have intergenerational activities in nursing homes, but it's not the place to have children see the elderly. We're not in nursing homes. Unfortunately, a big thing that's happened is that families are going out different directions, and they're not with their grandparents. So you have to find a way to help the young people see the older people who are not necessarily their grandparents and not in nursing homes.*

COTÉ: *What are the things we share with the children? We share dietary problems. None of the age groups exercise enough. We all suffer at times from lack of self-esteem. These are not just generational things. But when hospitals send out their literature they have page after page of all these courses that they offer—some free, some with a charge—and it seems that they're aimed at seniors. For instance, if there's a class on diabetes, have children and adults and seniors there. If it's on dieting, if it's on yoga, if it's on nutritional matters, exercise, walking—just make sure that people realize that it's open to all ages. They would all meet there, do the same thing, and learn the same thing. I think that's a doable thing: Find the things you have in common and treat all ages together. Maybe the people who put on the program have never even heard the suggestion and would be open to it.*

MCGUIRE: *We all like to hang out with kids. I think that's part of it. You can't isolate yourself from the rest of society.*

BURACK: *I don't think you can legislate relationships.*

MCGUIRE: *No, but you can legislate that schools interact with older people and adults more. I just read about a program in one town in which they had a class of high school seniors who called up elderly people in the community—these weren't people that were ill or anything else, they were just, maybe, a little lonely—and they had a telephone conversation with them at least once a week for several months. Then they all met and talked about all kinds of things. They were so interested in meeting each other and saying, "Gee, I'm so glad to meet you. I thought you'd look like this or that" or whatever. It's pretty minimal cost to doing something like that, and timewise it isn't too big, either; but it got them to relate to each other.*

TAYLOR: *That program has been going on for several years. Some of the comments from the kids were "I didn't know an old person was like that." They were surprised. I think it's important for a kid to realize that "Hey, there is a gap here, and it could be closed." It's sponsored by the town senior center and the schools.*

MCGUIRE: *You can't legislate togetherness, but you can legislate more awareness of each other by making the school curriculum include learning about other segments of society, not just themselves. And get to know who your legislators are and what they stand for. And if they don't stand for the things we want, don't vote for them. It seems that we have a lot of people that are elected to office that really don't have the best interests of society as a whole at heart.*

BURACK: *At every level.*

MCGUIRE: *An educational program about Social Security is taking place at the university. It's being put on for the benefit of our students there. So this is something we're trying to do to reach out to younger people to educate them about this issue of importance to those who are older adults now and will be in the future.*

SUMMERS: *They don't want to come, that's the problem.*

MCGUIRE: *No, that isn't true. We had one session already and there were a lot of younger people there. I think one of the things we're missing in our society today is a community consciousness, looking out for the good of the whole community. People got too interested in what's good for the individual. When the society all works together, it's good for the whole society.*

TAYLOR: *One of the biggest stumbling blocks in our American culture is that we do not prepare for the end of life in any aspect of our culture. We think we're gonna live forever, be healthy forever, and we never teach the young people that there is a time to end things. That's unfortunate. It's not an easy subject to talk about, not in the American culture. But it has to be addressed and it has to be prepared for. You say to yourself, "A kid doesn't want to know that. Let a kid have some fun in his young life. He's gonna be faced with that when he gets old." But I think it's wrong to adopt that type of attitude. If we can learn about the end of life, we will be more prepared to accept retirement, Social Security, health care, and all this other stuff that goes along with it.*

SUMMERS: *My children don't live near me, so they don't have opinions about my advocacy work.*

MCGUIRE: *My kids think it's great. My oldest daughter is a high school English teacher, and she's an advocate for older people. For children, too—she's very interested in children. They live out in Oregon, and the place we like to go to visit is called Bandon by the Sea. They have built a beautiful assisted living and nursing facility there in conjunction with the Kokil Indians—it's Native American land. The high school burned down just before the kids were going to have their prom, so the older people invited them all to have their prom at the facility, where they had a big ballroom. And the older people got up and danced, too; it was fabulous! This is just an example of something we could do. And my second daughter, Cathy, is a nurse who works in a nursing home-assisted living facility, and she's very interested in the elderly. I think their interest is in part because all my kids had a part in taking care of my dad. My three sons were living at home at the time, and they would help my dad take a shower till he needed a home health aide. They would do all kinds of things for him. My little granddaughter would bring him his walker. They got used to seeing an older person.*

SUMMERS: *That's because the children lived near the grandparent. That's the unfortunate situation in America today: Grandparents do not live near their grandchildren and the grandchildren can't see the aging process on a regular basis. They come on a weekend and see me one weekend a month.*

MCGUIRE: *The grandparents have to make an effort, too. We make an effort to go to Oregon to visit my daughter, and we make an effort to go to my grandchildren's basketball and baseball games, and things.*

SUMMERS: *Not everybody can afford to make that kind of effort.*

MCGUIRE: *But I'm also talking about maybe a 20-minute ride to a neighboring town, or even a 2- or 3-hour ride.*

SUMMERS: *A 3-hour ride is not the easiest thing in the world.*

MCGUIRE: *In your own neighborhood the older people could seek out the younger kids and try to become friendly with them. And the younger people could visit an elderly person who has a hard time getting out of their house, right in their own neighborhood.*

SUMMERS: *It's happening slowly. The councils on aging are working on those things.*

MCGUIRE: *I know it's very sad and very upsetting if people are not able to see their own grandchildren. But if you can't be with your own grandchildren, there are plenty of kids around that need a substitute grandmother or grandfather.*

BURACK: *Adopt a grandparent.*

MCGUIRE: *I had an extended family close to me. My grandfather lived with me when I was younger. My grandmother came and lived with us when she couldn't live alone anymore. So I've been used to an extended family. I don't want you to think that we're leaving out the middle ages of people, from say 30 to 50. And one thing that these 30 to 50-year-olds should realize is that grandparents can be a great babysitting asset and stuff like that. We do that. My husband and I went down and spent a weekend so my son and daughter-in-law could go away for a few days, and we stayed with their 7- and 9-year-old children. It works both ways: We had the kids all to ourselves and were in seventh heaven, and their parents had a chance to get away and do things. I think everybody can benefit. Those 30 to 50-year-olds with a teenage son can say, "Mrs. Smith next door, that 80-year-old woman, why don't you share a walk with her?" Then Mrs. Smith will inevitably invite him in to sit and have hot chocolate. And then a relationship forms. There's a parent that's teaching to look out for other people.*

SUMMERS: *Parents are the ones that should be doing this. We hope that we taught our children to teach our grandchildren, but we don't know.*

BURACK: *There is another responsibility of that age group: The parents of these little kids are also the children of the elders, and they go through a double transition in their lifetime. They have to deal with the growing up and teaching of the children, and they have to assume the role of parenting the parent. And the parent has to assume the role of allowing them to do this. This is a point in the process of growing old that is probably the most difficult, I think you'll all agree with me: making the transition easy for yourself and for your children to relieve you of some of the responsibilities, to take over jobs and responsibilities and powers that they had up to that point not been permitted. They're the middle generation, these 50-year-olds. They have a huge responsibility.*

Another thing that I wanted to address: When I was a child every household had a grandparent and the children were not products of mechanical things like television. People visited, and that made it a whole different world. Now there's a new concept: the facility. Think about how many facilities we've been talking about: a nursing home facility, an assisted living facility. We turn to facilities for help. We graduated from an informal family neighborhood existence to facilities.

MCGUIRE: *We lived together communally. Today, we send children to camps.*

BURACK: *It's not easy to bring the experiences and habits of our earlier lives into these facilities and expect them to thrive under the circumstances of institutional living. This brings us back to aging at home. There are so many avenues to pursue.*

SUMMERS: *We didn't talk about the issue of grandparents raising grandchildren. I was a part of a program that was grandparents raising grandchildren. There were wonderful, wonderful people.*

PRINCE: *And the grandparents who are raising their grandchildren, they take it as a love commitment. They say, "What else am I going to do?" I mean, especially in our African American culture that is nothing new. It has always been and I think it will always be.*

SATIN: *You have covered a wide range of topics and still not come to the end of the issues about the health of older adults. And you have not come to the end of your experience and ideas for improvement. Thank you for your expertise and recommendations. And, most of all, thanks for this promising picture of older adulthood with its vigor, wisdom, and caring about people. This gives a realistic context within which younger health professionals learn an interdisciplinary approach to health management for older adults.*

3

The Older Adult Care, Training, Research, and Planning Program

DAVID G. SATIN

The following case study incorporates the various planning, research, education, and health care–provision issues addressed in this text. It also involves a spectrum of health disciplines and institutions. It will help integrate the topics presented in the various chapters by having each chapter apply its perspective to this same example.

It should be noted that this case is entirely fictional, though it incorporates real experience with real projects, institutions, and disciplines at various times.

The Older Adult Care, Training, Research, and Planning Program

A university medical center, recognizing opportunity in the increasing social and funding focus on the aging population, embarked on a project in community health care for older adults. Its missions are multiple:

1. To develop and test theories about the planning, funding, and provision of health care in a community setting
2. To provide community-based, multispecialty clinical care for the local community, but also to feed the parent tertiary-care academic medical center with referrals

3. To provide training for students in various health-care disciplines, supported by fees for service or grants
4. To study the factors that affect health, functional status, and need for and use of health services; these include economic, social, cultural, biological, and attitudinal factors

It is administered under the academic medical center, with a project director and administrative staff responsible for its overall management but not for program planning and administration for service, research, and education.

It is funded in part by a large "unrestricted grant" from HealthCo, Inc. (which develops and markets medications and devices for older adult health), and by smaller research and demonstration grants from the federal Center for Medicare and Medicaid Services (CMS) and the state Department of Health and Social Services. Special projects may be supported by smaller grants. In addition, clinical services may be reimbursed by Medicare, several private health insurance programs, or out-of-pocket payments. There are problems in accessing Medicaid funds due to Medicaid reimbursement rates and contract negotiations with the academic medical center and the Older Adult Care, Training, Research, and Planning Program (OACTRPP).

Several public interest groups are involved in monitoring, critically evaluating, and lobbying the OACTRPP. They include the local community improvement association, the Gray Action Coalition (a state older adult advocacy group), the city Health Department, the state Department of Elder Services, the federal CMS, and the National Institute on Aging.

The OACTRPP is located on the second floor of an office/apartment complex in a mixed commercial/residential area, a section of the city which was formerly working- and lower middle-class multifamily houses but has gradually been encroached on by upper-class condominiums and apartments, stores, and offices, as well as the expansion of the local academic medical center. The residential population is partly gentrified but with sections of working-class population. The ethnic character is very mixed—older second- and third-generation descendents of the immigrant groups; staff and employees of local businesses and institutions; and upper middle-class, Americanized business and professional childless and small family groups.

The OACTRPP service, research, and education programs are staffed by faculty members, consultants, and students from a broad range of disciplines:

Business
Dentistry
Epidemiology
Health-care administration and management
Health-care planning

Health education and physiology
Law
Medicine
Nursing
Nutrition and dietetics
Occupational therapy
Pastoral counseling
Pharmacy
Physiatry
Physical therapy
Political science
Psychiatry
Psychology
Social work
Speech and language sciences
Urban planning

4

The Structure and Financing of the Health-Care System: Reality and Consequences

LAURENCE G. BRANCH AND KATHRYN H. PETROSSI

A health-care system has two basic components—the delivery of health and medical services to those who need them and the payment for those delivered services. The current health-care system in the United States is a by-product of several factors. First, access to and payment for health care in the United States has never been recognized officially as a right of citizenship and a responsibility of the government, as it has in virtually every other industrialized country. Therefore, health care in the United States is appropriately viewed as a consumer good/service in a capitalistic society. Second, health insurance, the dominant form of payment for health-care services, is generally a benefit for the worker and his or her family as a result of participating in the labor force. Third, federal and state governments have legislated responsibility for access and payment for health care of those retired from the labor force (via Medicare, a responsibility of the federal government alone but limited), the poor (working or not, Medicaid, a joint responsibility of the federal and state governments), and children (Children's Health Insurance Program [CHIP], a joint responsibility of the federal and state governments).

However, the current health-care system for older people in the United States—Medicare—reflects a fundamental flaw in the process of social legislation. As noted by former secretary of Health, Education, and Welfare Wilbur J. Cohen, the basis of any legislation has to be an "idea," which is the "irreplaceable, irreducible, first essential in the political process."[1] Unfortunately for the older recipients of health care in the United States, there was either no underlying idea or, at best, an unstable, fragmented, and contradictory one. The original charter of Medicare called for hospital insurance to cover the catastrophic costs of hospitalization for those over age 65, which was the leading cause of impoverishment for older people at the time. Medicare was not intended as comprehensive health care. This absence of a cohesive, widely agreed-upon "idea" behind national health insurance programs has impacted/distorted public perception of these programs over the years and the manner in which the charters are being implemented.

Therefore, the authors suggest that trying to address health care from two divergent philosophical perspectives means that we live up to the expectations of neither very well. Any successful reform efforts must concentrate not only on issues of the budget but also on "regrouping" to solidify the underlying philosophy of medical care and health insurance in America, followed by intensive dissemination of these ideals to the public.

How the Health-Care System Came About

To help us understand the virtues, strengths, and complex problems of the American health-care system, it is important to know how and why it came about and the multiple social and legal iterations that brought it to where it is today.

Early Beginnings

Internationally, the origins of a health-care system can be traced back to ancient Greece, where societies of individuals were formed to help pay for the costs of funerals and the city-states supported physicians' medical practices. Germany (under the leadership of Chancellor Otto von Bismarck in 1883) was the first country to institute a nationwide, compulsory health insurance program.[2] Britain's passage of a national program of social insurance in 1911 had a direct and powerful impact on the leaders of the United States and broad-based attempts to provide national health insurance, though efforts were already under way in America on a smaller scale.

Modern industrialization began in the mid-1800s and created new standards through machine production, bringing more and more people into growing cities from their self-reliant farms to work in centralized factories. Such advances also brought about the concept of "retirement," whereby able-bodied people provided a pension for those who were no longer working. Labor unions, made legal by *Commonwealth v. Hunt* in 1842,[3] were another product of industrialization. Labor unions first championed safety bene-fits and then health benefits (sick/vacation days). After the notion of work-related benefits was established, there was a shift in responsibility for health insurance from labor unions to employers. By 1915, 30 states had passed laws that required employers to provide safety benefits.[2] By 1917, bills were sponsored in 12 states to extend benefits to cover hospital and medical ben-efits for workers and their dependents.[2] Passage of the War Risk Insurance Act in 1917, which gave employment benefits (including health insurance) to military servicemen, seemed to be consistent with a movement toward employment-based support for health insurance. Ultimately, the popularity of Jeffersonian politics, laissez-faire economics, and social Darwinism dur-ing this time prevailed and the campaign for national health insurance died in 1919, not to revive again until the late 1920s.[2] Despite the failure, many interest groups remained organized and instead transferred their energies to increasing knowledge of health insurance not only as a benefit of employ-ment but also for retirement.

It is important to keep in mind that legislative tradition at this point in American history was concentrated at the state level. Therefore, the struggle to legislate benefits pressed for by labor unions and then provided by employ-ers varied from state to state. It was not until the Great Depression in the late 1920s and early 1930s that economic strife changed Americans' belief systems. Prior to the Great Depression, the United States was a country founded on rugged individualism, where hard work alone was believed to produce gains. This belief system came under doubt as the country was trying to pull out of the Depression and Franklin Delano Roosevelt's New Deal, which called for a more activist government, made the climate ripe for a new debate on national health insurance, this time at the federal level. Among many policies and actions, the New Deal led to the passage of the Social Security Act of 1935, which called for government support for the elderly to prevent abject poverty. President Roosevelt initially favored including national health insur-ance as an amendment to the Social Security Act (based on public opinion favoring the idea) but eventually tabled the proposition due to fierce oppo-sition by the American Medical Association (AMA), which threatened the passage of the entire Social Security Act.[2] In the months and years after the Social Security Act was passed, efforts were concentrated on old-age insur-ance, unemployment insurance, and public assistance ("welfare"), although the issue of national health insurance was not completely tabled.

Just prior to World War II, the Wagner Bill of 1939 proposed the creation of a general medical care program known as the National Health Program, which sought to provide expansion of the existing child–maternal health programs, federal payments for disability, grants for hospital construction, and grants to states to encourage medical care programs for the needy and health insurance for all. While multiple versions of the bill failed from 1939 to 1948, it laid important groundwork for the establishment of Medicare and Medicaid.

The 1950s, McCarthyism, and the continued opposition by the AMA further buried initiatives for a national health-care system. However, major advances were made when it was suggested the national health-care system be limited to Social Security beneficiaries. Numerous bills were proposed, at least one in every congressional session, between 1952 and 1965.[4] It was the Kerr-Mills Bill, which eventually passed in 1960, that legislated a program of federal grants to be matched by the states for hospital insurance for the elderly. Several revisions and two presidents later, the final passage of national health insurance for the elderly came in 1965 as the Mills Bill (H.R. 6675), officially dubbed "Medicare."[2] Although Medicare as enacted was not really health care for older people but actually only hospital insurance (under Part A and with enrollee premiums) and physician outpatient care (under Part B but with enrollee premiums), it was a start. In the same year, Medicaid was also passed; and with this legislation, the United States had finally joined the rest of the industrialized world by providing a national system of health care for its poor citizens (though it has not expanded this benefit to all citizens, nor would it officially be recognized as a right of citizenship).

Reforms Since Conceptualization

The passage of Medicare in 1965 did not create the health insurance system for older adults that we have today. Much reform has taken place in the past 40+ years, to provide additional services as well as different reimbursement and practice protocols. In the 1970s, President Richard Nixon passed the Health Maintenance Organization Act, which provided $375 million to begin endorsing, certifying, and subsidizing health maintenance organizations (HMOs), which provided fixed, prepaid capitation rates to providers for the health care of individuals.[5] Another wave of Social Security amendments passed in 1972, adding the disabled and those with end-stage renal disease as Medicare beneficiaries. Rising health-care costs, multiple mandates revising services covered by Medicare, technological advances, and the Vietnam War caused many policy makers to ponder the cost–benefit ratio of a national health-care system for the elderly. The result was a focus on cost containment rather than expansion of access throughout the 1970s and 1980s.

Under President Ronald Reagan, Medicare stopped making payments on the basis of treatment; instead, payments were based on diagnosis-related groups (DRGs), with the intent to eliminate fee differences among providers. Previously, Medicare would reimburse providers based on their bill; consequently, the same procedure or service was reimbursed in different amounts to different providers. With DRGs, the same procedure or service was reimbursed in the same amount (with some geographic variation allowed) throughout the country. Other legislation enacted in the 1980s brought drastic cuts to federal health programs and attempted to stimulate competition among health-care providers and lower the costs of health care. It was also during the 1980s that federal assistance for HMOs was repealed, generic drugs became available, portable health insurance was made available for those changing jobs, and the first (unsuccessful) attempts were made to legislate a prescription drug benefit. Medicare's coverage of preventive health services is legislated on a condition-by-condition basis as evidence-based medicine demonstrates the effectiveness of the various tests and procedures. Coverage for mammograms and prostate cancer screening began in the late 1980s, and now a variety of additional procedures, including flu vaccinations, bone density measurements, colorectal cancer screening, diabetes services, glaucoma screening, Pap tests and pelvic examinations, and other vaccinations, are covered.

During the 1990s, health-care costs rose at double the rate of inflation[5] and the economy slowed dramatically. President Bill Clinton assigned First Lady Hillary Clinton to address the daunting task of reforming Medicare. The clash between employer- and individual-mandated insurance was unreconcilable, and reform efforts died. Despite this failure, important legislation in this decade allowed for health insurance portability and managed care within Medicare.

The Medicare Prescription Drug Improvement and Modernization Act of 2003 (passed by President George W. Bush) provides a drug benefit for Medicare enrollees as well as a modification of the Medicare + Choice Plans to allow for regional preferred provider organizations (PPOs), subsequently renamed "Medicare Advantage." The legislation also improved preventive care by allowing for a one-time initial preventive physical exam within 6 months of enrolling in Medicare, coverage for blood screenings to detect cardiovascular disease, and diabetes screening tests for those at high risk. The Medicare Modernization Act of 2003 also added two forms of Medigap coverage.[6] Additionally, this legislation slightly increased Medicare Part B premiums, and beginning in 2007, Medicare Part B premiums were adjusted for income (those with higher incomes pay a higher premium). As of June 2003, more than 3 million people had enrolled for stage I of the prescription drug benefit.[7] Recent studies from the Center for Medicare and Medicaid Services (CMS) indicate that the average savings on name-brand drugs will be 11%–18%, while savings on generic drugs will be 37%–65% in stage II of the benefit.[7]

Structure and Function of the Current Medicare System

What Is Medicare?

Now that we have discussed how Medicare came about, how does it operate? Essentially, what "is" Medicare? Medicare is federally administered by the CMS as a hospital insurance program for people over the age of 65, for those under 65 who have certain disabilities, and for people with end-stage renal disease. As of 1995, there were 33 million people, nearly all the adults aged 65 and older at the time, enrolled in Medicare. Additionally, there are over 4 million disabled Americans under the age of 65 receiving Medicare benefits.[8] There are four components to Medicare: Part A provides hospital insurance generally without premiums to the enrollee, Part B adds physician service insurance under an insurance model administered by the CMS and funded jointly by enrollee premiums and federal subsidies, Part C gives beneficiaries more options for coverage and service delivery under a variety of managed care organizations, and Part D adds prescription drug benefits.

Medicare Part A

Medicare Part A provides insurance for hospitalization and skilled nursing facilities (for rehabilitative purposes after at least a 3-day hospital stay, not long-term care). It also covers hospice services, some home health care, and inpatient psychiatric care (190 days maximum per lifetime) (see Table 4.1).

Medicare Part A is funded through payroll taxes from when the individual was working. Nonworking spouses are eligible to receive benefits, and those who never contributed via payroll taxes have the opportunity to pay a premium and receive Part A.

Medicare Part A is traditionally a fee-for-service program, where a set fee is charged for each individual medical service or procedure as it is needed. The beneficiary pays a deductible before Medicare pays its benefit, and the beneficiary also pays a copayment or coinsurance after meeting the deductible level.

Medicare Part B

Medicare Part B picks up where Part A leaves off, providing medical insurance to cover the costs of medically necessary doctor's services and outpatient care. Nearly all of the 37 million Americans receiving Medicare Part A also opt to receive Part B.

Unlike Medicare Part A, Medicare Part B benefits are not earned over time via payroll taxes. Instead, Part B is mostly paid for by general tax revenues (65%),[8] with the remaining costs being borne by beneficiaries via monthly premiums ($58.70 in 2003).[9] The cost of Medicare Part B can vary depending upon the date of enrollment relative to the first date of eligibility (the longer one waits, the more it costs). However, premiums for Medicare Part B are automatically deducted from your Social Security payment at age 65 unless you indicate that you do not want to receive the benefit at that time.[4] Medicare Part B is also traditionally a fee-for-service program, where a set fee is charged for each individual medical service as it is needed. The beneficiary pays a deductible before Medicare pays its benefit as well as a copayment or coinsurance. For example, based on Table 4.2, if a Medicare patient received

TABLE 4–1. Detailed description of Medicare Part A benefits, 2007

MEDICARE PART A BENEFIT	WHAT IS INCLUDED	CORRESPONDING INDIVIDUAL RESPONSIBILITY
Hospital stays	Semiprivate room, meals, general nursing, and other hospital services and supplies	Up to $992 total for 1–60 days of hospitalization; $248 per day for days 61–90; $496 per day for days 91–150; all costs after day 150
Skilled nursing facility care	Semiprivate room, meals, skilled nursing and rehabilitative services, other supplies and services	Nothing for the first 20 days; up to $124 per day for days 21–100; all costs after day 100
Home health care	Part-time or intermittent skilled nursing care and home health aide services, physical therapy, occupational therapy, speech- language therapy, medical social services, durable medical equipment, and medical supplies	Nothing for home health-care services; 20% of Medicare-approved amount for durable medical equipment
Hospice care	Symptom control and pain relief medications, medical and support services for those with terminal illness, also short-term hospital and inpatient respite care	Copayment of $5 for outpatient prescription drugs; 5% of Medicare-approved amount for inpatient respite care
Blood	Pints of blood received during a covered hospital or skilled nursing facility stay	100% of cost for first three pints of blood; 20% Medicare-approved amount cost thereafter

Source: U.S. Department of Health and Human Services. Centers for Medicare and Medicaid Services. Medicare & You: 2007. Available at http://www.medicare.gov/Publications/Pubs/pdf/10050.pdf (accessed 7/08).

TABLE 4–2. Detailed description of Medicare Part B benefits, 2007

MEDICARE PART B BENEFIT	WHAT IS INCLUDED	CORRESPONDING INDIVIDUAL RESPONSIBILITY
Medical and other services	Doctor services (although routine physicals are not covered), outpatient medical and surgical services and supplies, diagnostic tests, ambulatory surgery center fees, limited chiropractic services, clinical trials, and durable medical equipment; also surgical second opinions, outpatient mental health care, outpatient occupational and physical therapy	20% of the Medicare-approved amount for most doctor services, outpatient therapy, most preventive services, and durable medical equipment; there may be limits in physical therapy, occupational therapy, and speech–language pathology services
Clinical laboratory services	Blood tests, urinalysis, some screening tests	Nothing for Medicare-approved services
Home health Care	Part-time or intermittent skilled nursing care, home health aides, physical and occupational therapy, speech–language therapy, medical social services, and durable medical equipment	Nothing for Medicare-approved services; 20% of Medicare-approved amount for durable medical equipment
Outpatient hospital services	Hospital services and supplies received as part of care provided as an outpatient	Your coinsurance or copayment amount, which varies by service
Blood	Pints of blood received during covered Part B services	100% of cost of first three pints; 20% of Medicare-approved amount for additional pints (after deductible)
Preventive services (for those who are qualified)	Bone mass measurements, colorectal cancer screening, diabetes self-management supplies and services, flu shots, glaucoma screening, mammogram screening, one-time "welcome to Medicare" physical exam, PAP test and pelvic examination, pneumococcal shots, prostate cancer screening, smoking cessation counseling, and vaccinations	Generally 20% of Medicare-approved amount after deductible

(continued)

TABLE 4–2. Continued

MEDICARE PART B BENEFIT	WHAT IS INCLUDED	CORRESPONDING INDIVIDUAL RESPONSIBILITY
Other services	Medically necessary ambulance services, artificial limbs, braces, chiropractic services for spinal subluxation, emergency care, eye exams, eyeglasses, hearing and balance exams, immunotherapy for transplant patients, kidney dialysis, diabetic foot exams, prescribed nutrition therapy, medical supplies, telemedicine, organ transplant services, and limited travel expenses for medical services provided in Canada	Your coinsurance or copayment amount, which varies by service

Source: U.S. Department of Health and Human Services. Centers for Medicare and Medicaid Services. Medicare & You: 2007. Available at http://www.medicare.gov/Publications/Pubs/pdf/10050.pdf (accessed 7/08).

a bill for $300 for an outpatient surgical procedure and it was the first bill of the year, the Medicare beneficiary would owe $100 for the deductible plus 20% of the remaining $200 (another $40), for a total of $140 out-of-pocket for the $300 bill. If that same person receives another bill in the same year, the person owes 20% of the subsequent bill and CMS will reimburse the provider the other 80%.

Although Medicare Parts A and B are quite comprehensive, there are many services and supplies they do not cover, such as routine physicals, acupuncture, dental care and dentures, cosmetic surgery, custodial care in the home or nursing home, health-care costs incurred while traveling outside of the United States, hearing aids and exams to fit a hearing aid, long-term care (assisted living or nursing home for the purpose of providing custodial care), orthopedic shoes, routine foot and eye care, eyeglasses, routine/annual physical exams, and some diabetic supplies such as syringes and insulin.[9] There are several options for getting these services covered, including private insurance (often referred to as "Medigap" policies because they cover the gaps in Medicare), veterans' benefits (if the beneficiary qualifies as a veteran), Medicare savings programs, Medicaid (if the Medicare beneficiary is also poor enough to qualify for Medicaid), long-term care insurance, and Medicare Managed Care Organizations.

Supplemental coverage Medicare Parts A and B, covering hospitalization and outpatient doctor care, are commonly referred to as the "original Medicare plan." While Parts A and B cover many services, they do not cover everything a beneficiary might need for health care, nor are the services it does cover fully reimbursed. Therefore, according to Medicare,[9] most Medicare enrollees choose to carry additional coverage. The traditional choice has been Medigap policies, whereby private health insurance companies sell policies that fill in both the gaps of coverage and the gaps in payment for the original Medicare plan. While private companies offer Medigap policies, federal and state laws regulate them. Additional coverage can be provided in several other forms, such as supplemental retiree coverage from previous employers or veterans' benefits.

Medicare Part C

Medicare Part C (Medicare + Choice) allows beneficiaries to choose a nontraditional mechanism for receiving their benefits. While the "original Medicare plan" (Parts A and B) provides services on a fee-for-service basis, beneficiaries can choose to get their benefits through Part C, which offers health care through managed-care organizations. While much media and academic attention is spent on the issue of managed care, estimates indicate that only 14% (5.5 million) of beneficiaries received their care via managed care in 2002.[10] You must be eligible for and enrolled in Medicare Part A as well as paying premiums to receive Medicare Part B to join a Medicare + Choice plan.

Medicare + Choice allows beneficiaries to choose how they receive their care, with each plan having different levels of out-of-pocket costs, benefits, doctor choice, and convenience.[4] While the original Medicare plan is a fee-for-service plan, Medicare + Choice plans allow you to receive care through their managed-care plans, private fee-for-service plans, PPO plans, or specialty plans.

Medicare managed-care plans are distinctly different from fee-for-service plans in two ways. First, rather than charging a set fee for each individual service incurred at the time it is provided, Medicare pays providers a set amount per year (capitation rate) for the care of each enrollee, and it is up to the provider to use this predetermined money to cover any services an individual needs; and second, managed-care plans limit the number of doctors and hospitals that the beneficiary can receive services from to those participating in the plan's network. This helps management keep costs down by restricting the network to include only doctors who agree to the preferred treatment guidelines.[8] For providers, while they may earn less compensation per patient visit, they anticipate receiving more revenue in the long run, either through the vast number of referrals (if the provider receives a fee for each visit) or through a fixed price for seeing a predetermined number of patients. For the beneficiary, limiting the pool of providers may lead to receiving additional benefits such as choosing their primary-care physician and possibly prescription drug coverage.[9] The disadvantages to this type of plan are the limited number of providers, referrals being required to see specialists, and the additional out-of-pocket cost for services received outside of the networks (which are generally not covered at all).

Medicare private fee-for-service plans are similar to the original Medicare plan as they allow the flexibility of seeing any provider approved by the plan, but in the private fee-for-service arrangement it is the private company, rather than the federal government, that sets the reimbursement rates.[9] By choosing this plan, a beneficiary may receive benefits above those offered by the original Medicare plan but may be subject to premiums and larger copayments or coinsurance due to the fact that private companies, rather than the federal government, set the payment schedule.

Medicare PPO plans are a variant of the managed-care plans in that a beneficiary can see any of the doctors and hospitals in the plan's network but have the added flexibility of not requiring a referral to see a specialist. Seeing a provider outside the network will likely still be covered but at a higher cost to the patient. This Medicare + Choice plan may also offer some additional benefits above those of the original Medicare plan.[9]

Medicare specialty plans are most appropriate for individuals who require focused health care to manage a specific disease or condition, while still receiving the basic Medicare health-care benefits. While new specialty plans are being created every day, these plans are currently offered for treatment and management of congestive heart failure, diabetes, and end-stage renal disease.

While there are some subtle differences in the coverage provided by supplemental forms of health insurance coverage and Medicare Part C, the main difference between the two is that Medigap policies are provided by private companies and offer benefits outside of the Medicare program, whereas Medicare + Choice involves private companies formally contracting with the Medicare program to provide benefits as part of the Medicare program.[9] It is not necessary to purchase both a Medicare + Choice plan and a Medigap policy.

Medicare Part D

Medicare Part D was created as a result of the Medicare Prescription Drug, Improvement, and Modernization Act of 2003, which provides a drug benefit for Medicare enrollees. The drug benefit involves a $35 monthly premium with a $250 annual deductible. Coverage is 75% up to $2250 total costs, no coverage between $2250 and $5100, and 95% coverage over $5100. There is an annual out-of-pocket limit of $3600/year. Enrollment in Medicare Part D is voluntary.

The program implements the drug benefit in two stages. Stage I allows seniors to pick one of several drug discount cards, which cost on average $30 per year and provide a 10%–15% discount on prescription drugs. It makes those with limited incomes eligible to have the annual fee waived and receive up to $1200 credit on their card in 2004 and 2005. The plan schedules stage II of the drug benefit to be implemented in 2006. Medicare beneficiaries also enrolled in state Medicaid programs are not eligible to receive the Medicare drug benefit.[11]

Critical View of How the System Affects the Care of Older Adults and the Practice of Health Professionals

How does the past and present structure of the Medicare system influence the care that older adults receive? How does the system influence health-care professionals?

The series of political compromises that resulted in the creation of Medicare and Medicaid is a fundamental example of trying to ride two horses at the same time. One horse represents the dominant philosophy of developed countries in the last half of the twentieth century that comprehensive health care is a right of citizenship and therefore a responsibility of government to provide to its citizens. The other horse represents the prior philosophy of a capitalistic society that health care represents a consumer good/service and that it is available in the marketplace like any other good or service. With the passage of Medicare, the federal government created a single federal agency to pay for the single most serious threat to the economic security of retirees at that time, namely, the catastrophic costs of hospitalization. Although not quite a right of citizenship, enrollment in Part A of Medicare did not cost the retiree any money and was available to all those who had participated in Social Security and were therefore eligible for Social Security benefits. It is important to bear in mind that Medicare was never charged with providing comprehensive health care for older people in the beginning, nor has its charter been changed to embrace comprehensive health care for older people. Part A pays for hospital care and the services associated with hospitalization; Part B pays for physician and outpatient care based on an insurance model, with one-third of revenues coming from enrollee premiums and two-thirds coming from the general revenues of the federal government. Both Part A and Part B are entitlement programs for retirees participating in Social Security.

Medicaid, on the other hand, was established as a federal–state partnership (hence, there are different Medicaid programs in each of the 50 states and participating territories) to provide comprehensive health care for poor people. Medicaid for the poor in the United States is similar to the world's approach to health care as a right of citizenship in that it is intended to provide comprehensive health care to all eligible citizens, albeit still subject to the political process that determines the breadth and depth of services provided.

Medicare continues to try to ride two horses, one horse racing under the banner of comprehensive health care as a right of age and citizenship with the federal government as the single payer and the other horse under the banner that health care is just another good or service to be purchased in the marketplace of a capitalistic society by individuals or by nongovernmental third parties on behalf of those individuals. Without actually changing the charter to embrace comprehensive health care, we have periodic acts of Congress to expand coverage under both Part A and Part B (with 1991 being a banner year with the authorization of certain preventive services under Part B). The continual incremental expansion of authorized Medicare services can be argued to cause the operation of Medicare to resemble a comprehensive health-care system that is similar to some national health insurance systems, but the tax structure that supports it is still based on the idea that health care is a commodity. As fiercely independent Americans with some of the lowest taxation rates in the world, we are unlikely to want to change tax rates dramatically to cover such comprehensive services for all retirees, let alone for all Americans.

Such an inconsistent policy has impacts at every level of society. For health professionals, let us consider the example of the ethical dilemma that physicians, the vast majority of whom have practiced only in the post-Medicare era, have in trying to get Medicare home-care benefits for their patients. Under Part B, the CMS has determined that the home-care benefit would be available to only the frailest Medicare beneficiaries, defined by Medicare as being homebound. What if the physician judges that her patient's health status would be improved with home-care services but the patient does not meet the strict definition of "homebound" as offered by CMS? What can the Medicare provider do when there are differences among the legal, ethical, and moral codes which govern her conduct? Whose responsibility is it when the law or the regulations do not reflect the value system of the majority? Who is qualified to determine this?

Since the passage of Medicare and Medicaid in 1965, many older people in the United States have accepted the popular misconception that Medicare will provide for any comprehensive health care that they should need. Many of these older people were rudely surprised to learn that Medicare (until quite recently) would not pay for evidenced-based preventive practices demonstrated to reduce illness and health care among older people. Many older people have been rudely surprised to learn that Medicare generally does not pay for nursing home care. Many older people have been rudely surprised that Medicare would pay the much higher bill for an inpatient procedure but would not pay for the same procedure to be performed on an outpatient basis.

Over the years, a large portion of Medicare beneficiaries have accepted the premise that Medicare is a government program designed to provide them with comprehensive health and medical care. Notwithstanding that Medicare was never established to provide comprehensive health care for seniors and Medicare's charter has never been changed, some older beneficiaries and some Medicare providers have been reported to be in silent collusion to provide comprehensive care. Before an act of Congress (Omnibus Budget Reconciliation Act of 1993) authorized certain prevention services, many older people were reported to have received them and their physicians filed for reimbursement under a claim as a general office visit. Is that fraud? Does hospitalizing a frail older person for a procedure that could be safely and effectively carried out in a physician's office or a day-surgery center make any sense at any time, particularly when there are concerns about insufficient funds in Medicare?

Years ago, Supreme Court Justice Abe Fortas wrote insightfully about rights in conflict. Right vs. wrong represents the easy choice for health-care providers; rights in conflict offer the difficult choices. The payer has the right to specify what it will pay for and what it will not pay for under the policy that health care is a commodity in a capitalistic society. But the provider has a responsibility to provide the best care available for his or her client. Or should we say the provider has the responsibility to provide the best care "authorized" for the client? Clearly, the payer's right to limit what it will pay for and the clinical provider's right (and responsibility) to provide the best care available can be in conflict. The resolution of rights in conflict in health care has not received systematic attention.

Possible Solutions to the Problems of Riding Two Horses: Reforming Medicare

Politicians and the media spend much time discussing Medicare reform. It is a hot topic during every election year, and everyone seems to have an opinion about it. Maybe that is because Americans value Medicare so much: In 1994, three-fourths of Americans said Medicare is an important program in their lives.[12] This opinion is held among both old and young, but young people are more likely than older adults to agree that the federal government has a basic responsibility to guarantee health insurance for the elderly and disabled.[12] Before we can "solve" the problems of Medicare, let's discuss the many issues involved.

The Heart of the Debate: The Cornerstones of Health-Care Policy

The cornerstones of health-care policy, certain to be at the heart of the reform debate, are access, quality, and cost. *Access* refers to determining who qualifies for benefits and what medical services are provided. Health-care *quality* pertains to the following questions: Was the appropriate care provided, and did it achieve the desired outcome? Was it as positive an experience as possible for the beneficiary? Who should monitor quality? *Cost* is the third cornerstone of health-care policy: How much does a service cost the provider and the beneficiary?

At different times throughout recent history, each of these cornerstones has been the center of action and, therefore, debate. At some times it has even been possible to consider two of these cornerstones as the same. As examples, from the 1930s until the mid-1960s, the focus of health-care policy for older people was on access and cost. From the mid-1960s through the 1970s, the focus was primarily on access. In the 1970s and 1980s, the predominant discussion was cost as gerontologists and policy makers realized that Americans are living longer and longer and that the pay in/pay out balance would quickly become askew. History tells us, however, that as one set of issues is addressed and reforms are implemented, another area for improvement becomes apparent. This can be seen in the debate throughout the 1990s, which continues today. Again, the focus is on access or cost, depending somewhat on one's political philosophy on the role of government in providing health care.

What Is Good About Medicare?

The Twentieth Century Fund[8] provides a reasonable framework for examining Medicare reform by breaking down the issues into two categories: (1) What is good about Medicare? and (2) What does not work in Medicare?

Despite the constant onslaught of criticism surrounding the program, Medicare has evolved to the point that it now provides health insurance for millions of older adults who otherwise would not have it if private insurance was the only option. As of 2004, Medicare covered 41 million elderly and disabled Americans. This is a dramatic increase from pre-Medicare 1965, when only 56% of the elderly had hospital insurance.[8] It is reasonable to suggest that without Medicare today's uninsured would be at least 50%, given the rising costs of health care and prescription drugs. Furthermore, Medicare covers many older Americans who otherwise could not afford private insurance of the same quality, depth, and breadth. As of 1995, nearly 80% of beneficiaries had incomes less than $25,000 per year.[8]

Since Medicare was created in 1965, nearly 3 years have been added to the average life span. It can be argued that this increase is due in part to Medicare's facilitation of greater access to health car, and its financing of innovations to treat common medical conditions such as heart disease and cancer.[8] Furthermore, the structure and financing of Medicare have fostered the growth of home health and hospice organizations, which did not even exist 40 years ago.[8] Services offered by these organizations can be less expensive than hospitalization and provide comfort and quality at the end of life. Medicare, along with many of the advances of the late twentieth century, in all likelihood has extended the length and quality of American lives.

Because of its size and resultant power in influencing payment schedules, Medicare is a value compared to private insurance. As the payer of about 30%–35% of all health-care bills through Medicare and Medicaid, the CMS and its predecessor organization, the Health Care Financing Administration (HCFA), have been able to implement more uniform (and lower) payment schedules than most private insurance companies.

The widespread acceptability of Medicare by doctors coupled with numerous options for how to receive care (including Medicare Part C) provides beneficiaries with a network of doctors, hospitals, and other services that far surpasses the options of any private health insurance company. In addition to greater access to care, Medicare's system of premiums, deductibles, and copayments (see Tables 4.1 and 4.2) is far more generous than most private plans.[8]

The CMS prides itself on its very low administrative costs to beneficiary service costs ratio. Administrative costs include overhead, salaries, computers, etc.—essentially costs other than medical care for beneficiaries. While the insurance industry in the United States maintains an average of approximately 17% in administrative fees to total premiums (and that figure does not include the profit margin for the for-profit insurance companies), the comparable figure for the CMS is approximately 2%.[8] In addition to keeping administrative costs low, Medicare has managed to keep benefit cost increases at or below those of private insurers for the majority of years since 1979.[8] This cost containment is noteworthy, given that many Medicare beneficiaries use more services than their younger counterparts enrolled in private insurance plans.

As previously mentioned, the periodic customer satisfaction surveys of Medicare beneficiaries demonstrate a continued high level of satisfaction among those receiving care. As of 1993, 94% of Medicare beneficiaries report being satisfied with the ease of seeing their physician. Ninety-seven percent said they had no trouble getting care during the past year.[8]

Beyond the benefits of Medicare for older adults, it is also important from a societal perspective to acknowledge the role of Medicare in the support of medical institutions across the country. For example, Medicare provides almost all revenue for home health-care agencies, hospices, and renal dialysis facilities[8]: 25%–75% of the revenue for clinics, laboratories, and ambulance services. As of 2001, Medicare funded almost 30% of all hospital expenditures.[12] Furthermore, Medicare provides higher payment rates to teaching hospitals,

hospitals that serve disproportionately higher levels of low-income Americans, and hospitals in rural areas. Medicare does good not only for its beneficiaries but also for the development of medical technology and the training of new practitioners.[8]

What Is Bad About Medicare?

Also worth mentioning are the faults of the Medicare system, including financial troubles, waste, fraud, the lack of emphasis on preventive care, and the lack of coverage for total health care, including the specific lack of coverage for long-term care in nursing homes beyond short rehabilitation stays following hospitalization.

Many Americans receive more benefits than what they actually contributed via payroll taxes throughout their working years. For example, it has been estimated that the average working couple who retired in 1994 will receive roughly $117,000 more in benefits than they contributed; the benefit surplus is valued at over $65,000 for a single woman and at just over $40,000 for a single man.[8] The financial solvency of Medicare (as well as the financial solvency of the whole Social Security system in the United States) is of recurring concern to many health-policy experts. These experts are dealing with a complex problem with multiple etiologies: the rising costs of medical care, the anticipated increase in beneficiaries, the decreasing ratio of beneficiaries to workers, and longer life spans that increase the number of years benefits are received. Those who contend that deficit spending cannot endure over the long run are especially concerned.

Another concern about Medicare is waste and fraud. It is estimated that 10% of Medicare expenditures are wasted—by the private contractors that process Medicare claims and the private health-care providers that bill Medicare for services that they did not perform or that were performed inappropriately.[8]

As described in the previous section, the limitation inherent in Medicare to cover inpatient care through Part A and outpatient care through Part B and several acts of Congress to expand coverage into certain preventive services create serious ethical dilemmas for many providers. The standard of health care in the United States underscores comprehensive care, yet nearly one-third of Medicare's expenditures are paid to individuals who have less than 1 year to live.[8]

Preventive care was virtually nonexistent in the Medicare system before the early 1990s, and the number of people taking advantage of the added benefits has been lower than expected. Until Medicare expands its basic narrow charter to the broader responsibility of comprehensive health care for older Americans, it will continue to be limited.

The basic charter of Medicare—to pay for hospital coverage and related expenses under Part A and some specified outpatient services under Part B—has never been changed to allow for total health care according to the current art and science of medicine and health care. It literally takes an act of Congress to add specific benefits to Medicare. This approach hinders the ability of Medicare providers to meet the total health-care needs of beneficiaries.

Extended nursing home care in the future is a necessity for nearly half of Medicare enrollees. Yet, Medicare only pays for limited rehabilitation stays in nursing homes. The need for extended nursing home care is a fundamental part of total health care for many people at the end of life.

Proposals to reform Medicare are numerous, including options for reducing payments for providers, increasing premiums and/or copayments for beneficiaries, use of a voucher system, medical savings accounts, and reducing the benefits that Medicare covers. Some advocate overhauling the entire health-care system in the United States, not just Medicare. There are strengths and weaknesses of each of these approaches, but the authors fundamentally believe that the U.S. government and the American people will need to decide which horse—right of citizenship or commodity—that they want our country to ride before any reform measure will be successful and long-lasting.

The recent health policy debates over drug benefits and catastrophic care highlight an important public health policy issue, namely, whether Medicare should provide first-dollar coverage or last-dollar coverage. In first-dollar coverage, the third-party payer typically commits to pay the initial costs up to a specified maximum, while the beneficiary has responsibility to pay for the costs beyond that specified maximum. The initial costs are traditionally easier to forecast and, therefore, more predictable, and predictability is a value to payers. The costly tail of the utilization or cost curve is much less predictable; therefore, government budget planners, especially in an era of legally required balanced budgets, are more drawn to first-dollar coverage. However, the cornerstone of group insurance programs—health and otherwise—is to pool resources to pay for precisely the high-cost, unpredictable expenses that catastrophes can bring. Last-dollar coverage is more consistent with the philosophy that government is designed to provide a safety net once an individual's private resources are gone. Many older people value economic security very highly and will go to great lengths to have insurance for the unpredictable last-dollar costs. Medicare would be more valuable to them if it met this need for economic security from unpredictable and high medical care costs (see Table 4.3).

TABLE 4–3. Pros and cons of Medicare

PROS	CONS
1. Medicare provides health insurance for people who would likely be uninsured without it.	1. Medicare hospital insurance is running out of money.
2. Medicare extends lives and improves quality in later life.	2. Retiring Baby Boomers will greatly increase the Medicare-eligible population.
3. Medicare is a good deal for seniors.	3. Health-care costs continue to rise.
4. Medicare costs are increasing no faster than that of private insurance.	4. Medicare is continually vulnerable to dramatic budget cuts due to the size of the program.
5. Medicare is more efficient than private insurance.	5. The current Medicare system still leaves many beneficiaries without medical services.
6. Older Americans are satisfied with Medicare.	6. Medicare wastes some of its money.
7. Medicare supports many community agencies and vital medical institutions.	7. Medicare does not do enough to encourage prevention.

Source: Twentieth Century Fund. The Basics: Medicare Reform. A Twentieth Century Guide to the Issues. New York: Twentieth Century Fund Press, 1995.

Statements About the Application to Health Management and Professional Practice

The U.S. health-care system can be quite complex. Health-care professionals need to be well versed in how the system works and thus able to provide the best possible (and covered) care to patients. A studied consideration of the principles of "Rights in Conflict" can be instructive. Older people often think they have comprehensive health care in Medicare, but at present they do not.

For those who work closely with the elderly in a nonmedical capacity, understanding the health-care system is also important because the prevalence of medical conditions in this age group, as well as the financial burden of health care, can potentially impact every aspect of life.

It is interesting to note that Medicare now requires providers, doctors, and suppliers to submit claims electronically and that some beneficiaries are able to view their Medicare Summary Notice online. However, only a minority of people over age 65 has ever used the Internet; the Kaiser Family Foundation estimated that 31% of people over age 65 had used the Internet in 2004. In their report they noted that if we are to take advantage of the potential the Internet offers as a useful tool for seniors, then health providers, advocates, and the entire public health community will need to help seniors learn to be proficient in cyberspace.[13]

The Kaiser Family Foundation survey, conducted through 1450 random telephone interviews, reported that about one in five (21%) seniors had gone online to find health information, including information about prescription drugs (13%); nutrition, exercise, and weight issues (9%); and cancer (7%). This study also reported that income was a major factor in determining Internet usage among seniors. Internet use among seniors with annual household incomes of $50,000 or more was reported at 65%, while only 15% of older people with incomes under $20,000 a year used the Internet.[13]

Facts and Figures of Health Policy Importance

Medicare spending has grown from $3.3 billion in 1967[14] to $300 billion in 2004[15] and was estimated to increase by 30% from 2005 to 2007 with the introduction of the drug benefit (see Table 4.4 and Fig. 4.1). The CMS projects Medicare spending to exceed $530 billion by 2013.[6]

Learning Exercises

CASE STUDY: *Description of senior—decide which Medicare plan (original A, +B, Medicare + Choice) is best.*

CASE STUDY: *Description of senior—decide whether drug benefit will help or hurt financially.*

Case Study 1 (adapted from AARP: Medicare Changes that Could Affect You, www.aarp.org)

Marie and Evan are a middle-income married couple. Evan has heart disease and Marie takes medicine for arthritis. Their drugs cost $6810 a year—$1960 for her, $4850 for him. In 2006, under the Medicare drug benefit, Marie would save 44% but Evan, with higher costs, would save only 22%. That's because he'd fall partly into the coverage gap. Remember, the coverage gap is all drug costs above $2250 until your out-of-pocket drug costs equal $3600. Together, the couple would pay $4868 out-of-pocket and save $1942 (see Table 4.5).

Questions

1. What is the average amount spent, per individual, on prescription drugs per year?

TABLE 4–4. Summary of health-care expenditures in the United States, 1965–2002

	1965 (pre-Medicare)	1970 (full federal involvement in health care)	1980	1990	2000	2003
		TOTAL POPULATION				
National health expenditures (billions)	$41.0	$73.1	$245.8	$696.0	$1,309.4	$1,678.9
Private	$30.80	$45.4	$140.9	$413.5	$714.9	$913.2
Public	$10.21	$27.6	$104.8	$282.5	$594.6	$765.7
Federal	$4.67	$17.6	$71.3	$192.7	$416.0	
State and local	$5.54	$10.0	$33.5	$89.8	$178.6	$224.0
Health services and supplies		$67.3	$233.5	$669.6	$1,261.4	$1,614.2
Personal health care		$63.2	$214.6	$609.4	$1,135.3	$1,440.8
Hospital care		$27.6	$101.5	$253.9	$413.2	$519.9
Professional services		$20.7	$67.3	$216.9	$426.5	$542.0
Nursing home and home health		$4.4	$20.1	$65.3	$125.5	$150.8
Retail outlet sales of medical products		$10.5	$25.7	$73.3	$170.1	$232.1
Prescription drugs		$5.5	$12.0	$40.3	$121.5	$179.2
Other		$5.0	$13.7	$33.1	$48.5	$52.9
Government administrative and net cost of private health insurance		$2.8	$12.1	$40.0	$80.3	$119.7
Government public health activities		$1.4	$6.7	$20.2	$45.8	$53.8
Investment (research and construction)		$5.7	$12.3	$26.4	$48.0	$64.6
		PER CAPITA (TOTAL POPULATION)				
National health expenditures	$205	$348	$1,067	$2,738	$4,670	$5,671
Private		$216	$612	$1,627	$2,550	$3,084
Public		$131	$455	$1,111	$2,121	$2,586
Federal			$310	$758	$1,483	
State and local			$146	$353	$637	

Source: U.S. Department of Health and Human Services, Centers for Medicare and Medicaid Services. Available at: http://www.cms.hhs.gov.

2. Which person, Marie or Evan, will save more (in dollars and/or percent of expenses) under the new drug benefit?

3. What are the benefits and pitfalls of the "doughnut hole" (that intermediate interval of spending on drugs not covered by Medicare D) for consumers, providers, and the federal government?

Application to the Case Study: The Older Adult Care, Training, Research, and Planning Program

The Older Adult Care, Training, Research, and Planning Program (OACTRPP) describes an attempt to make the Medicare and Medicaid programs more effective in the provision of health and medical services to older adults. The OACTRPP model is based on community-based multispecialty care. We address the following issues:

How does the OACTRPP reflect the structure and funding of health care?
Is the project likely to improve the health-care system in the future?
How does the OACTRPP reflect the structure and funding of health care?

It is entirely consistent with the observation that the delivery of services stems from interactions between patients and providers of care and that the payment for health care results from interactions between payers and providers but that our current health-care system does not encourage any three-way interactions among provider, patient, and payer. Perhaps some forms of quality control are missing when we have interactions among two components at a time but not all three at once.

The OACTRPP also reflects the current structure and funding of health care in that the CMS has already authorized some Medicare Part B payments for services provided by OACTRPP professional staff. This is an accurate reflection of how the system currently operates—the provider of health care must assure that he, she, or they will be compensated for services by the insurance carrier before providing the service. Providing a service without prior authorization coupled with subsequent denial of payment leaves the provider in the difficult position of either asking the patient to pay directly for the services out-of-pocket (which is not customary for older people at this time) or forgoing any payment for the service. Forgoing payment is not a long-term solution for a health-care provider like the OACTRPP—even if the physicians have a source of income other than the medical center, the receptionists, nurses, physical therapists, occupational therapists, speech therapists, and all the other clinic workers need to get paid in order to pay rent and buy groceries. Delivering health care without compensation is rarely a long-term solution.

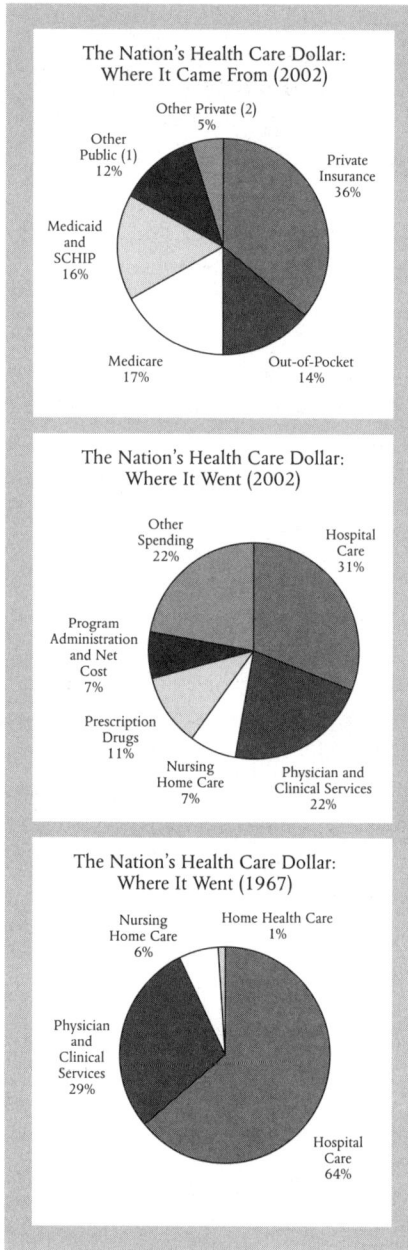

The Nation's Health Care Dollar: Where It Came From (2002)

- Other Private (2) 5%
- Other Public (1) 12%
- Private Insurance 36%
- Medicaid and SCHIP 16%
- Medicare 17%
- Out-of-Pocket 14%

The Nation's Health Care Dollar: Where It Went (2002)

- Other Spending 22%
- Hospital Care 31%
- Program Administration and Net Cost 7%
- Prescription Drugs 11%
- Nursing Home Care 7%
- Physician and Clinical Services 22%

The Nation's Health Care Dollar: Where It Went (1967)

- Nursing Home Care 6%
- Home Health Care 1%
- Physician and Clinical Services 29%
- Hospital Care 64%

FIGURE 4.1 The nation's health-care dollars.
SCHIP, State Children's Health Insurance Program.

TABLE 4–5. Health-care costs for Marie and Evan, 2006

MARIE	$ PER YEAR IN 2006	EVAN	$ PER YEAR IN 2006
Total drug costs	$1,960.00	Total drug costs	$4,850.00
Total out-of-pocket spending (with premium, which does not count toward $3600 out-of-pocket)	$1,097.50	Total out-of-pocket spending (with premium, which does not count toward $3600 out-of-pocket)	$3,770.00
Savings	$862.50	Savings	$1,080.00
Out-of-pocket spending counted toward Medicare drug benefit		Out-of-pocket spending counted toward Medicare drug benefit	
Annual premium (estimated $35/month)	$420.00	Annual premium (estimated $35/month)	$420.00
Annual deductible	$250.00	Annual deductible	$250.00
25% copay on next $2000 in total drug spending after $250 deductible	$427.50	25% copay on next $2000 in total drug spending after $250 deductible	$500.00
Full cost of drugs above $2250 in total drug spending and below $3600 in out-of-pocket drug spending (coverage gap)	$0.00	Full cost of drugs above $2250 in total drug spending and below $3600 in out-of-pocket drug spending (coverage gap)	$2,600.00
5% copay above $3600 in out-of-pocket drug spending	$0.00	5% copay above $3,600 in out-of-pocket drug spending	$0.00

Is the project likely to improve the health-care system in the future? We should have ample reason for optimism, stemming primarily from the well-intentioned, thoughtful approach of the planners. However, there are also a few reasons for concern. From one perspective pertaining to the integrity of health services and medical outcomes research, we would be leery that, as stated in Chapter 3 several public interest groups are involved in monitoring, critically evaluating, and lobbying OACTRPP, which include a local community improvement association and the Gray Action Coalition (a state older adult advocacy group). The integrity of science is better served when the investigators have no stake or involvement in the outcome of the study. It is for this reason that innovators typically do not evaluate their own innovations;

unbiased third parties are required. In the present example, a local community improvement association and an older adult advocacy group may not have the correct training to implement an unbiased, scientifically sound, and defensible evaluation of the OACTRPP innovation. An unbiased third party with training in evaluation research methods would be a better choice.

Glossary of Terms (adapted from U.S. Department of Health and Human Services[6])

Access: One of the four cornerstones of health-care policy, access refers to who has the ability to receive needed services and procedures.

Adjusted Average Per Capita Cost: The average amount estimated that Medicare would spend on a single beneficiary in a year.

Assignment: The agreement between Medicare and providers to accept the Medicare-determined amount of payment (as full payment) for a particular service.

Beneficiary: The name for a person who is receiving health-care benefits through Medicare.

Capitation Rate: A specified amount of money paid to a health plan or doctor. This is used to cover the cost of a health plan member's health-care services for a certain length of time.

Coinsurance: The percentage of the charge for services that you may have to pay after you pay any plan deductibles. Often, the coinsurance payment is a percentage of the cost of the service (like 20%).

Cost Sharing: The cost for medical care that you pay yourself like a copayment, coinsurance, or deductible.

Deductible: The amount a beneficiary must pay for health care before Medicare begins to pay, either for each benefit period for Part A or each for year for Part B. These amounts can change every year.

Diagnosis Code: The first of these codes is the *International Classification of Diseases*, ninth edition, *Clinical Modification* (ICD-9-CM) diagnosis code describing the principal diagnosis (i.e., the condition established after study to be chiefly responsible for causing this hospitalization). The remaining codes are the ICD-9-CM diagnosis codes corresponding to additional conditions that coexisted at the time of admission or developed subsequently and which had an effect on the treatment received or the length of stay.

Diagnosis-Related Groups (DRGs): A classification system that groups patients according to diagnosis, type of treatment, age, and other relevant criteria. Under the prospective payment system, hospitals are paid a set fee for treating patients in a single DRG category, regardless of the actual cost of care for the individual.

Dual Eligibles: Persons who are entitled to Medicare (Part A and/or Part B) and who are also eligible for Medicaid.

Durable Medical Equipment: Items such as wheelchairs, hospital beds, oxygen, and walkers which are covered by Medicare Part A. Also items such as wheelchairs, hospital beds, walkers, and oxygen which are covered by Medicare Part B.

Excess Charges: In the original Medicare plan, this is the difference between a provider's actual charge and the Medicare-approved payment amount for that service.

Exclusions: Items or services that Medicare does not cover, such as long-term care and custodial care in a nursing or private home.

Federal General Revenues: Federal tax revenues (principally individual and business income taxes) not earmarked for a particular use.

Fee-for-Service: The type of payment arrangement for the original Medicare plan, where providers are paid for each health-care service or procedure performed. This is in contrast to the managed-care payment arrangement, where a set amount is paid per beneficiary per year, regardless of what services or procedures are performed.

Fee Schedule: A complete listing of fees used by health plans to pay doctors or other providers.

First-Dollar Coverage: The third-party payer typically commits to pay the initial costs up to a specified maximum, while the beneficiary has responsibility to pay for the costs beyond that specified maximum. The initial costs are traditionally easier to forecast and therefore more predictable, and predictability is a value to payers. The costly tail of the utilization or cost curve is much less predictable, but "high-cost, unpredictable expenses" are the cornerstone of group insurance programs. See **Last-Dollar Coverage.**

Generic Drug: A prescription drug that has the same active-ingredient formula as a brand-name drug. Generic drugs usually cost less than brand-name drugs and are rated by the Food and Drug Administration to be as safe and effective as brand-name drugs.

Health Insurance Portability and Accountability Act (HIPAA): A law passed in 1996, which is also sometimes called the "Kassenbaum-Kennedy law." This law expands health-care coverage: If you have lost your job or moved from one job to another, HIPAA protects you and your family if you have preexisting medical conditions and/or problems getting health coverage and you think it is based on past or present health. HIPAA also limits how companies can use preexisting medical conditions to keep someone from getting health insurance coverage; usually gives you credit for health coverage you have had in the past; may give special help with group health coverage when you lose coverage or have a new dependent; and generally guarantees your right to renew your health coverage. HIPAA does not replace the states' roles as primary regulators of insurance.

Health Maintenance Organization (HMO): A type of Medicare managed-care plan where a group of doctors, hospitals, and other health-care providers agrees to give health care to Medicare beneficiaries for a set amount of money from Medicare every month. A beneficiary usually must get care from the providers in the plan.

Last-Dollar Coverage: The third-party payer typically commits to pay the remaining costs after the beneficiary pays a deductible. The deductible can be low, such as the first $100 of the hospital bill, or high, such as the first $5000 of medical expenses in a year. The remaining costs after a deductible are difficult to forecast for an insurer. See **First-Dollar Coverage.**

Limiting Charge: When enrolled in a Medicare + Choice program, a beneficiary may choose to receive services outside of the plan. Limiting charges set an upper limit for fees providers can charge if they do not choose assignment (the Medicare-set reimbursement rate), usually 15% over the approved assignment amount.[4]

Medicaid: A federally and state-administered program that provides health insurance for low-income and limited-resource persons.[4]

Medically Necessary: Services or supplies that are proper and needed for the diagnosis or treatment of a medical condition; are provided for the diagnosis, direct care, and treatment of a medical condition; meet the standards of good medical practice in the local area; and are not mainly for the convenience of a beneficiary or his or her doctor.

Medicare: The federal health insurance program for people 65 years of age or older, certain younger people with disabilities, and people with end-stage renal disease.

Medicare Approved Amount: The amount a health-care professional is paid by Medicare for a service or supply. This may or may not coincide with the amount the physician charges for this service or supply otherwise. Also known as the "approved charge."

Medicare Summary Notice (MSN): A summary form that lists all of the services or supplies billed to Medicare in your name in the past 30 days. Medicare is currently pilot testing an e-MSN, which allows beneficiaries to view MSNs online and print copies. This can be accessed at www.medicare.gov.

Medigap Policy: A Medicare supplement insurance policy sold by private insurance companies to fill "gaps" in original Medicare plan coverage. Except in Massachusetts, Minnesota, and Wisconsin, there are 10 standardized plans, labeled Plan A through Plan J. Medigap policies work only with the original Medicare plan.

Network: A group of doctors, hospitals, pharmacies, and other health-care experts hired by a health plan to take care of its members.

Nonparticipating Physician: A doctor or supplier who does not accept assignment on all Medicare claims. See **Assignment.**

Preferred Provider Organization (PPO): A Medicare + Choice coordinated care plan that (*a*) has a network of providers that have agreed to a contractually specified reimbursement for covered benefits with the organization offering the plan, (*b*) provides for reimbursement for all covered benefits regardless of whether the benefits are provided with the network of providers, and (*c*) is offered by an organization that is not licensed or organized under state law as a health maintenance organization.

Provider: Any Medicare provider (e.g., hospital, skilled nursing facility, home health agency, outpatient physical therapy, comprehensive outpatient rehabilitation facility, end-stage renal disease facility, hospice, physician, nonphysician, laboratory, supplier, etc.) supplying medical services covered under Medicare Part B.

Risk Adjustment: The way payments into health plans are changed to take into account a person's health status.

Social Security Administration: The federal agency that, among other things, determines initial entitlement to and eligibility for Medicare benefits.

Usual and Customary Rates: Early in Medicare's history, health-care (hospitalization) costs were reimbursed based on the average cost of the procedure in the previous year, as reported by individual hospitals.

References

1. Cohen, W.J. What every social worker should know about political action. Social Work 1966;11(3):3–11.
2. Corning, P.A. The Evolution of Medicare: From Idea to Law. Research report 29. U.S. Department of Health, Education, and Welfare (Social Security Administration, Office of Research and Statistics). Washington, DC: Government Printing Office, 1969.
3. American industrialization. Available at: http://home.earthlink.net/~gfeldmeth/lec.indust.html.
4. Gluck, M.G., Reno, V. (eds.) Reflections on Implementing Medicare. Washington, DC: National Academy of Social Insurance, 2001.

5. Mayo, T. Health care law: U.S. health care timelines. Available at: http://faculty. smu.edu/tmayo/health%20care%20timeline.htm. 2002.
6. U.S. Department of Health and Human Services. Centers for Medicare and Medicaid Services. Available at: http://www.cms.hhs.gov.
7. U.S. Department of Health and Human Services. Centers for Medicare and Medicaid Services. Medicare: today's issue—June 8, 2004.
8. Twentieth Century Fund. The Basics: Medicare Reform. A Twentieth Century Fund Guide to the Issues. New York: Twentieth Century Fund Press, 1995.
9. U.S. Department of Health and Human Services. Centers for Medicare and Medicaid Services. Medicare & You: Available at http://www.medicare.gov/Publications/Pubs/pdf/10050.pdf (accessed 7/08).
10. U.S. Department of Health and Human Services, Centers for Medicare and Medicaid Services. 2003 CMS Statistics (CMS publication 03445), June 2003.
11. www.aarp.org.
12. Bernstein, J., Stevens, R.A. Public opinion, knowledge, and Medicare reform. Health Affairs 1999;18:180–193.
13. Kaiser Family Foundation (2005, January). E-health and the elderly: how seniors use the internet for health information. January 2005. Available at: http://www.kff.org/entmedia/upload/e-Health-and-the-Elderly-How-Seniors-Use-the-Internet-for-Health-Information-Key-Findings-From-a-National-Survey-of-Older-Americans-Survey-Report.pdf. Accessed March 2, 2007.
14. National Center for Health Statistics, Centers for Disease Control and Prevention. Data warehouse on trends in health and aging. Available at: http://www.cdc.gov/nchs/agingact.htm. Accessed November 29, 2004. July 28, 2008
15. Pear, R. Bush nominee wants states to get Medicaid flexibility. January 19, 2005. Available at: www.nytimes.com. Accessed February 15, 2005.

Additional Resources

Social Security Administration: 1-800-772-1213.

www.medicare.gov, to find information about eligibility, benefits, premiums, which personal plan is best for you, and quality information.

5

Elder Autonomy and
Consumer-Directed Care

MARK SCIEGAJ

The provision of health-care and long-term care services often raises a number of issues of elder autonomy. The sections that follow describe current theoretical models for understanding individual autonomy and the primary conflict that often occurs in providing elder care services between the elder's preferences and the professional's judgment. The chapter also covers the emergence and evolution of consumer-directed care models for older adults and people with disability. *

Definition and Theoretical Models of Autonomy

Since the nineteenth century, individual autonomy has been a major theoretical concept in the Western philosophical literature.† This literature defines

---

* There's a difference between consumer-directed care for elders and emerging consumer-directed health-care plans. The latter focus on the creation of insurance products for young adults, aged 18–24, to enable them to purchase health-care insurance. Consumer-directed care for elders and people with disabilities focuses primarily on their ability to exercise greater choice or control with respect to their care.
† Two classic philosophical texts that influenced modern discussion of individual autonomy are John Stuart Mill's *On Liberty* and Immanuel Kant's *Critique of Practical Reason*.

autonomy as the individual's ability for self-governance. In general terms, autonomy is understood as an individual's independence from controlling influences and the capacity for intentional action (i.e., to possess agency). With the emergence of biomedical ethics in the late twentieth century, respecting the autonomy of patients and clients has been recognized as a major guiding principle for the conduct of health-care professionals.[1] Capitman and Sciegaj[2] have described three distinct theoretical models of individual autonomy: ideal autonomy, real autonomy, and contextual autonomy.

Ideal autonomy has had dominance in Western philosophical and legal traditions, and is viewed as the traditional model for understanding autonomy. Ideal autonomy models are abstract descriptions of autonomy. These models focus on the rational free will of separate individuals. To be autonomous in the ideal model requires that an individual possess rational capacity and sufficient knowledge about the situation as well as the absence of internal or external constraints. People who do not satisfy these criteria are said to have a reduced sense of autonomy. A major research initiative on the concept of autonomy in the late 1980s challenged this assumption.

In the late 1980s, the Retirement Research Foundation in Chicago sponsored the Autonomy in Long-Term Care initiative and provided grants to scholars across disciplines to examine whether the traditional ideal autonomy model applied to older adults. The outcome of this initiative was the creation of a range of real autonomy models. In real autonomy models, all individual autonomy is reduced autonomy. These models understand autonomy as a complex configuration of the individual's physical, psychosocial, and spiritual dimensions. The fact that everyone possesses a reduced autonomy requires more sophisticated conceptual frameworks.

One example of a real autonomy model was created by Bart Collopy[3] and suggests that the concept of autonomy embodies many different dimensions beyond rationality, with each dimension possessing polarities. For example, one dimension he discusses is decisional vs. executional autonomy. While autonomy would perhaps be best described where individuals could make decisions and execute these decisions, people with disabilities can be physically unable to do things for themselves. Does this mean they possess a reduced sense of autonomy? Collopy would argue that in fact individuals who have physical disability could be extremely autonomous because they maintain the ability to make their own decisions and express their own preferences. Indeed, at the time of Collopy's work it was being reported that people with even moderate forms of mental retardation could consistently express preferences and desires, leading some to believe that, while they lacked the rational capacity of the typically developed person, they actually still possessed an element of decisional capacity and, therefore, had decisional autonomy.

The research sponsored by the Retirement Research Fund autonomy initiative[*] advanced our understanding of individual autonomy within frail and disabled populations. While real autonomy models were certainly an improvement over the ideal autonomy dominance in thinking about the provision of health and long-term services for elders and people with disabilities, a real shortcoming of the models was that they continued to focus on individuals in isolation.

For this reason, in the 1990s a refinement of real autonomy took place, with the proposal by Capitman and Sciegaj of a contextual autonomy model.[2] The contextual autonomy model focuses on the relationships between individual interpretations and social/institutional contexts. The particulars of an individual's situation, according to this model, influence the range of choices that are available, how the person understands his or her ability to make a decision, and how the person's autonomy is defined and respected by others. Attention within this model is directed to the range of meaningful choices that individuals may have in any given system of care. To adequately assess individual autonomy, one must also assess the relationship and context between the individual, the informal care network, and the social institution.

As listed in Table 5.1, in this contextual autonomy model, there are a number of variables that influence the individual's range of meaningful choices. These include the individual's health and functional status. Health and functional status influence the range of choices that individuals can make for themselves. We recognize that populations with diminished cognitive status still have the ability to express preferences and desires; this does not mean that they are left to live and/or fend for themselves. Also, within the individual sets of variables that could influence their ability to make autonomous choices with respect to health and long-term care, their financial capacity and their knowledge about different care options certainly would make a difference. Also, the absence of a family or informal support networks might change their attitudes with respect to the kinds of care that they are seeking.

TABLE 5–1. Client-level determinants affecting ability to make meaningful choices

Individual	Health/functional/cognitive status
	Financial capacity
	Knowledge about options
Family/informal caregiver	Presence of support
	Competing demands

[*] The majority of the research sponsored by the Autonomy in Long-Term Care initiative can be found in the June 1988 volume 28 supplement of *The Gerontologist* and the 1990 volume 14 supplement of *Generations*.

Table 5.2 identifies a number of health-care and long-term care system features that can either support or hinder elder autonomy. One example of an institutional feature prevalent in the provision of long-term care for elders or people with disability is the professional agency person known as the "care manager." The care manager is responsible for meeting with the individual, conducting an assessment of his or her abilities or care needs, and then developing a plan of care to address those needs. While it is true that in some systems care managers solicit the opinion of the elder client, this is totally dependent upon the whim of the care manager. There is no requirement that the care manager consult extensively with the client and/or his or her family. In care systems where the care manager is solicitous of elder and/or family opinion, that would be a supportive element for individual autonomy. In systems where the care manager is not, the individual would have a reduced sense of autonomy which is based upon the actual circumstances of the care delivery system.

Conflict Between Autonomy and Beneficence

In any of these models, certain conflicts are inherent in the provision of care for elders and/or adults with disability. The central conflict that occurs in the provision of care is when elder preferences conflict with professional judgment. Historically, the philosophical literature has described this as the principle of autonomy conflicting with the principle of beneficence.

TABLE 5–2. System features that support or hinder client ability to make meaningful choices

FEATURES	SUPPORTS	HINDERS
Entry circumstances	Professional support for decisions	Health insurance counseling programs do not include long-term care
Care manager	Multiple service options	Lack of information on service choices
Care plan	Programs that assist elders in identifying and considering preferences for care	Narrow care manager authority over service options
Caregiver	Lack of multiple providers	Voucher systems with options
Daily routine	Inflexible schedules	Negotiated schedules
Exit circumstances	Reentry exclusions	Follow-up commitment

Beneficence is often described as the act of promotion of an individual's welfare. Those in the helping professions, be it health or long-term care provision, certainly see part of their obligation as the promotion of the individual's welfare—to do good to them or at least do no harm. When autonomy conflicts with beneficence, it creates a condition described as "paternalism."

Paternalism refers to the intervention in another person's preferences or actions with the intention of either avoiding harm to that individual or benefiting that individual. Paternalism is justified if we think that, left to her or his own, the individual poses a potential harm to her- or himself or others.[4] We also justify paternalism if we feel that our actions or our judgments are in the individual's "best interests." How this conflict of paternalism is played out or how it is justified determines whether we feel that the intrusion on the individual's autonomy is balanced by the provision of major benefit or the prevention of major harm.

Paternalism is also justified if it is seen as being only a minor violation of an individual's autonomy (i.e., the person's direction in life is not drastically altered). If it is a minor intrusion, then paternalism is seen as being justifiable. Finally, we justify paternalism using the principle of proportionality. In other words, elder-care professionals make decisions on a case-by-case basis, as opposed to creating a uniform policy for all elders despite their individual circumstances.

Consumer-Directed Long-Term Care

Consumer direction represents both a philosophical and a new orientation to service delivery of long-term care to elders.[5] The philosophical departure is that, whereas existing systems of care might emphasize beneficence as the operational principle, a consumer-directed model focuses on enhancing consumer choice, control, and decision making. The consumer-directed model orientation differs in service delivery from the traditional service delivery model, which focuses upon the use of professional judgment in making managerial or service decisions. In the consumer-directed model, the orientation of services is in the creation of opportunities to make meaningful decisions about one's service package. Such decisions include the amount of services received, the type of services received, or who is the provider of the services.

These are important issues because of the nature of long-term care service provision. Long-term care, unlike acute care, is typically given for indefinite periods of time, so the indignities often associated with professional care are even harder to endure. In a hospital setting, elders will be willing to forfeit their ability to do things on their own because of the demands of the treatment regimen. However, in long-term care settings, because they are being assisted with activities of daily life, elders typically have long histories of making decisions and performing self-care. In the context of long-term care, policy and program planners need to find ways to foster the ability of elders to take greater control of and make decisions with respect to their care needs.

This is not to say that there have not been a number of barriers to the development of consumer-directed long-term care for elders. One barrier historically has been that of professional training. Those who work in the elder care delivery system today have been trained with the principle of beneficence—the promotion of an individual's welfare. This has often led to autonomy being diminished in the name of either protection or the provision of benefit.

A second major barrier to the development of consumer-directed care was concern about quality assurance. Initially, there was great concern that elders would be the victims of fraud or that they themselves would perpetrate fraud. The concerns with respect to elder fraud would be that the elder and/or the family would accept monies or reimbursement and not actually use them for the services that the elder needed. There were also concerns with respect to elder abuse; that is, whether family members would take shortcuts or would not prescribe or utilize the full amount of services the elder needed.

A last quality-assurance issue, which was expressed not from elder advocates but, in fact, from the long-term care system itself, was that of worker exploitation. It was feared that consumer-directed models would put workers in a position of having to accept and/or work in conditions that were not of the same level and quality as the existing agency-based models.[6]

The Trend Toward Consumer-Directed Long-Term Care

However, even given these concerns and potential barriers, consumer-directed care options emerged in the 1980s. Two reimbursement mechanisms enabled the development of consumer-directed care models. Both of these came from the Medicaid program.[*] In the 1980s, the Medicaid program created two Medicaid waivers. A Medicaid waiver enables a state to propose to the Medicaid program an alternative system of care that is not institution-based (i.e., not skilled nursing–based). The first of these waivers that Medicaid allowed states to apply for was the 1915C Home and Community–Based Waiver. Under the 1915C waiver, states could create home and

[*] Medicaid is the primary payer of long-term care services in the United States. For this reason, the Medicaid program has been, since the early 1980s, looking for more cost-effective ways of delivering care. Historically, Medicaid has been directed only to the delivery of care in nursing homes. However, nursing home care is very costly. In 2006 the average cost of nursing home care was $75,000 a year. So Medicaid has been trying to find ways to keep people who don't necessarily need to have skilled nursing care out of nursing homes.

community–based services for elders who met the Medicaid financial aid eligibility and who, without such services, would end up in an institution. Again, the focus of the waiver was to divert unnecessary institutionalization of elders. The goal of the 1915C waiver was to allow elders to receive care at home and remain engaged in their communities. A second waiver developed by Medicaid for states was the 1115 Research and Demonstration Waiver. The 1115 waiver allowed states to create unique care options for elders to allow different kinds of services to be delivered. And it was under the 1115 Research and Demonstration Waiver that the first consumer-directed care models were formed.

In addition to a financial mechanism and philosophy of diverting elders from nursing homes and remaining in the community, the Retirement Research Foundation's autonomy initiative in the late 1980s gave impetus for the emergence of consumer-directed care. As discussed earlier in this chapter, the Retirement Research Foundation's Autonomy in Long-Term Care Initiative led to the redefinition of the concept of "autonomy." As well as creating new conceptual models of real autonomy, the Retirement Research Foundation initiative proposed how long-term care would adapt its practices and goals for elder-care services. Many of the initiative pieces adapted practices and goals of the disability community: to provide services in the least restrictive environment and that an individual had a right to self-determination. Together, the financial mechanisms of Medicaid and the reconceptualization that came out of the Retirement Research Foundation's autonomy initiative, gave a basis for the creation of consumer-directed care.

In addition to those elements of the 1980s, the passage of the Americans with Disability Act of 1990 gave impetus for the creation of consumer-directed care models for elders. The Americans with Disabilities Act guaranteed opportunity for individuals with disabilities in the areas of public accommodations, employment, and transportation.[7] In short, the Americans with Disabilities Act enables people with disabilities to be active and connected in their community. Namely, social institutions needed to make reasonable accommodations to support the disabled individuals' preferences, choices, and autonomy. The passage of the Americans with Disabilities Act encouraged elder advocates to demand more choice and control of elder-care services. The Americans with Disabilities Act had an invigorating effect on elder advocates, to demand increased support for elder autonomy.

In 1994 the 104th Congress was elected in part based on the "contract with America." While many argue that the 104th Congress had a negative impact on social welfare services, its increased emphasis on personal responsibility had a beneficial effect on the development of consumer-directed care models for elders. Members of the 104th Congress introduced the Medicaid Community Attendant Services and Supports Act (MiCASSA). If passed, MiCASSA would have been a radical reformulation of the Medicaid program. The Medicaid program, which historically focused on funding of elder-care services with money that would flow to an agency that then would be responsible for providing individual care, would now have the funding actually flow to the individual, with the individual being responsible for the creation and management of the care package.

Both conservative and liberal elements of Congress supported MiCASSA. However, it was not passed in 1994, nor has it been passed subsequently, although it was an active bill in the last legislative cycle for 2006. Even though it did not pass, MiCASSA also reinvigorated elder-care advocates to seek and create new forms of service delivery that would enhance an elder consumers' ability to direct their own care.

In the mid-1990s, after the Americans with Disability Act and the MiCASSA introduction, the Robert Wood Johnson Foundation had a series of requests for proposals around the delivery of care for elders that was focused on enhanced autonomy. There were three major initiatives that the Robert Wood Johnson Foundation funded in the mid-1990s. The first of these was its Self-Determination Program. The Self-Determination Program was a series of grants that would be given to states to develop consumer-directed care systems for persons with intellectual disabilities. As noted earlier, research began to document the ability of people with intellectual disabilities to consistently state preferences and opinions with respect to their care.

The Self-Determination Program allowed 28 states initially and 38 states currently to create consumer-directed care for this particular population. A second major initiative of the Robert Wood Johnson autonomy initiative was the Cash and Counseling Demonstration and Evaluation Program. Cash and Counseling is a radical departure from the traditional service-delivery system for elders. Under the Cash and Counseling model, elders would be assessed for a care plan, but, instead of the agency delivering that care plan, the agency would provide the elder with a cash allowance to implement and manage his or her own care.

In the initial Cash and Counseling program, there were three states selected to participate. The states were selected based upon their willingness to contribute to a substantial amount of their own resources as well as their willingness to conduct a statewide experiment on Cash and Counseling. The experiment would be that the states randomly enroll 1500 people in Cash and Counseling and an equal number in a traditional agency-based service-delivery system. Those who were selected for Cash and Counseling would be evaluated, have a care plan drawn up, and receive a percentage of the total cost of that care. Depending upon the state, it could be 90% or 85% of the total care package. States reduced the total amount from 100% to 90% or 85% because they removed the cost of the care package that they would attribute to the agency's administrative overhead.

As part of the program, 1500 individuals who received Cash and Counseling would be evaluated against 1500 counterparts who received care in the traditional model. All 3000 participants in each of the states had to express a willingness to accept Cash and Counseling. This certainly led to, in some states, people not being happy about Cash and Counseling and then being assigned to the traditional model; however, it was this randomized selection that enabled the evaluators of the program to have a true experimental design. The experimental design would compare the experiences of the Cash and Counseling recipients vs. their traditional counterparts. Some of the areas that the participants were asked to focus on were level of satisfaction, extent of unmet need, existence of fraud or abuse situations, and overall health and well-being. In each of these areas, Cash and Counseling recipients demonstrated better outcomes than the recipients of traditional agency-based care.[6,8–10] The success of the three-state demonstration prompted an expansion to 15 states which either have established or are in the process of establishing Cash and Counseling programs.[11]

The final initiative of the Robert Wood Johnson Foundation in the 1990s was its Independent Choices Program. Independent Choices was mandated to look at other alternative consumer-directed care models short of Cash and Counseling. For example, the Robert Wood Johnson Foundation was interested to know whether the existing system could be altered or adapted short of developing Cash and Counseling. The Independent Choices Program contained 13 research projects and eight demonstration projects. The demonstration projects made alterations to existing programs to enhance consumer choice and control, while the 13 research projects focused on understanding what the implications for service delivery were if elders possessed greater choice and control.[12] The findings of the projects and research funded under Independent Choices confirmed the emerging evidence from the Cash and Counseling program; consumer-directed care provided its recipients better outcomes with respect to satisfaction, fewer unmet needs, and care quality.[5]

Does Consumer Direction Work?

From the Cash and Counseling Demonstration and Evaluation Program as well as the Independent Choices Program and a number of independent studies with respect to consumer-directed care, there is a growing body of evidence of its utility for the provision of elder-care services. In a meta-analysis funded by the National Council on Disability, researchers examined whether people enrolled in consumer-directed care models have greater levels of satisfaction, a greater sense of control, fewer unmet needs, fewer safety concerns, and enhanced quality of life. Along each of these parameters in the three Cash and Counseling states as well as eight large-scale national representative studies, it has been found that people enrolled in consumer-directed care models have greater levels of satisfaction, greater feelings of control, fewer unmet needs, higher quality of life, and fewer issues with respect to their own safety.[13]

With external evaluations of consumer direction documenting positive outcomes of those enrolled in the program, the Department of Health and Human Services in 2002 announced the Independence Plus initiative. The purpose of Independence Plus is to simplify the Medicaid waiver application process in order to facilitate the creation of programs like Cash and Counseling-like programs. By 2007 there were 11 approved Independence Plus waivers in 10 states, with several more working with the Centers for Medicare and Medicaid Services on proposed waivers.[14]

The Reauthorization of the Older Americans Act in 2006 firmly incorporated consumer-directed care and elder autonomy as a part of its mission. The Reauthorization of the Older Americans Act of 2006 created Choices for Independence.[15] Under Choices for Independence, the Administration on Aging has committed $28 million to demonstration projects to promote consumer-directed and community-based long-term care options. In the Older Americans Act of 2006 explicit language under Choices for Independence focuses and redirects long-term care for elders to promote the dignity and independence of older people. The justification or rationale for the Choices for Independence Demonstration Program is to meet the challenges associated with the aging of the baby boom generation. The baby boom generation, it is believed, will be more demanding with respect to systems of care that promote their autonomy and their ability to make their own decisions. With the creation of the New Freedom Initiative and the Reauthorization of the Older Americans Act, consumer-directed long-term care will be a prominent feature in the delivery of long-term care services for elders in the United States for decades to come.

Application to the Case Study: The Older Adult Care, Training, Research, and Planning Program

With respect to the case, the Older Adult Care, Training, Research, and Planning Program, the focus on elder autonomy and consumer direction is most applicable to the fourth part of the stated mission, states that one of the goals of the training program is to study the factors that affect health, functional status, and need for and use of health services including economic, social, and cultural factors. In thinking about elder autonomy, particularly from a contextual autonomy model, it is important to recognize that individuals are enmeshed in different social structures, institutional structures, and familial structures and that those structures really have an impact on individuals' understanding of what their care needs may be, the options that they may have to meet those needs, and their ability to obtain the necessary resources to maintain or improve their health.

A training and research planning program, as proposed in the case, particularly given its social location, would need to be sensitive with respect to the various institutional, social, and cultural networks that may shade the vision or shape the worldview of the elder recipients whom they are seeking to work with. As the case notes, the ethnic character is very mixed in older second- and third-generation immigrant groups. For this reason, having a greater understanding of racial and ethnic differences with respect to autonomy for health-seeking behavior is important. While race has been commonly understood as a dichotomous variable (i.e., either you were a member of a particular race or you weren't), researchers and service providers now recognize that there is great heterogeneity within as well as between racial and ethnic groups. Thus, understanding how these elements manifest themselves would be critical for fulfilling the mission of this proposed research and education entity.

Because the proposed center has a number of health-planning, health education, restorative care, occupational therapy, physical therapy, mental health with psychological counseling, and social work elements, the trainees and other service professionals will need to consider possible conflicts between autonomy and beneficence, especially when professional judgment is used to preempt elder preferences. In each of these areas of service delivery, understanding why people may not be inclined to use a particular service or why they may deviate from a service plan and whether those reasons or preferences are legitimate should limit professional judgment in certain instances.

Finally, we seek not only to understand elder autonomy in terms of ideal, real, or contextual models, but within these broad frameworks we seek opportunities for professionals to enhance an elder's ability to exercise choice and control with respect to health care. In a training program like the proposed comprehensive model that provides education, services, and training of future health-care professionals, as well as having an element of research itself, it seems that those elements lend themselves to understanding elder autonomy in all of its many different facets as a way of enabling elders to become greater participants in the receipt and provision of care. It also would create opportunities for partnerships between service providers and care recipients.

Bibliography

Brown, B., Dale, S. The research design and methodological issues for the Cash and Counseling evaluation. Health Services Research 2007;42(1 part 2):414–445.

Capitman, J., Sciegaj, M. A contextual approach for understanding individual autonomy in managed community long-term care. The Gerontologist 1995;35: 533–540.

Carlson, B., Foster, L., Dale, S., Brown, R. Effects of Cash and Counseling on personal care and well-being. Health Services Research 2007;42(1 part 2):467–487.

Dale, S., Brown, R. How does Cash and Counseling affect costs? Health Services Research 2007;42(1 part 2):488–509.

National Council on Disability. Newsroom. Consumer-directed health care: how well does it work? Available at: http://www.ncd.gov/newsroom/publications/2004/consumerdirected.htm. Accessed May 23, 2007.

Schore, J., Foster, L., Phillips, B. Consumer enrollment and experiences in the Cash and Counseling program. Health Services Research 2007;42(1 part 2):446–466.

Squillace, M., Firman, J. The myths and realities of consumer-directed services for older persons. Available at: http://www.ncoa.org/Downloads/Myths_and_Realities.pdf. Accessed May 22, 2007.

References

1. Beauchamp, T., Childress, J. Principles of Biomedical Ethics, 5th ed. New York: Oxford University Press, 2001.

2. Capitman, J., Sciegaj, M. A contextual approach for understanding individual autonomy in managed community long-term care. The Gerontologist 1995;35:533–540.

3. Collopy, B. Autonomy in long-term care: some crucial distinctions. The Gerontologist 1988;28(Suppl.):10–17.

4. Mill, J.S. On Liberty. New York: Dover Publications, 2002.

5. Squillace, M., Firman, J. The myths and realities of consumer-directed services for older persons. Available at: http://www.ncoa.org/Downloads/Myths_and_Realities.pdf. Accessed May 22, 2007.

6. Schore, J., Foster, L., Phillips, B. Consumer enrollment and experiences in the Cash and Counseling program. Health Services Research 2007;42(1 part 2):446–466.

7. Americans with Disabilities Act of 1990. Available at: http://www.ada.gov/pubs/ada.htm. Accessed May 23, 2007.

8. Brown, B., Dale, S. The research design and methodological issues for the Cash and Counseling evaluation. Health Services Research 2007;42(1 part 2):414–445.

9. Carlson, B., Foster, L., Dale, S., Brown, R. Effects of Cash and Counseling on personal care and well-being. Health Services Research 2007;42(1 part 2):467–487.

10. Dale, S., Brown, R. How does Cash and Counseling affect costs? Health Services Research 2007;42(1 part 2):488–509.

11. Cash and Counseling. About us. Participating states. 2007. Available at: http://www.cashandcounseling.org/about/participating_states.

12. Robert Wood Johnson Foundation. Independent Choices: enhancing consumer direction for people with disabilities. June 2004. Available at: http://www.rwjf.org/reports/npreports/indchoices.htm.

13. National Council on Disabilities. Newsroom. Consumer-directed health care: how well does it work? Available at: http://www.ncd.gov/newsroom/publications/2004/consumerdirected.htm. Accessed May 23, 2007.

14. Centers for Medicare and Medicaid Services. Independence Plus overview. Available at: http://www.cms.hhs.gov/IndependencePlus/. Accessed May 7, 2007.

15. Administration on Aging. Choices for independence: modernizing the Older Americans Act. 2006. Available at: http://www.aoa.gov/about/legbudg/oaa/Choices_for_Independence_White_Paper_3_9_2006.doc. Accessed May 23, 2007.

6

Prevention

SARITA BHALOTRA AND JOHN ORWAT

> The role of (acute) medical care in preventing sickness and premature death is secondary to that of other influences; yet society's investment in health care is based on the premise that it is the major determinant. It is assumed that we are ill and made well, but it is nearer the truth that we are well and made ill.
>
> —T. McKeown (1979) The Role of Medicine: Dream, Mirage, or Nemesis? Princeton, NJ: Princeton University Press

> It is our duty, my young friends, to compensate for (aging) by a watchful care; to adopt a regimen of health, to practice moderate exercise, and take just enough food and drink to restore our strength and not to over-burden it...
>
> —Cicero, 106–43 BC. In: Porter, R., The Greatest Benefit to Mankind: A Medical History of Humanity. New York: WW Norton and Co., 1999, p. 69.

Over 45 years ago Leonard W. Larson, MD, then president of the American Medical Association, called for a "revolution in aging" in which medicine is reformulated to emphasize a proactive approach to addressing healthy behavior in the individual throughout the life course rather than reactively treating disease.[1] Since then, the U.S. population has continued to age as better living conditions and technological advances have increased life expectancy dramatically and normative expectations around functionality have increased, making prevention throughout the life course even more important. The potential for improved quality of life accompanied by cost savings due to compression of morbidity,[2] i.e., optimizing aging so that disability is minimized, is significant. However, the U.S. health-care system remains structured and financed in a manner most responsive to the treatment of acute conditions rather than prevention throughout the life span or the treatment of chronic and disabling illness.

Research continues to demonstrate that much of the decline traditionally attributed to the aging process can be prevented by reducing risky behaviors and increasing healthy behaviors.[3-5] By shifting the emphasis from treating symptoms to the prevention of illness and reducing its progression, health-care providers can be more effective at improving not only the length of life but also the quality of life, by encouraging health-promotion efforts in their patients. Despite their proven effectiveness and potential for savings, barriers to providing these services remain for patients and physicians in utilizing them, and for health care delivery and financing systems for implementing them. Many of these barriers are grounded in the myth that aging is a process of intractable decline due to factors such as genetics which are not affected by behavioral change. This chapter focuses on health promotion and primary prevention in older adults by reviewing the natural history of aging, the factors which cause ill health and functional decline, models of health promotion, and the policy implications for delivery and financing of care.

Demography and Epidemiology of Older Adults in the United States: Age, Gender, Ethnicity, Health Status, Functional Status, and Projections

As a result of advances in medical sciences and improved living conditions in the United States, Americans are living longer and older adults constitute a growing proportion of the population. The U.S. Census Bureau estimates that in 2004 over 36 million people were 65 or older.[6] This group now makes up just under 13% of the U.S. population, up from 4% in 1900 and projected to increase to 20% by 2030.[6] Life expectancy has increased to 77.8 years in 2004 (80.4 years for women and 75.2 years for men).[7] Moreover, in 2004 life expectancy for those who reach age 65 was 18.7 years, and it was 11.9 years for those reaching 75.[7] As life expectancy increases, those over 85, often referred to as the "oldest old," have become the fastest-growing segment of the elderly population, comprising just under 2% of the population in 2004 and projected to increase to 5% by 2050. In fact, the number of centenarians, or those 100 or older, has continued to grow from 37,000 in 1990 to over 70,000 in 2005.[7]

The elderly are a racially and socially diverse segment of the population. In 2003, non-Hispanic whites were the largest elderly racial group at 83%; blacks made up 8%, Asians 3%, and Hispanics 6%.[7] Projections indicate increasing diversity: by 2030, non-Hispanic whites will make up 72%, Hispanics 11%, blacks 10%, and Asians 5%.[7] In 2005, women made up a majority of those 65 or older at about 58% and almost 70% of those over 85.[6] With regard to marriage, in 2003 71% of men over 65 were married compared to approximately 41% of women.[6,7] This trend continues into the oldest old, among whom 56% of men and 13% of women were married.[6,7] Widowhood was experienced by 44% of women who were 65 and older but only 14% of men; for the oldest old, 78% of women and 35% of men were widowed.[7]

As people age, the risk of chronic conditions and disability increases (Table 6.1): 87% of adults over 65 years old and 92% of those 80 and older have at least one chronic condition.[8] The most common chronic conditions in this age group are hypertension (51%), arthritis (37%), heart disease (29%), and eye disorders (25%).[8] Among those over 65, 67% have multiple chronic conditions, that puts individuals at greater risk for disability and functional limitations.[8] Fully 73% of those who are 80 or older have two or more chronic conditions.[8] Women are more likely than men to have one or more chronic conditions (Fig. 6.1).

Activity limitations are often caused by chronic conditions, and these limitations disproportionately impact people of color. For Americans 65 or older, 34% reported any activity limitation, with 6.1% reporting a limitation in activities of daily living (ADL) and 11.5% reporting limitations in instrumental ADL.[7] Asian Americans are the least likely to have activity limitations due to chronic illnesses, followed by whites (11.6%), African Americans (15.3%), and American Indians/Alaskan Natives (17.1%).[7] When considering ethnicity, Hispanics are less likely to report limitations (10.2%) than non-Hispanics (12.3%).[7]

TABLE 6–1. Prevalence of chronic conditions, disability, and functional limitations, 1996

	AGE (YEARS)			
	50–64	65–74	75–84	85+
None of the three problems	30%	17%	10%	4%
Chronic conditions only	47%	51%	37%	17%
Disability only	2.3%	2.1%	2.1%	3%
Functional limitations only	0.1%	°	0.4%	°
Any two of the three problems	16%	22%	32%	32%
All three problems	5%	8%	19%	44%

°Cell size too small to report

Source: Partnership for Solutions. Johns Hopkins University analysis of MEPS, 1996. Available at: http://www.partnershipforsolutions.org/index.html.

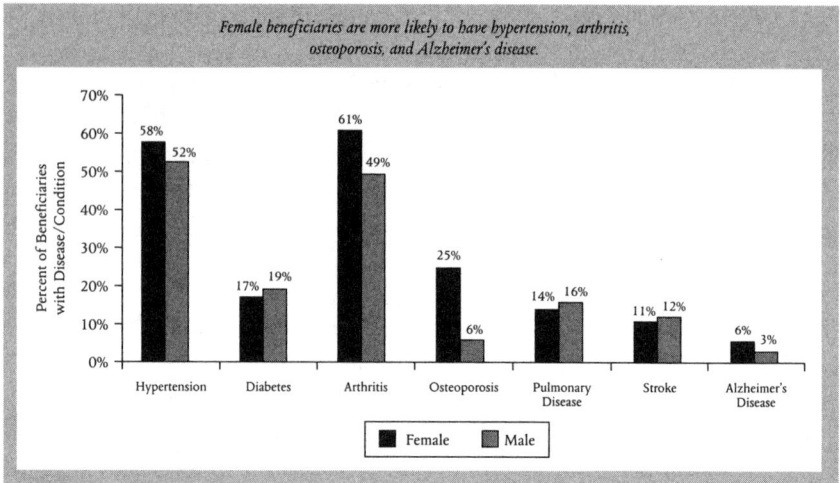

Female beneficiaries are more likely to have hypertension, arthritis, osteoporosis, and Alzheimer's disease.

FIGURE 6.1 Medicare beneficiaries' self-reported diseases and conditions by gender, 2000.
SOURCE: CMS, Office of Research, Development, and Information.
Data from the Medicare Current Beneficiary Survey (MCBS), 2000.
Access to Care File. Available via http://www.cms.hhs.gov/LimitedDataSets/
11_MCBS.asp#TopOfPage

The elderly are likely to have limitations in ADL (Figs. 6.2 and 6.3). Across all age groups, chronic conditions account for significant direct and indirect costs. The treatment of chronic conditions accounts for 83% of health-care spending in the United States.[8] Further, people with chronic conditions are the heaviest users of health-care services.[8] Patients who have poorer health and more disabilities are more likely to be on Medicaid. The average per capita spending increases with the number of chronic conditions; furthermore, the cost of care for chronic illness rises exponentially with the number of chronic conditions, for both insured services and out-of-pocket costs, as Tables 6.2 and 6.3 illustrate.[8] Indirect costs include not only the costs related to lost workdays of the individual but also caregiver costs.

Topping the list of leading causes of mortality for those 65 years old and over are diseases of the heart (30%), malignant neoplasms (22%), cerebrovascular diseases (7%), and chronic lower respiratory diseases (6%) (Table 6.4).[7] The development of these conditions is often affected by modifiable risk factors, including the use of tobacco, alcohol, and illicit drugs; the consumption of high calorie foods with minimal nutritional value; inadequate physical activity; the misuse of toxic agents, firearms, and motor vehicles; and risky sexual behaviors.[9] Yet, primary intervention efforts begin only when clinical conditions manifest themselves, usually in old age after years of engaging in

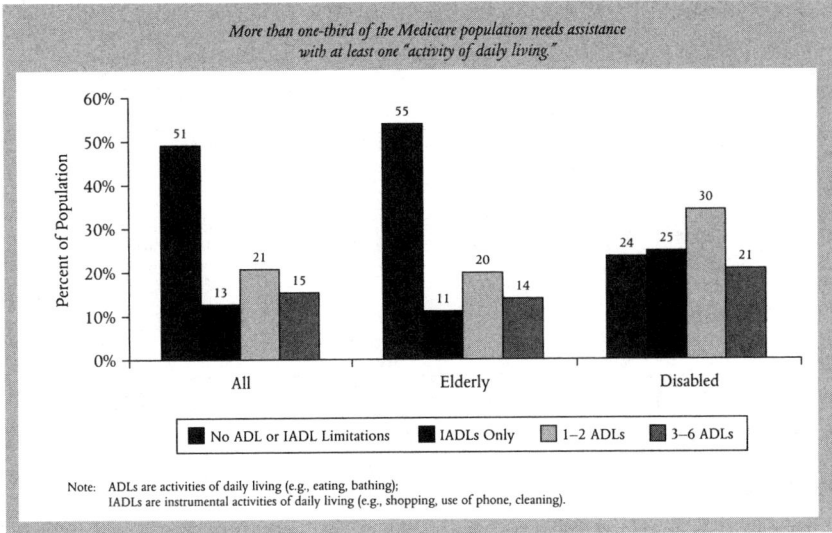

FIGURE 6.2 Distribution of Medicare enrollees by functional status, 2000.
SOURCE: CMS, Office of Research, Development, and Information: Data from
Medicare Current Beneficiary Survey (MCBS). 2000. Access to Care File.

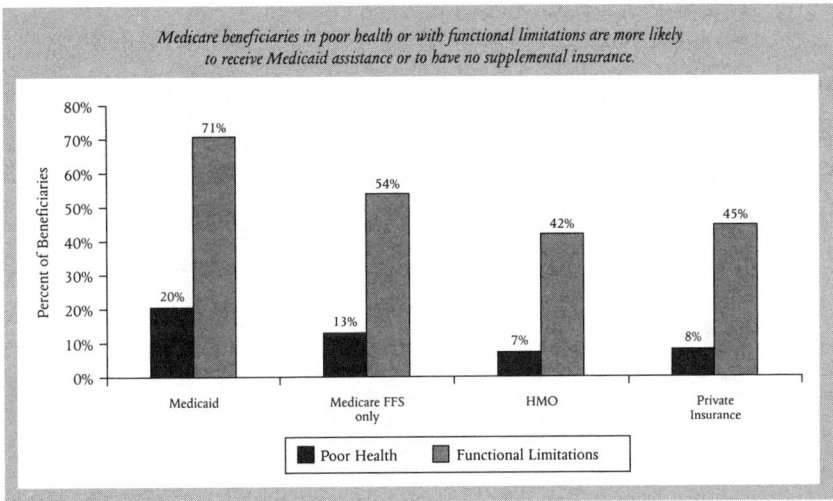

FIGURE 6.3 Beneficiaries with poor health and functional limitation by insurance
status, 2000. FFS, fee-for-service.
SOURCE: CMS, Office of Research, Development, and Information: Data from
Medicare Current Beneficiary Survey (MCBS). 2000. Access to Care File.

TABLE 6–2. Chronic conditions in the United States

	2000	2020
Prevalence	125 million	157 million
Direct cost	$520 billion	$1.07 trillion
Multiple chronic conditions	60 million	81 million

Source: Partnership for Solutions. Johns Hopkins University analysis of MEPS, 1996. Available at: http://www.partnershipforsolutions.org/index. html. Accessed March 3, 2007.

TABLE 6–3. Costs of chronic illness

NUMBER OF CHRONIC CONDITIONS	OUT-OF-POCKET COSTS	TOTAL ANNUAL COSTS
None	$182	$1,105
One	$369	$6,032
Two	$621	$10,908
Three or more	$1,106	$16,245

Source: Partnership for Solutions. Johns Hopkins University analysis of MEPS, 1996. Available at: http://www.partnershipforsolutions.org/index.html. Accessed March 3, 2007.

TABLE 6–4. Leading causes of death and numbers of deaths, 65 years and over: United States, 2004

All causes	1,755,669
Diseases of heart	533,302 (30%)
Malignant neoplasms	385,847 (22%)
Cerebrovascular diseases	130,538 (7%)
Chronic lower respiratory diseases	105,197 (6%)
Alzheimer disease	65,313 (4%)
Diabetes mellitus	53,956 (3%)
Influenza and pneumonia	52,760 (3%)
Nephritis, nephrotic syndrome, and nephrosis	35,105 (2%)
Unintentional injuries	35,020 (2%)
Septicemia	25,644 (1%)

Source: National Center for Health Statistics. Health, United States, 2006. In: Statistics NCHS. Washington, DC: U.S. Government Printing Office, 2006.

risky behavior, rather than forestalling the occurrence of these conditions through prevention. Furthermore, once chronic conditions become apparent, we fail to make use of ongoing prevention efforts to slow their progression and to improve the functioning of older adults. For example, Figure 6.4 shows that the rates of flu shots have gone up, albeit with disparity by race and ethnicity, but Table 6.5 shows the discrepancy between preventive services

TABLE 6–5. U.S. Preventive Services Task Force (USPSTF)-recommended preventive services and Medicare-reimbursed preventive services

USPSTF-RECOMMENDED PREVENTIVE SERVICES, ADULTS[1]	MEN	WOMEN	MEDICARE-REIMBURSED PREVENTIVE SERVICES[2]
Abdominal aortic aneurysm screening	X		
Alcohol misuse screening and behavioral counseling interventions	X	X	
Aspirin for primary prevention of cardiovascular events	X	X	
Breast cancer chemoprevention		X	
Breast cancer screening		X	Screening mammography
Breast and ovarian cancer susceptibility, genetic risk assessment and BRCA mutation testing		X	
Cervical cancer screening		X	Screening Pap test and pelvic examination
Chlamydial infection screening		X	
Colorectal cancer screening	X	X	Colorectal cancer screening
Depression screening	X	X	
Diabetes mellitus in adults, screening for type 2	X	X	Diabetes screening; diabetes self-management, supplies, and services
Diet, behavioral counseling in primary care	X	X	Medical nutrition therapy
Gonorrhea screening		X	
High blood pressure screening	X	X	
HIV screening	X	X	
Lipid disorders screening	X	X	
Obesity in adults screening	X	X	
Osteoporosis in postmenopausal women screening		X	Bone mass measurement
Syphilis infection screening	X	X	
Tobacco use and tobacco-caused disease, counseling to prevent	X	X	Smoking cessation

(continued)

TABLE 6–5. Continued

USPSTF-RECOMMENDED PREVENTIVE SERVICES, ADULTS[1]	MEN	WOMEN	MEDICARE-REIMBURSED PREVENTIVE SERVICES[2]
Recommended immunizations for adults 65 and older: TD booster every 10 years Measles-mumps-rubella, 1 dose Influenza annually Pneumococcal, 1 dose Hepatitis A Hepatitis B Meningococcal	X	X	Influenza immunization Pneumococcal vaccination Hepatitis B vaccination

[1] USPSTF recommends that clinicians discuss and prioritize these services with eligible patients. These services have received an "A" (strongly recommended) or a "B" (recommended) grade from the USPSTF. See http://www.ahrq.gov/clinic/ for specifics.

[2] Medicare reimburses for a "Welcome to Medicare Visit." Medicare preventive services that are reimbursable but do not meet USPSTF's A or B grade: prostate cancer screening, cardiovascular disease screening, and glaucoma screening.

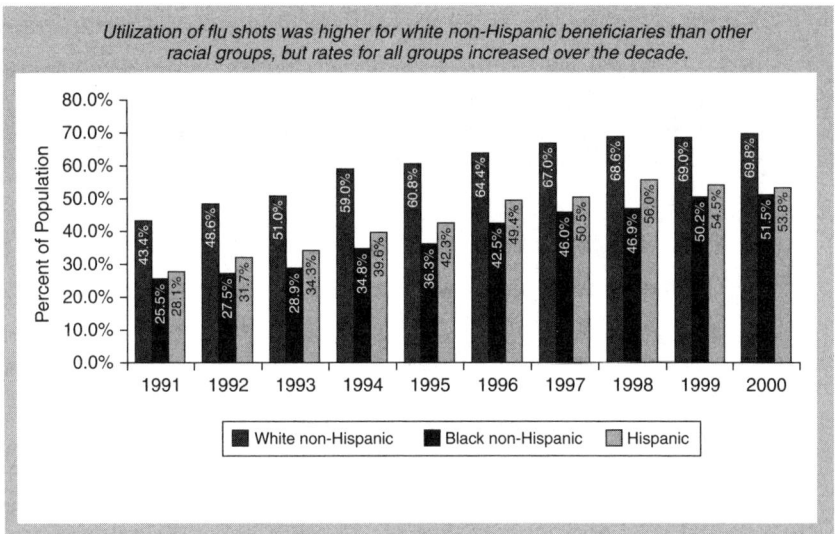

FIGURE 6.4 Medicare beneficiaries who received flu shots by race, 2000.
Note: Data reflect beneficiaries who reported receiving flu shots. The MCBS survey includes fee-for-service and managed care enrollees as well as aged and disabled beneficiaries; it does not include beneficiaries in facility care.
SOURCE: CMS, Office of Research, Development, and Information: Data from Medicare Current Beneficiary Survey(MCBS). 1999–2000. Access to Care Files.

recommended by the U.S. Preventive Services Task Force and what is covered as a benefit by Medicare.

Clearly, those over 65 years of age are quickly becoming a larger segment of the population and increasingly diverse. In fact, the population of the elderly will probably grow at rates that far exceed projections as unforeseen advances in technology advance life expectancy beyond what is considered possible today.[10] Further, the elderly are more likely to expect to be active and functional. The aging of the population as well as the changing nature of aging has and will continue to have an effect on the organization, delivery, and financing of the health-care system and, specifically, Medicare, the primary payer for the elderly.

Models of Aging: Natural History of Aging, including the Psychology of Aging as well as the Physiology–Pathology Continuum

Two schools of thought which conceptualize "successful aging" have gained prominence over the years.[11] The psychosocial school defines *successful aging* in terms of mental states such as life satisfaction and the acceptance of aging and eventual mortality. The biomedical school focuses on the avoidance of disease and disability. However, successful aging is not an "either–or" phenomenon but rather a "both–and" process. There is growing recognition that quality geriatric care involves not only the treatment of acute illness but also the promotion of both physical and psychological health by addressing lifestyle and risk factors.

Rowe and Kahn[3,12] define *successful aging* as growing old in the domains of health, strength, and vitality by avoiding disease and disability, engaging with life, and maintaining high cognitive and physical functioning. They expand on pathological/nonpathological models of aging by defining successful aging as the intersection of the three aforementioned domains and not just the absence of disease. Their model differentiates two pathways for nonpathological aging: *usual aging*, defined as high-risk and tenuous functioning, and *successful aging*, or low-risk and high function. These distinctions are important as historically "normal" aging was only defined as the absence of disease, leading many practitioners to conclude that decline and illness in old age were related to the genetically predetermined aging process, thus missing opportunities to prevent morbidity or mortality. However, research continues to demonstrate that many "usual" aging characteristics are related to behavior and lifestyle that, although age-related, are not age-dependent.[12]

Allostatic load is a measure of how well the adaptive systems of the body—the neuroendocrine system, autonomic nervous system, and immune system—have been able to maintain stability through change and has emerged as a factor in the resilience of the aging organism.[13] In their review of the literature Rowe and Kahn[12] identify three overall findings that influence the resilience of the aging organism. First, intrinsic factors alone, while highly significant, are not predominant in successful aging. Rather, extrinsic environmental factors and lifestyle play a highly significant role. Second, the relative contribution of genetic factors decreases with advancing age, and the impact of nongenetic factors increases. Third, and most importantly for the purposes of this chapter, most usual aging characteristics are modifiable.

"Normal Aging"

Research continues to demonstrate that decline during the aging process may have less to do with genetics and more to do with behavior.[4] *Normal aging* or *successful aging* is defined as the physiological attributes of aging uncomplicated by disease, environmental exposures, or lifestyle changes.[4] This is contrasted with the agingassociated with changes in the elderly that is caused by disease and adverse environmental and lifestyle factors.

Normal aging involves several physiological changes in organ systems (Table 6.6). Heart, lung, and bladder capacities decrease; neurons in the brain are either lost or damaged; and the kidneys become less efficient at removing waste from the blood, usually declining 30% by age 70. Eyesight, hearing, and muscle mass also decline. By 70 years of age, only 50% of the smells identifiable at 40 are recognized. Mental decline before the age of 80 is usually due to disease and not the normal aging process. Overall, personality, mood, and happiness/life satisfaction remain stable over the last half of life.[14] Over the past 20 years, the number of years spent in active retirement has increased dramatically. There are two clear conclusions: The population is aging, and the elderly as a group not only are more diverse than ever before but also expect a better quality of life as they age.

Factors in the Causation of Ill Health and Functional Decline of Older Adults: Impact of Lifestyle, Needs of Older Adults Based on These Factors

Sultz and Young[15] offer a concise model of the natural history of aging and its relationship to prevention that describes two periods: prepathogenesis and pathogenesis. In the prepathogenesis period, people need primary prevention, including such health-promotion activities as health education, wellness promotion, good nutrition, exercise, adequate housing, stress reduction, and the avoidance of alcohol, drugs, and tobacco. Specific protections are

Table 6–6. Normal aging

What is normal aging?

Individuals age at varying rates. Even within individuals, organs and organ systems show different rates of decline. However, some generalities apply as follows:

Heart: It grows slightly larger with age. Maximal oxygen consumption during exercise declines in men by about 10% with each decade of adult life and in women by about 7.5%. However, cardiac output stays nearly the same as the heart pumps more efficiently.

Lungs: Maximum breathing (vital) capacity may decline by about 40% between the ages of 20 and 70.

Brain: With age, the brain loses some cells (neurons) and others become damaged. However, it adapts by increasing the number of synapses and regenerating dendrites and axons.

Kidneys: These become gradually less efficient at extracting wastes from the blood. Bladder capacity declines. Urinary incontinence, which may occur after tissues atrophy, can often be managed through exercise and behavioral techniques.

Body fat: The body does not lose fat with age but redistributes it from just under the skin to deeper parts of the body. Women are more likely to store it in the lower body (hips and thighs) men tend to store fat in the abdominal area.

Muscles: Without exercise, estimated muscle mass declines 22% for women and 23% for men between the ages of 30 and 70. Exercise can slow this loss.

Sight: Difficulty focusing may begin in the 40s; the ability to distinguish fine details may begin to decline in the 70s. From 50 on there is increased susceptibility to glare, greater difficulty in seeing at low levels of illumination, and more difficulty in detecting moving targets.

Hearing: It becomes more difficult to hear higher frequencies with age. Hearing declines more quickly in men than in women.

Personality: After about age 30, personality is generally stable. Sudden changes in personality sometimes suggest disease processes.

Source: Adapted from "In Search of the Secrets of Aging", National Institute of Aging Booklets, NIH Publication 93–2756, http://www.healthandage.com/html/min/nih/content/booklets/in_search_of_the_secrets/p2.htm (last accessed 8/27/08).

also required, such as immunizations, accident prevention, seat belts, and the reduction of risk factors. The early period of pathogenesis requires secondary prevention involving early diagnosis and treatment as well as disability prevention. Beyond this period, tertiary prevention is needed, which involves rehabilitation and long-term support.

However widely used, the model is most useful in considering the development of a single acute condition in a linear process. As mentioned earlier, the elderly often have multiple chronic conditions that develop in an iterative fashion. Thus, activities considered "primary prevention" under the traditional model should persist through and beyond the occurrence of sentinel events requiring medical care. How can prevention be reframed so that what is traditionally considered "primary," in that it addresses risk factors before disease is precipitated, also applies once pathogenesis has been initiated, disease has progressed, and medical interventions are occurring? We propose the term "postevent prevention" (PEP) to stress the fact that prevention need not stop but in fact is essential to optimize aging. This term recognizes the ongoing importance of primary, secondary, and tertiary prevention to optimize aging.

Health status outcomes, including morbidity, mortality, quality of life, and satisfaction with care, are determined by a wide-ranging and not completely understood spectrum of factors including genetics. Historical, socioeconomic, and cultural factors not only shape the complex and interrelated meanings of social location (race/ethnicity, gender, social class, region and community) but also determine the resources available for health care and the environments in which one receives them. Where one is located socioeconomically is associated with lifetime cumulative and current effects of potentially modifiable health-related behaviors and risks. Community norms relating to lifestyle factors, for example, smoking, have a great influence on individual behavior; community availability of health services and healthy options for food and exercise vary considerably. What this reveals is that much of what impacts health status is modifiable, even postevent, and into aging.

Lifestyle

Lifestyle includes the behaviors in which one engages such as diet, exercise, substance use (including tobacco), and stress management. These behaviors continue to influence the health status of those over 65, and behavioral changes can improve the quality of life and reduce morbidity for those in this age group.

Research has repeatedly demonstrated the benefits of exercise, even when started in old age. It has a significant, positive impact on both psychological and physical health. It is known to reduce the severity and symptoms of depression and to slow the reduction of muscle loss associated with normal aging, thus possibly reducing the frequency and/or intensity of falls that lead to disability.[16] A review of the literature on strength training and older adults provides conclusive evidence of its efficacy, even when initiated in old age, in combating the weakness and frailty that occurs with aging as well as in reducing the risk of osteoporosis.[17] The literature also shows that exercise ameliorates the signs and symptoms of such chronic diseases as diabetes, hypertension, and heart disease.

Other lifestyle factors are also important contributors to health. Body fat is a significant risk factor for chronic illness and disability, and much attention has been paid recently to the epidemic of overweight and obesity in the United States. Up from 59% in the period 1988–1994, 68% of Americans 65 and older were overweight (39%), obese (29%), or severely obese (3.2%) in the 1999–2002 period.[7] Several factors play a role in this growing epidemic including the consumption of processed food with low nutritional value; only 31% of those aged 65 and older report eating more than five servings of fruits and vegetables daily.[7] Further, only 39% of adults 65 years and older report engaging in moderate physical activity.[7]

Smoking also continues to be one of the leading causes of preventable morbidity and mortality. Smoking has a cumulative effect and can lead to several types of cancers and various cardiovascular diseases. In 2005, just over 20% of Americans reported smoking cigarettes. For adults 65 years or older, 8.8% are current smokers and 41.6% are former smokers.[7] Smoking status, functional status, and health outcomes are related, which has important implications for the delivery and financing of health-care services. Smoking in old age contributes not only to increased mortality but also to morbidity (e.g., causing reduced bone density). Nonsmokers live longer and may be exposed to more disability, but their capacity to "maintain and restore health compresses their years of actual disability."[18] The benefits of quitting smoking in old age are significant. Long-term quitters have better functional status than those who still smoke. Clearly, smoking cessation at any stage has implications for improving both survival and functional status.

Substance use is one of the most significant yet underreported issues among the elderly. Estimates of alcohol abuse among the elderly range 4%–20% of those living in the community and 25% of those who are hospitalized.[19] The biggest barrier to treating geriatric alcoholism is its underdiagnosis, even though there are screening tools and treatment interventions that are known to be effective.[20] While fewer dual-diagnosis adults (those with concurrent psychiatric and substance use) survive into old age, those who do survive consume far more health services,[21] which suggests an increased need to promote behavior change.

Finally, the fact that a growing number of adults acquire human immunodeficiency virus (HIV) in their latter years suggests that risky sexual behavior prevention and intervention efforts also need to be included in this population.[22]

Needs of Older Adults in the United States Based on the Natural History of Aging

There is a significant association between functional decline, physical disability, and chronic disease, with the average older person having two or more chronic conditions including hypertension, stroke, diabetes, arthritis, heart disease, and lung disease. Fried et al.[23] show that disability in the elderly can be reduced, if not prevented, through health-promotion efforts. There is also increasing evidence that prevention and health promotion in older adults can lead to lifestyle changes and improved health status. Comprehensive, integrated education programs for the elderly who reside in the community are effective at improving health-promotion knowledge and behaviors. DeVito et al.,[24] for example, demonstrate that implementing a low-intensity exercise program for a clinically defined population of deconditioned elders at high risk of falling and sustaining serious injury leads to improvements in physical functioning that are retained over the long term. Prevention of disability in elders who are already symptomatic is vital in order to prevent further progression of disease and the development of functional limitation and disability.[25] This type of prevention targets elders who may have impairments and some functional limitation but have not yet developed any disability. Significant advances in health promotion and disease prevention could lead to the next cohort of elders being healthier, thus also decreasing health-care costs.[26] Since disabled elders incur on average five times as much in Medicare costs than the non-disabled do, a decline in disease and disability due to improved prevention would reduce costs. It is clear that practices and systems to meet the needs of older people must alter the basic acute-care orientation of primary care and address the preventive and psychological needs of elders, as well as enhance the patient's role in the self-management of illness.[27,28] However, the health care delivery system and financing mechanisms create obstacles to preventive initiatives so that the potential for providing preventive strategies remains underdeveloped.[3,29]

Models of Care: What Medicare Provides and What Other Models Exist—the Continuum of Patient Self-Management

The passage of Title XVIII of the Social Security Act in 1965 authorized Medicare to offer a range of medical benefits, thus reducing the percentage of the elderly uninsured from over 50% in 1963 to just under 1% in 2003.[30] Subsequent amendments to Medicare have extended coverage to apply not only to those age 65 and over but also to the disabled and those with end-stage renal disease. Medicare was designed to cover acute medical care, not prevention services. However, research on the prevention and management of chronic disease demonstrates their effectiveness and cost savings, an area of increasing importance in light of the extensive demands placed on Medicare. Medicare began covering pneumococcal vaccination in 1981; it made provisions for the development of prevention initiatives to promote early diagnosis and prevention in the Balanced Budget Act of 1997, and in the Medicare Modernization Act of 2003 it authorized a "Welcome to Medicare" visit, a one-time physical exam screening for those new to Medicare that covers heart disease and diabetes screening tests.[30] The new prescription drug benefit under Medicare (Part D) may also improve prevention efforts.

Medicare is not yet a sufficient resource for the health-care services required by elders, as Table 6.5 shows with regard to the utilization of Medicare-reimbursed clinical preventive services.[31] These needs will continue to be a growing burden and a major societal concern for the United States due to the increased number of elders. In this section, we discuss the literature on the need for prevention programs for elders with chronic disease and various models shown to manage chronic illness, slow progression of illness, and prevent disability for elders with chronic disease.

Wagner's Chronic Care Model

Wagner's model emphasizes high-quality chronic disease management at the community, organization, practice, and patient levels, with a focus on improving collaboration and partnerships between the community and the health-care system as a means to effectively manage chronic illness.[32]

This chronic care model addresses health-care system changes necessary for improving chronic illness care and recommends evidence-based interventions in six areas known to improve the processes of care and patient outcomes: delivery system design, decision support, information systems, linkages to the community, self-management support, and organization of the health-care system with proactive patients and providers.[32]

Chronic Disease Self-Management

Successful self-management programs rely on collaboration between patients and providers to define problems, set priorities, establish goals, create treatment plans, and solve problems.[27,33] Self-management support is a central feature of the chronic care model since the informed, active patient is central to productive patient–provider interactions.[34]

The patient–provider partnership embraces two primary components— collaborative care and self-management education.[35] Collaborative care implies patient–physician relationships in which patients and physicians make health-care decisions together.[33] Self-management education provides patients with problem-solving skills which enhance their lives and improve their ability to reduce risky behaviors. Both collaborative care and self-management education frameworks emphasize the role of patients as principal caregivers, but great responsibility remains with health professionals, who need to use their expertise to inform, activate, and assist patients in their self-management.[33]

Chronic Illness Care Breakthrough Collaboratives

Chronic illness care breakthrough collaboratives are designed to address disease management limitations and to provide effective models for improving care across a variety of chronic illnesses.[34] Collaboratives involve health-care teams from multiple health-care settings who use a longitudinal and iterative process designed by the Institute of Health Care Improvement and Associates in Process Improvement, using the chronic care model to implement system changes shown to improve care. These collaboratives focus on diabetes, asthma, depression, and cardiac disease.

Lorig's Chronic Disease Self-Management Programs

Since elderly patients often have more than one chronic condition, disease-specific patient education may not be the most efficient or most effective means of dealing with the growing problems associated with chronic disease. The Stanford University Patient Education Research Center addresses this issue with Lorig's Chronic Disease Self-Management (CDSM) program, which is a community-based intervention built on self-efficacy theory focused on helping seniors with goal setting; problem solving; exercise; nutrition; medication use; coping with anger, fear, frustration, and depression; management of pain, fatigue, and shortness of breath; and improving communication with friends, family, and health-care professionals.[36,37]

Senior Wellness Projects

Senior centers have long provided a place for social interaction and health-related programs, although the diversity and efficacy of such programs vary markedly.[38] The Northshore Senior Center of Seattle/King County in Bothell, Washington, has a Senior Wellness Project that is a good prototype of various interventions shown to decrease disability risk and/or improve function in elders in one interconnected program.

Diabetes Self-Management Programs

Medicare now pays for diabetes chronic disease self-management programs. Due to reimbursement support, hundreds of these programs exist all over the country. Medicare guidelines also dictate substantive aspects of these programs, such as the need for them to be run by a diabetes education specialist.[39] The programs must also follow self-management clinical guidelines published by the American Diabetes Association.

Arthritis Self-Management Programs

The Arthritis Foundation bought the rights of Dr. Kate Lorig's CDSM programs and sponsors these programs all over the country.

Program of All-Inclusive Care for the Elderly

The Program of All-Inclusive Care for the Elderly (PACE) is a national demonstration model integrating care for frail elders who are eligible for nursing facilities but who prefer to live at home. The 1997 Balanced Budget Act established PACE as a permanent program, and more than 90% of PACE participants (members) are eligible for both Medicare and Medicaid. The PACE programs are excellent examples of linkages of medical care with community settings like elder housing sites or federally assisted housing sites and senior centers. They often partner with hospitals or other health-care organizations that take responsibility for the medical aspects of care. At the heart of the PACE model of care is an interdisciplinary team of physicians, nurses, social workers, therapists, dietitians, and transportation and home-care workers who focus on each member. The team makes service allocation decisions based on member and caregiver input and continuously assesses member needs, treatment plans, and services.[40]

Social Health Maintenance Organizations

Social health maintenance organizations (HMOs) integrate community-based services, acute care, and long-term care services, thus improving the ability to respond to the medical needs of frail members with acute and long-term care needs.[41] The social HMO model has an advantage over the PACE model because it is open to all Medicare beneficiaries rather than only to those who are disabled. Social HMO benefits include all Medicare-covered services as well as community care services ranging from in-home aides, transportation, adult day care, and non-Medicare durable equipment to personal emergency response services.[42]

Geriatric Assessment Programs

The literature suggests that comprehensive geriatric assessments produce substantial benefits, including reduced mortality rates and nursing home admissions.[43] Comprehensive geriatric assessments, developed in the United Kingdom, delineate an elder's medical, psychosocial, functional, and environmental resources and problems and link these to an overall plan for treatment and follow-up. Comprehensive geriatric assessment programs that combine geriatric evaluation with strong long-term management improve survival and function in elders.

Policy Implications for the Interdisciplinary Delivery and Financing of Health Care

A prevention model in health care is clearly understood when applied to children and younger adults. Preventive measures are often ignored, however, when providing care for elders due to popular misconceptions that prevention may no longer be effective for older adults or that they will be nonresponsive to such efforts. Health policy, and therefore the service-delivery system and its financing mechanisms, should reflect the fact that prevention activities can effectively improve the quality of life and decrease the cost of care for older adults. This is an essential first step toward effective programmatic intervention. It is clear that prevention activities such as lifestyle modifications around diet, exercise, and smoking cessation contribute immensely to health, even "if adopted late in life."[3] We need to develop a system that has the flexibility, credibility, and resources necessary to encourage and support these services for older adults. Rowe[3] has suggested that the Medicare program would be a natural leader for initiating a model such as this, which he refers to as a "preventive geriatrics" program that can improve elders' health and quality of life. Moreover, an expanded, population-based approach by Medicare, emphasizing prevention of chronic disease, may well have a favorable impact on Medicare program costs.[26]

Medicare is an obvious avenue for actively initiating this policy. Indeed, the Centers for Medicare and Medicaid Services' proposed and current demonstration programs indicate how much attention is being directed to this issue. These include, for example, the Chronic Illness Disease Management Program, including end-stage renal disease management, smoking cessation, healthy aging, senior risk reduction, care management, a lifestyle modification program for patients with established coronary artery disease, and voluntary chronic illness care. As the recent debate around providing drug benefits showed, any provision for increasing benefit levels under Medicare can be expected to be met with great scrutiny and political resistance. There is persuasive evidence, however, that preventive measures can actually save Medicare costs in the long run and may therefore be both politically and financially viable. As a single illustrative example, patients with arthritis, cardiovascular disease, parkinsonism, stroke, depression, and sleep disorders can all show improvement with exercise; and exercise can prevent hip fractures from falls by increasing bone density and muscle strength, even in frail and very old adults.[44] Such preventive measures can have an impact on the over billions of dollars expected to be spent in direct costs for treating fall injuries in adults 65 years and over.[45]

Of course, even the universal adoption of preventive measures and lifestyle changes would not guarantee improvements in the health of older adults. As Blum[46] proposed, four major domains, or "force fields," simultaneously influence health: genetics, environment, lifestyle, and access to tertiary-care services. Health-care workers often experience frustration with the apparent intractability of addressing health behaviors through preventive health interventions and health-promotion activities. This may be exacerbated when managing older patients, in whom such behaviors are presumably far more firmly entrenched. And yet, the evidence continues to build that these interventions are effective. In fact, the desire to remain as fully functional as possible in the face of declining physiological function, as well as the shock of experiencing a potentially life-threatening condition at least partially precipitated by modifiable health behaviors, may make older adults more amenable to such interventions. The fact of aging should not prevent patients, providers, and the health care–delivery system from planning for, implementing, and practicing prevention for older adults.

We should not expect that raising awareness and providing enhanced services will automatically result in universal adoption of healthier lifestyles and preventive behaviors. The burgeoning health education and behaviors literature attests to the challenges faced by past and current lifestyle modification approaches. Neither can the health-care system be expected to assume full responsibility for broader social problems such as poverty and social isolation. However, a shift in the way an issue is viewed can itself result in gains on both the health and social fronts.

Application to the Case Study: The Older Adult Care, Training, Research, and Planning Program

One Academic Medical Center's Response

The Older Adult Care, Training, Research, and Planning Program (OACTRPP) was started by the university medical center (UMC) because of a felt need to expand the services offered to older adults within its catchment area beyond health-care services. This resulted from a growing recognition that acute-care services meet only a fraction of the needs of older adults and that serving the continuum of needs would improve both quality of life and clinical outcomes. Many clinicians had observed patients with, for example, congestive heart failure or diabetes cycling in and out of the hospital because of inadequate community services. Others had observed poorer clinical outcomes associated not with the quality of acute-care services but with inadequate attention to social or mental health needs. Lack of education about and awareness of self-care or doubts about self-efficacy in partnering in one's own care were also common observations. Thus, during the planning phase, the advisory committee of the OACTRPP reviewed research evidence in the area of prevention and health promotion for elder adults. Their review substantiated the fact that prevention and health promotion are effective at all stages of life and along the continuum of disease. A planning subcommittee was convened to review best practices in these areas. A report outlined the structure and features of a program that would best meet the needs of the elderly as well as achieve the goals of the OACTRPP. This was the PEP program, launched shortly after the opening of the OACTRPP.

The goal of the PEP program is to improve the quality of life for older adults who have one of several chronic conditions and to slow the progression of their clinical condition. In doing so, the PEP program is responsive to the OACTRPP's tripartite mission of adult education, research on aging, and planning programs for elder care. It will test whether participation in such a program improves the clinical condition and reduces the utilization of health-care services such as ambulatory care. Older adults will learn how to become more efficacious in the management of their condition through participation in a multimodal lifestyle modification program consisting of nutrition management, exercise, stress management, group support, and chronic condition-specific education. This program fulfills two of the OACTRPP's missions:

- To develop and test theories about planning, funding, and provision of health care in a community setting
- To study the factors that affect health, functional status, and need and use of health services, including economic, social, cultural, biological, and attitudinal factors

Initially, participants in the PEP program will be recruited from patients admitted to the UMC with a cardiac diagnosis, including acute myocardial infarction, coronary artery bypass grafting, and percutaneous transluminal coronary angioplasty. Later, eligibility criteria for participation will be broadened to include diabetes, hypertension, chronic renal failure, and major joint replacement. Staff for the PEP program will be drawn from the OACTRPP's multidisciplinary research, education, and service staff. A protocol for the multimodal program will be drawn up based on material available in the literature about its various components. Education staff will prepare a manual detailing the implementation of the various modalities of the PEP program. The UMC's information technology staff will provide the PEP program with a list of eligible patients, and the PEP service staff will contact these patients before discharge to introduce them to the program. They will follow up with interested patients and enroll them in the PEP program. An evaluation plan will be developed by the OACTRPP's research staff.

With the changing demographics and epidemiology in the United States reflecting a greater numbers of older adults and a greater prevalence of chronic conditions, it is imperative to shift the paradigm for managing this population from a reactive, acute-care model to a community-based, patient-centered model. Research has demonstrated that a passive approach to aging and the presence of chronic conditions, which is predicated on an inevitable model of precipitous decline, is not optimal and that models of self-care involving attention to nutrition, exercise, stress management, group support, and medication protocols can improve clinical outcomes. The PEP program will further test this theory.

Cases for Class Discussion

Mrs. Freeman and the Health-Care System

Bertha Freeman is a 67-year-old woman who lives in an inner-city area of Anytown. She is widowed and has three grown children. Two of her children live out of state, and the third lives in a suburban town 60 miles away. Bertha worked off and on as a store clerk until her diabetes and arthritis forced her to retire at the age of 54. Since then, she has been on Medicaid and Social Security disability. Lately, her problems have been further exacerbated by hypertension. She lives on the third floor of a walk-up six-unit apartment building. Her street has a series of similar buildings, most dating from the 1930s and 1940s and all in a run-down state. There is a convenience store on one corner of her street, that stocks everyday needs, including canned goods and occasional fresh produce. At the other end of the street is a liquor store. Mrs. Freeman does not drive or own a car. There is public transportation to downtown areas that are 2 miles away as well as to the imposing new UMC, which is 9 miles away. Mrs. Freeman is grateful that her church is just 1 block away because she likes to attend Sunday services regularly and to go out with "the ladies" afterward for the senior chicken-fried steak special at the local diner. The church has been instrumental in getting glasses for Mrs. Freeman since her eyesight deteriorated, but it has had less success in finding a hearing aid for her.

At 5 feet 4 inches, Mrs. Freeman weighs 210 pounds. She has never smoked, but her husband Billy did until he died of lung cancer just a few years ago. She receives her medical care at the local community health center 3 blocks away. This center was converted from a small community hospital and is now funded through the city council, the state, and some federal funds. It is staffed by a family practitioner and medical residents from the UMC. There are health education classes on some evenings, but Mrs. Freeman does not like having to walk back home at night. There are basic lab and radiology services. The nearest pharmacy on the bus route is 3 miles away. She is supposed to go to the health center once a month to have her medications checked but sometimes misses an appointment if she has run out of funds to pay for a taxicab and is not feeling well enough to walk. Since she is dual-eligible for Medicare and Medicaid and her state's Medicaid plan allows some prescription drug benefits, she has not had to pay much out-of-pocket until recently, when her hypertension became harder to control and the number and quantity of her prescription drugs increased. She heard that Medicare would pay for some of her drugs, but she does not know how to get the forms. Mrs. Freeman gets most of her information from television. Recently, she has seen several advertisements for new drugs and wonders whom she can ask about them.

When she goes for her checkups, there is usually a new resident who sees her. A few years ago, the center hired two nurse-practitioners. Three months ago, the nurse-practitioner noticed that Mrs. Freeman's ankles were swollen. Since she had not had any blood tests for almost a year, the resident ordered some tests. When Mrs. Freeman appeared for her visit 2 months later, the resident informed her that her kidneys were failing and that she would eventually need dialysis. She explained the procedure briefly to Mrs. Freeman and told her that she would set up a visit with the nephrologist at the UMC. She informed her that the dialysis center was located 15 miles away in the opposite direction and that she would eventually have to travel there three times a week to receive dialysis and to check in with the nephrologist at the UMC. Mrs. Freeman went home feeling so depressed that she did not go for her nephrologist visit. Since then, she has been feeling worse. She is nauseated much of the time and does not feel like eating. She can tell that her swelling is getting worse, and she hardly has the energy to walk to the corner store to buy her staple diet of macaroni and cheese and doughnuts.

Five days ago, Mrs. Freeman called her son, who lives 60 miles away, and in a weak voice told him that she had been vomiting steadily and could not get out of bed. An ambulance was called to transport her to the UMC, where she was acutely dialyzed. For several days specialists, including a nephrologist, a cardiologist, a rheumatologist, an endocrinologist, and a surgeon, came to see her every day to examine her and adjust her medications. She was told that she would need to start regular dialysis treatments after discharge. She was also told they would discharge her as soon as she had completed a number of dialysis treatments in the hospital. She would need to come back several times to the hospital to create a permanent access for dialysis. Mrs. Freeman is very nervous about going home.

Question

You are the leader of the PEP program interdisciplinary team managing Mrs. Freeman's care. What is your assessment of the services Mrs. Freeman needs? How will you help her get these services?

Mrs. Watkins and the Health-Care System

Mary Watkins is a 67-year-old woman who lives in a suburb of Anytown. She is widowed and has three grown children. Two live out of state, and the third lives in another suburban town 60 miles away. Mrs. Watkins helped with the books in her husband's business until her husband retired when she was 58. Mrs. Watkins is on Medicare and has supplemental insurance. Lately, Mrs. Watkins has needed increasingly expensive dental work, and her overall health-care costs have been creeping up. She thinks she may have to cut back on lawn maintenance in order to meet her monthly Medigap (Medicare supplement insurance) payment. She has smoked regularly since she was in high school, although lately she has cut back to a pack a day. She gets frequent upper respiratory infections, suffers from chronic sinusitis, and was hospitalized with pneumonia last winter. She lives in a four-bedroom, two-story home full of memorabilia, knickknacks, and oriental rugs on a tree-lined street in a quiet neighborhood. She drives her trusty Volvo wagon to the suburban malls and grocery stores, where she does all her shopping. Most of her friends have moved away to be near their children or to warmer climates, so she does not have much of a support network left. Mrs. Watkins spends her evenings watching television and sipping martinis just like she and her husband Fred did before he died. She had considered volunteering at the gift shop at the UMC, 2 miles away from her home, but decided it would be too boring.

At 5 feet 4 inches, Mrs. Watkins weighs 118 pounds. She was always the same height as her daughter but now appears to be a couple of inches shorter. Mrs. Watkins' daughter works in an adult day-care center. She purchased a monitoring system for her mother costing $69 per month that alerts the company when she presses the button concealed in a pendant worn around her neck. Mrs. Watkins thinks it is silly but wears it to humor her daughter. She receives her medical care at a multispecialty clinic located next to the mall where she usually shops. She has been with the same practice for 27 years, since her obstetrician referred her to an ear, nose, and throat specialist there for her frequent attacks of sinusitis. She was then referred to a pulmonologist when she came down with an upper respiratory tract infection. The next time she needed care was when her wrist and hand started hurting, and the pulmonologist referred her to a neurologist, who sent her to a hand surgeon for treatment of carpal tunnel syndrome. After that, she was referred to an orthopedic surgeon for painful bursitis in her big toe. When her husband's firm switched to a managed-care plan, she was allowed to choose her primary-care physician from the same group. He provided her with care when she called with a problem, most often a respiratory infection, for which she was prescribed antibiotics. Her regular physician was on vacation 2 months ago when Mrs. Watkins developed a cold, swollen glands in her neck, and a low-grade fever. She was seen by a young, newly hired female internist. Expecting to be examined and prescribed antibiotics as usual, Mrs. Watkins was surprised when this physician also told her to take calcium, follow the food pyramid, exercise every day, lift weights, and stop smoking, and admonished her gently for missing her scheduled mammography and annual flu shot, all in the 15 minutes she was allotted per patient. She also recommended a bone density scan some-time soon.

Mrs. Watkins did not know how she could accomplish all this by her next visit and went home feeling so confused that she did not go in for her follow-up visit. Since then she has been feeling worse. Her chest feels tight, and she gets breathless walking up the stairs. She gets fatigued carrying gro-ceries, so she buys smaller quantities and then finds herself running out of food faster than before. Mrs. Watkins finds it a chore to carry the laundry up from the basement laundry room and now makes several trips to bring up one load at a time, resting between loads.

Five days ago, when Mrs. Watkins began to prepare her usual light dinner of white bread with scrambled eggs, she discovered there were no more eggs and settled for bread with strawberry jelly. She had become absorbed in the Miss America pageant over her martinis that evening and realized with a start that her warm flannel robe was still in the dryer. As she came up with the laundry hamper, she tripped on the rug on the landing and fell down the stairs. Fortunately, she was able to press the button on her pendant, and the company alerted her son, who lives 60 miles away. An ambulance was called to transport her to the hospital, where she was found to have broken her hip. Several specialists came to see her every day for several days to examine her and adjust her medications: an orthopedic surgeon, a pulmonologist, a cardi-ologist, a rheumatologist, and an anesthesiologist. She was told that she would need a hip replacement, but it was not clear what degree of surgical risk her damaged lungs and weakened heart could bear, nor how well her healing would proceed given the severity of her osteoporosis. They would need to dis-charge her promptly from the hospital in any case. Furthermore, she would need weeks of physical therapy and outpatient rehabilitation after that. Mrs. Watkins is very nervous about going home.

Question

You are the leader of the interdisciplinary PEP program team managing Mrs. Watkins' care. What is your assessment of the services Mrs. Watkins needs? How will you help her get this care?

Bibliography

Bassett, R., Bourbonnais, V., McDowell, I. Living long and keeping well: elderly Canadians account for success in aging. Canadian Journal on Aging 2007;26(2):113–126.

Bhalotra, S.M., Mutschler, P.H. Primary prevention for older adults: no longer a paradox. Journal of Aging and Social Policy 2001;12(2):5.

Fries J.F. Reducing disability in older age. Journal of the American Medical Association 2002;288(24):3164–3166.

Jette, A.M. Disability trends and community long-term health care for the aged. In: Satin, D.G., Blakeney, B.A., Bottomley, J.M., Howe, M.C., Smith, H.D. (eds.) The Clinical Care of the Aged Person: An Interdisciplinary Perspective. New York: Oxford University Press, 1994, chapter 12.

Partnership for Solutions. Johns Hopkins University analysis of MEPS, 1996. Available at: http://www.partnershipforsolutions.org/index.html.

Reichstadt, J., Depp, C.A., Palinkas, L.A., Folsom, D.P., Jeste, D.V. Building blocks of successful aging: a focus group study of older adults perceived contributors to successful aging. American Journal of Geriatric Psychiatry 2007;15(3):194–201.

Rowe, J.W., Kahn, R.L. Successful Aging. New York: Pantheon Books, 1998.

Vaillant, G.E. Aging Well. Boston: Little Brown, 2002.

References

1. Larson, L.W. The revolution in aging is here. Journal of the American Geriatrics Society 2003;51(6):874–876.

2. Fries, J.F. Reducing disability in older age. Journal of the American Medical Association 2002;288(24):3164–3166.

3. Rowe, J.W. Geriatrics, prevention, and the remodeling of Medicare. New England Journal of Medicine 1999;340:720–721.

4. Rowe, J.W., Kahn, R.L. Successful Aging. New York: Pantheon Books, 1998.

5. Vaillant, G.E. Aging Well. Boston: Little, Brown, 2002.

6. U.S. Census Bureau. Table 1: Annual estimates of the population by sex and five-year age groups for the United States: April 1, 2000 to July 1, 2005 (NC-EST2005-01), 2006. Retrieved 8 August 2008 from http://www.census.gov/popest/national/asrh/NC-EST2005-sa.html.

7. National Center for Health Statistics. Centers for Disease Control and Prevention, United States, 2006. In: Statistics NCHS. Washington, DC: U.S. Government Printing Office, 2006.

8. Partnership for Solutions. Chronic Conditions: Making the Case for Ongoing Care. Available at: www.partnershipforsolutions.org/DMS/files/chronicbook2004.pdf. 2004.

9. McGinnis, J.M., Foege, W.H. Actual causes of death in the United States. Journal of the American Medical Association 1993;270(18):2207–2212.

10. Cassel, C.K. Successful aging—how increased life expectancy and medical advances are changing geriatric care. Geriatrics 2001;56(1):35–39.

11. lass, T.A. Assessing the success of successful aging. Annals of Internal Medicine 2003;139:382–383.

12. Rowe, J.W., Kahn, R.L. Successful aging. Gerontologist 1997;37(4):433–440.

13. McEwen, B.S. Interacting mediators of allostasis and allostatic load: towards an understanding of resilience in aging. Aging: Beneficial Effects on Patients From Recent Advances in Genetics, Neurobiology, and Physiology. Metabolism 2003; 52:10(Suppl. 2):10–16.

14. National Institutes of Health. In search of the secrets of aging. NIH Publication Number 93–2756, 1993.
15. Sultz, H.A., Young, K.M. Health Care USA: Understanding the Organization and Delivery. Gaithersburg, MD: Aspen, 2001.
16. Mazzeo, R.S., Cavanagh, P. Exercise and physical activity for older adults. Physician and Sportsmedicine 1999;27(11):115.
17. Seguin, R., Nelson, M.E. The benefits of strength training for older adults. Physical Activity: Preventing Physical Disablement in Older Adults American Journal of Preventive Medicine 2003 Oct;25:3(Suppl. 2):141–149.
18. Arday, D.R., Milton, M.H., Husten, C.G., et al. Smoking and functional status among Medicare managed care enrollees. American Journal of Preventive Medicine 2003;24(3):234–241.
19. Ondus, K.A., Hujer, M.E., Mann, A.E., Mion, L.C. Substance abuse and the hospitalized elderly. Orthopedic Nursing 1999;18(4):27–36.
20. Menninger, J.A. Assessment and treatment of alcoholism and substance-related disorders in the elderly. Bulletin of the Menninger Clinic 2002;66(2):166–183.
21. Prigerson, H.G., Desai, R.A., Rosenheck, R.A. Older adult patients with both psychiatric and substance abuse disorders: prevalence and health service use. Psychiatric Quarterly 2001;72(1):1–18.
22. Linsk, N.L. HIV among older adults: age-specific issues in prevention and treatment. AIDS Reader 2000;10(7):430–444.
23. Fried, L.P., Kronmal, R.A., Newman, A.B., et al. Risk factors for 5-year mortality in older adults. Journal of the American Medical Association 1998;279(8):585–592.
24. DeVito, C.A., Morgan, R.O., Duque, M., Abdel-Moty, E. Physical performance effects of low-intensity exercise among clinically defined high-risk elders. Gerontology 2003;49(3):146–154.
25. Stoller, E.P., Pollow, R. Factors affecting the frequency of health enhancing behaviors by the elderly. Public Health Reports 1994;109(3):377–389.
26. Tompkins, C.P., Bhalotra, S. Applying disease management strategies to Medicare. Milbank Quarterly 1999;77(4):461–484.
27. Wagner, E.H., Austin, B., Von Korff, M. Organizing care for patients with chronic illness. Milbank Quarterly 1996;74(4):1–34.
28. Wagner, E.H., Austin, B., Von Korff, M. Improving outcomes in chronic illness. Management Care Quarterly 1996;4(2):12–25.
29. Bhalotra, S.M., Mutschler, P.H. Primary prevention for older adults: no longer a paradox. Journal of Aging and Social Policy 2001;12(2):5.
30. American Association of Retired Persons. Medicare at 40: Past Accomplishments and Future Challenges. 2005. Available at: assest.aarp.org/rgcenter/health/medicare_40.pdf.
31. Agency for Healthcare Research and Quality. Guide to Clinical Preventive Services, 2006: Recommendations of the U.S. Preventive Services Task Force. AHRQ Publication 06-0588. Rockville, MD: AHRQ, 2006.
32. Wagner, E.H., Davis, C., Schaefer, J., Von Korff, M., Austin, B. Survey of leading chronic disease management programs. Are they consistent? Management Care Quarterly 1999;7(3):56–66.
33. Von Korff, M., Gruman, J., Schaefer, J., Curry, S., Wagner, E.H. Collaborative management of chronic illness. Annals of Internal Medicine 1997;127(12):1097–1102.
34. Glasgow, R.E., Funnell, M.M., Bonomi, A.E., Davis, C., Beckham, V., Wagner, E.H. Self-management aspects of the improving chronic illness care breakthrough

series: implementation with diabetes and heart failure teams. Annals of Behavioral Medicine 2002;24(2):80–87.

35. Bodenheimer, T., Lorig, K., Holman, H., Grumbach, K. Patient self-management of chronic disease in primary care. Journal of the American Medical Association 2002;288(19):2469–2475.

36. Lorig, K.R., Sobel, D.S., Stewart, A.L., et al. Evidence suggesting that a chronic disease self-management program can improve health status while reducing hospitalization—a randomized trial. Medical Care 1999;37(1):5–14.

37. Lorig, K.R., Ritter, P., Stewart, A.L., et al. Chronic disease self-management program—2-year health status and health care utilization outcomes. Medical Care 2001;39(11):1217–1223.

38. Archstone Foundation. 1999 Award for Excellence in Program Innovation. Retrieved 8 August 2008 from http://www.archstone.org/usr_doc/33535.pdf.

39. American Diabetes Association position paper. Standards of medical care in diabetes—2007. Diabetes Care 2007;30(Suppl.):S4–S41.

40. Williamson, J.D. Improving care management and health outcomes for frail older people: implications of the PACE model. Journal of the American Geriatrics Society 2000;48(11):1529–1530.

41. Leutz, W.N., Greenlick, M., et al. Adding long-term care to Medicare: the social HMO experience. Journal of Aging and Social Policy 1992;3(4):69–87.

42. Leutz, W.N., Capitman, J., Green, C.A. A limited entitlement for community care: how members use services. Journal of Aging and Social Policy 2001;12(3):43–64.

43. Stuck, A.E., Walthert, J.M. Risk factors for functional status decline in community-living elderly people: a systematic. Social Science and Medicine 1999;48(4):445–469.

44. Butler, R.N., Davis, R., Lewis, C.B., Nelson, M.E., Strauss, E. Physical fitness: benefits of exercise for the older patient. Geriatrics 1998;53(10):49–52.

45. Englander, F., Hodson, T.J., Terregrossa, R.A. Economic dimensions of slip and fall injuries. Journal of Forensic Sciences 1996;41(5):733–746.

46. Blum, H.L. Planning for Health: Geriatrics for the Eighties. New York: Human Sciences Press, 1981.

7

Justice in Community Care

JOHN A. CAPITMAN

Epidemiological Transition and Elder-Care Policies

In the United States, other established market economies, and some countries within Asia, Latin America, and the Caribbean, the epidemiological transition and associated changes in population age composition and causes of death had occurred to varying degrees by the 1990s.[1-3] The accelerating graying of the population expected in coming years stands out as a striking demographic force influencing individuals' lived experience in these countries. As populations age, policies and programs that promote public health and well-being face rapid growth in total demand (because of absolute and relative growth in the number of elders) and the need to direct services to managing co-occurring chronic disease and sociocultural challenges.[4,5] This rapidly changing medical and demographic context for elder-care practice has stimulated debate in many countries about social goals and the needed service systems, processes, and resource commitments.[6-9] This chapter explores a central theme in these debates: fairness in financing and provision of community-oriented supportive health services for elders. In this context, "supportive health services" references health and social services offered to elders to extend the period of active engagement in the community by preventing the progress of chronic disease and providing needed supports throughout the disablement process.

The unfolding of epidemiological transitions has drawn attention to socio-economic gradients in both health care and health outcomes. Cross-nationally, average health outcomes improve with country income and wealth.[10] Although national wealth may afford more accommodating physical and social environments, rich nations also have better health because they devote more resources to health care. For example, the Global Burden of Disease Study found that the most economically developed regions hold 11.6% of the worldwide burden from all causes of death and disability measured as disability-adjusted life years, yet they account for 90.2% of worldwide health expenditures. Further, increasing evidence suggests that both within and between countries increasing levels of socioeconomic inequality are associated with decreasing health.[10,11]

U.S. Health Inequalities and Elder Care

The consequences of socioeconomic inequality for health are particularly visible in the United States, where income, wealth, social status, educational attainment, and social capital have been linked to life-course differences in patterns of acute and chronic conditions, onset and progression of disability, quality of life, and satisfaction with the quality and respectfulness of services.[12–14]

Race, ethnicity, and gender further modify these economic effects. Among elders, African Americans, Latinos, and Native Americans/Alaska Natives face worse health challenges and less adequate care than other groups, as demonstrated by higher mortality in most age groups; higher prevalence of many chronic health conditions; earlier onset or more severe disabilities; lower use relative to disability of most forms of institutional and community long-term care; more difficulty accessing medical care; lower rates of supplemental insurance coverage; lower rates of Medicaid enrollment relative to financial status; more dissatisfaction with accessibility, quality, and responsiveness of care; and greater burden on informal caregivers.[12,14,15]

Although women outlive men, older women also face greater odds for inadequate insurance; more difficulties accessing appropriate medical care; longer periods of chronic disability, poverty, caregiving stress, and loneliness; and greater dissatisfaction with medical care accessibility and quality.[12,16–18]

In addition to racial/ethnic, gender, and other gradients in health, U.S. elder-care policies have created broad patterns of underinsurance, inadequate scope of insurance, and inadequate care access for older people, particularly those with chronic diseases and disabilities.[19–22] Many elders, particularly those with co-occurring disability and low income, face difficulties purchasing pharmaceuticals, nursing home care, and community-oriented services and, thus, report unmet needs for care with basic living tasks that often lead to more dramatic negative health outcomes.[23–26] These same elders often receive inadequate attention to self-management of chronic conditions and assistance in maximizing well-being through participation in health-promotion programs.[27–29] Elders face more out-of-pocket costs for health care than at any time since the passage of Medicare, including payments for long-term care.[30] In 1995, the average elder paid 19% or more of his or her income for health-related expenses not covered by Medicare or other insurance, with half of this expenditure for pharmaceuticals; those who had chronic diseases and disabilities had even higher uncovered costs. Out-of-pocket expenditures have risen sharply since then, especially for elders who joined managed-care plans despite the fact that these plans were intended to curb expenditure growth.[31] Out-of-pocket expenditures also rise with age, primarily because of long-term expenses, while nursing home and home-care costs out-of-pocket are closely linked with having supplemental insurance and socioeconomic status.[32] Even though the passage of Medicare Part D prescription coverage has created a complex and profitable new system of prescription drug coverage for elders and somewhat reduced the growth in out-of-pocket expenditures, many elders, particularly those with chronic conditions such as diabetes, face daunting costs for medications.[33,34]

In this chapter, I examine the value placed on fairness in the context of competing ethical frames for health-care policy. This discussion highlights a disconnection between the competitive market-based framework that dominates the elder-care policy debate in the United States and a framework based on the goals of security and solidarity. Next, I examine through these alternative ethical lenses the two dimensions of inequity noted above: inadequate and inconsistent accessibility of supportive health services and racial/ethnic disparities in elder health and health-related care. I note that despite differences between these examples, they actually raise similar challenges for policy makers and practitioners. I conclude by suggesting that new service financing and provision initiatives alone are unlikely to create values-based health systems and that changes in practitioner behavior and health system governance are also needed.

Fairness and Elder-Care Policies

Elder-care policies in the United States are primarily expressed by the Medicare and Medicaid financing of institutional and community-oriented health and long-term care services, the Older Americans Act, other social service funding of services for elders with disabilities, and public sector regulation of private long-term care financing and services. Both in their first enactment in the 1960s and in more recent modifications and expansion, these policies reflect a concern with ensuring elders fair access to appropriate supportive services. For example, in the years leading up to the passage of Medicare, findings that 44% of elders were poverty-stricken, without medical care, and "suffering from a downward spiral of sickness and isolation"[35] were viewed as unacceptable in an increasingly affluent country. The Older Americans Act, another pillar of elder-care policies, passed in 1965, also reflected a national commitment to equal opportunity and specifically targeted resources to states and communities on the basis of the proportions of elders who were poor, racial/ethnical minorities, or disabled. Yet, even at the time of this outpouring of beneficence toward the aged, market-oriented value frames were significant. As Stevens[35] notes, Medicare was designed to protect the status quo of private insurance for the working population and continued to focus public programs on insurance linked to work.

While the demographics and health-care needs of elders and the relative role of for-profit medicine in the United States have changed since the 1960s, the disconnect between the value frames used by health-care industry interests and their elite policy-making allies and the general public has not. Responding to the epidemiological transition and technological progress by bringing Medicare and related elder-care policies into alignment with current needs through more adequate coverage of pharmaceuticals and chronic care services has raised important questions about what counts as fair elder-care policies. As the national discussion about Medicare drug coverage culminated in controversial legislation in 2003, there initially appeared to be a consensus that it was unacceptable for Medicare beneficiaries to face growing uncovered medical care costs because of the increasing reliance on prescription medication by health-care providers. Pharmaceutical prices in the United States were found to be surprisingly higher than in other knowledge-economy democracies, and many came to view these pricing patterns as evidence of unfair business practices. Focus groups and surveys suggested that the public viewed the prospect of low- and moderate-income elders having to choose between the prescription drugs they needed and other survival expenses as unfair.[36] At the same time, many saw it as unfair for public programs to reimburse for professional services but not for medications: Persons who consume equal amounts (but different types) of health-care resources were not receiving equal benefits from the Medicare program. Policy action was needed to make the national elder-care financing system more fair by taming and covering costs for prescription drugs.

Yet, as the congressional debate progressed and a controversial reform plan emerged, the focus shifted to minimizing new expenditure through a complex set of limitations on coverage and copayment requirements, ensuring a private sector role in managing new pharmacy benefits and trying to entice seniors to leave traditional Medicare for private sector health plans. Rather than addressing how drug prices might be reduced, this legislation specifically blocks governmental negotiation with pharmaceutical makers to reduce prices.[36] In this debate, as in prior attempts to address the inequitable consequences of U.S. health policies, public value commitments to fairness were in a distant second place behind the commitment by industry and political elites to market-based competitive solutions in health care.[37] A new debate in 2007 on the Medicare Part D ban on national prescription drug formulary and pricing as well as the gaps in coverage for those with high-cost chronic conditions has already begun to focus on these same value distinctions.

The Medicare prescription drug debate underscores a disconnection between general public conceptions of the goals for health-care policy and the views of decision makers. The public tends to evaluate health-care policies by combining the value perspectives of beneficence, autonomy, and equity: Expert and kindly professional care for those in need, respect for individual choice, and equal help to those with equal needs are among the values that most people reference in assessing health policies and programs. By contrast, policy-making elites favor market-based competition solutions.[21,22,37,38] Schlesinger[37] found that nearly 60% of congressional staffers in 1995 were committed first to market solutions and viewed fairness in health care as maximizing individual choice of health insurance products that match their preferences and pocketbooks, while seeing the goals of equal treatment or access to as much care as professionals deemed necessary as relatively unimportant. (And the recent Medicare prescription drug debate would suggest that the political power of those fixated on health care as a commodity has only grown.) For that same year, Schlesinger's surveys of a representative sample of the U.S. public found that only 41% supported market solutions and that respondents were much less committed to maximizing choice of insurance plans than elites and overwhelmingly endorsed both the views that justice in health care was best expressed by equal treatment and access to needed care as judged by professionals.

For Churchill,[39] this focus on market solutions has created a health system primarily bent on maintaining professional prerogatives and ensuring the well-being of private insurers. Among the best evidence for this conclusion are findings that the United States, with its mix of profit-seeking insurers and providers, produces overuse of unnecessarily high-cost services and inefficiency and profits expressed as administrative costs that outstrip non-care-related expenditures in other countries.[21,22,40,41] Given the diversity of value judgments and analyses that characterize public opinion, Churchill concludes that the public might prefer security and solidarity as the value frames that shape health policy. By "security," Churchill means the freedom to live without fear that basic health concerns will go unattended and freedom from financial impoverishment from health care. By "solidarity," he means, a sense of community that emerges from recognition of shared benefits and shared responsibilities with others in the community. From this perspective, beneficence and justice are framed in communal terms, as in Hume's metaphor of a vault built by many hands that rises still with each addition. Justice in this context is a product of enlightened self-interest and policy-mediated cooperation. Just health policies create a network of reciprocal arrangements to cement separate acts (of greed and benevolence) into an enduring structure. The principal argument against this view is that individuals acting from self-interest might choose the health benefits and patterns of costs well-suited to their own needs and history, even though this might lead to important exclusions of groups of persons or groups of needs. Churchill argues from Hume, however, that in designing a system we would not "seek to exclude others" because if I support system features that I will not personally use, I can feel security that only by doing so can I expect them (other people in my community) to support system features I need but that they will not use.

In proposing the goals of security and solidarity, Churchill[39] is not espousing a "right" to health care in general or to any particular service. Thinking of health care as an individual entitlement could stimulate demand (as individuals compete to get their due) and thus produce as much inequity and inefficiency in care as a market-based model. Churchill argues that a right to health care should be understood as a right to equitable access based on need alone to a system that provides all the effective and efficacious care the society can afford. This view is consonant with more fully developed calls for single-payer national health insurance with comprehensive coverage for acute and long-term care services.[21,22] Individuals also have the responsibility to have realistic expectations and make wise use of resources. We build the vault through a response model—individuals have a right to access a fair health-care system and a responsibility to use only their fair share of its resources.

From the competitive market frame for just elder care, unequal care access and outcomes signal natural and appropriate working of the market. In this frame, some inequalities, however, are market failures that follow regulatory excesses or unfair and deceptive practices by insurers and providers. The needed national conversation is technical and focused on holding the health-care industry accountable for weeding out bad actors and practices and educating the public to make wiser choices for their own health and health-care consumption. The national conversation looks very different if just elder care is framed from the perspectives of security and solidarity. In this conversation, inequalities in health-care use and outcomes become central challenges for health policy. In addressing these challenges, the national conversation revolves around a thorny set of values questions, such as (1) How much health and health care can we afford given other social needs (education, defense, environmental quality)? (2) Which, among the seemingly inexhaustible array of human needs, will be secured under the health umbrella? (3) How do we hold individuals responsible for reasonable health expectations and health-care use? In the following sections, I underscore the differences between these two frameworks for addressing just elder care by using them to consider two dimensions of inequality associated with elder care in the United States.

Community-Oriented Long-Term Care in Justice Frameworks

As documented in other chapters in this book, elder-care policies in the United States offer unequal responses to various sequelae of illness and disablement.[42] That Medicare provided first-line coverage for physician and hospital services but not for pharmaceuticals is a well-known example of unequal response to diseases with diverse care requirements. Inconsistent responses to disablement are exemplified by the following:

- Medicare covers home health care and skilled nursing facility care on a postacute, time-limited basis for some patients but does not cover the same services in other settings (e.g., adult day health care, assisted living facilities), for longer time frames, or for patients who need similar services but have different likely outcome trajectories.
- Although Medicare provides coverage for some clinical preventive services, available coverage for health promotion and chronic disease self-management services is extremely limited (see Chapter 6).
- Medicaid programs fill gaps in Medicare coverage for qualified low-income persons, but these programs differ markedly from state to state with respect to income and asset standards for eligibility. Medicaid programs also differ between and within states with respect to the range of covered community long-term care services, conditions for eligibility, and care management/ quality assurance arrangements (see Chapter 4).
- Private elder-care financing options, such as long-term care insurance and continuing care communities, and privately financed services, such as assisted living facilities and home-care assistance, not only remain outside the financial grasp of most elders but also fail to provide reliable protection against impoverishment or reliance on public programs because of variable regulation across the states with respect to care quality and business practices.

From the competitive market-based frame for assessing just elder care, the fact that current public policies create highly variable access to institutional and community-oriented supportive services is examined from two perspectives. On the one hand, the market is seen as working almost appropriately: Communities (through the Medicaid program) and individuals are purchasing those long-term care services they desire and are able to afford. Nonetheless, that relatively affluent elders are not purchasing private long-term care options at the predicted rates suggests that more consumer education about the limits of Medicare and the need for private coverage would increase informed personal responsibility. On the other hand, inadequate and inconsistent coverage of community-oriented long-term care is viewed as the product of a technical problem: the failure to demonstrate that supportive community services are cost-effective alternatives to already covered services. From this perspective, increasing the accessibility of community-oriented supportive services for elders and others with chronic disabilities must wait until a pattern of eligibility restrictions and resource allocation rules that ensure cost neutrality can be demonstrated.

If framed from the perspective of security and solidarity, the unequal coverage for—and access to—community supportive services raises profound questions about the adequacy of elder-care policies. In this context, unequal care for co-occurring chronic disease, sociocultural challenges, and disabilities raises concern that these policies are not ensuring equitable access based on disablement-related need alone to a system that provides all of the effective and efficacious care the society can afford. "Disablement" as described by Verbrugge and colleagues[43–45] is the process that links diseases to impairments in functioning and to disabilities. Wolinsky et al.[46] describe "disablement" as patterns of serial transitions in context, with different combinations of diseases and limitations producing diverse patterns of stability or change in functioning over time as a function of social location and other factors. The trajectory from incompletely managed health condition through functional limitation to disability and thus need for various supportive services depends at least in part on contextual factors, including social location (gender, age, race/ethnicity, social class, availability of potential informal helpers), physical environments, and both cumulative lifetime and current access to appropriate care. Since our elder-care policies arguably do include a commitment, however shaky, to offering elders some security with respect to disease-related health-care costs, we can only justify unequal access to community-oriented supportive services if we conclude as a society that meeting the range of health-related needs that arise during the disablement process (1) is not possible or (2) requires resources beyond our consensually determined resource allocation to health care.

Given our emerging understanding of the disablement process, the security and solidarity frame looks for evidence that chronically ill elders are having daily personal care, household maintenance, social support, and communal participation needs. By contrast, the competitive market frame directs attention to evidence that meeting these needs produces additional benefits beyond promoting opportunities for age-appropriate normal function. Evidence from the 1115 Medicaid and 222 Medicare waiver community long-term care demonstrations, social health maintenance organizations, the Programs for All-Inclusive Care for the Elderly, and state Medicaid home- and community-based care programs consistently demonstrates that these programs can markedly reduce unmet needs for disablement-related care, support family and others in their informal caring role, and improve the health-related quality of life of elders within reasonable budgets.[19,47–49] These programs would satisfy the security and solidarity frame's focus on evidence for meeting daily needs within reasonable resource limits. Nonetheless, there is clear evidence that among those elders with fewer socioeconomic resources and in traditionally underserved racial/ethnic groups access to such potentially effective supportive services is interrupted and there are negative impacts on health conditions and medical care use.[12,50,51] From the solidarity and security value frame, unequal care for disabled elders is unfair since these needs are closely interwoven with already covered health conditions, it is technically feasible to meet these needs within reasonable budgets, and failure to meet these needs exacerbates socioeconomic health disparities.

Racial/Ethnic Health-Care Disparities and Elder-Care Policies

An impressive series of federal and private reports in recent years demonstrate a consensus that there are substantial racial/ethnic disparities in the accessibility and quality of health care for older people and others in the United States and that these disparities are an important factor in creating racial/ethnic disparities in mortality, morbidity, and quality of life.[12,13] Although some believe that we lack a good understanding of the causes of health-care disparities and their roles in health outcomes, an emerging conceptual frame points to important roles of elder-care policies in creating these disparities.

Clearly, health-care disparities are not the only cause of racial/ethnic health disparities. Krieger[52] concludes that from the perspective of social epidemiology, the fundamental cause of racial/ethnic health disparities is *racism*—institutional and individual practices that create and sustain a system of oppressive group relations that limit the opportunities and outcomes of targeted groups and individuals. One can trace at least five distinct pathways from societal racism to racial/ethnic health disparities: (1) economic and social deprivation; (2) exposure to toxic substances and hazardous conditions; (3) socially inflicted trauma (from verbal abuse to violent acts) and health consequences of social–psychological responses to discrimination; (4) targeted marketing of commodities that can harm health such as tobacco, alcohol, and high-fat foods; (5) inadequate and disrespectful health care.[53] Because elders in traditionally underserved racial/ethnic groups have been exposed to all of these factors, they enter old age with more chronic conditions and an accumulation of risk factors (both potentially individually modified behavioral risks and others) for disease and reduced capacity to resist new threats to their wellbeing. Life-course exposure to racism (and, for many, the comparable effects of poverty) for elders of color means that they approach the health-care system with reduced trust and lowered expectations for excellence in care[54,55] but also with greater needs for attention to both primary and preventive services and disease self-management services. Equal care means heightened attention to these consequences of social inequality.

Despite the heightened demands on health-care systems and practitioners in serving elders of color that flow from their accumulated diverse racism-related risk exposure, recent reports from the Institute of Medicine systematic evidence reviews and others have demonstrated that the care offered these elders is less comprehensive and appropriate.[13] Capitman et al.,[14] for example, show that racial/ethnic disparities in cancer mortality can be explained by elders of color being less likely to be offered or engaged in programs to manage primary behavioral risk factors; less likely to receive consistent primary care; less likely to participate in breast, cervical, colorectal, and prostate cancer screening services; less likely to receive appropriate follow-up services subsequent to a suspicious screening finding; and less likely to receive complete treatment and relapse prevention services. Similar points have been made about cardiovascular and cardiopulmonary disease prevention and treatment[56–58] and many other conditions. Notably, inequality in services provided reflects not only undertreatment of persons of color but overtreatment of dominant group members as a result of competitive pressures and perceived individual entitlement.

From the competitive market-based perspective on just elder care, the failure of health and chronic care systems to meet the heightened needs for comprehensive services in traditionally excluded racial/ethnic groups is viewed primarily as a question of irresponsible decision making by elder patient-consumers and as a technical challenge in the training of health practitioners. A focus on consumer education is demonstrated by ongoing attempts at social marketing about healthful lifestyles, dissemination of health care–provider performance data, and insurance/health plan decision-assistance programs. No body of research has demonstrated, however, that underserved groups have less motivation to make positive health-related choices or that any of these initiatives effectively addresses racial/ethnic disparities in the accessibility and quality of care.

The focus on improving the performance of practitioners was demonstrated by the Institute of Medicine report in its hypothesis that the primary mechanism in unequal care is the behavior of clinicians. Practitioners lack knowledge about how the cultural characteristics, beliefs, and behavior patterns of persons from diverse racial/ethnic groups combine with the uncertainties and pressures of medical encounters in ways that lead them to incorrectly apply race-based decision rules or fail to communicate adequately with patients. Practitioners, lacking training on cultural differences, are thought to rely too heavily on stereotypes or to simply forget to address all issues. For example, van Ryn and Burke[59] found that practitioners bring negative views of African American and low–socioeconomic status patients to encounters and, thus, spend less time and take fewer actions in these encounters. A recent review by van Ryn and Su[60] notes that while extensive literature demonstrates the role of practitioner behavior in unequal care, only two studies to date seem to explicate the process. In both cases,[61,62] the authors show how clinicians believe that a certain patient feature is crucial to adherence to treatment and that patients of color are less likely to have this feature—and that these beliefs in turn influence prescription behavior. In response to findings like these, many have called for culturally competent care and a small industry has evolved to teach cultural competence to clinicians.[63] No evidence has yet emerged that cultural competence training for practitioners is associated with greater equality in care.

From the security and solidarity perspective on just elder care, racial/ethnic disparities in treatment raise fundamental questions about the organization and financing of health services and the ways in which practitioners and patients share decision making. With respect to financing and organization of care, there is mounting evidence that elders of color are less likely to receive appropriate preventive and chronic disease management services as a result of financial barriers than as a result of preferences. Elders in traditionally underserved groups are less likely to have Medicare supplements, less likely to be enrolled in Medicaid (after controlling for income and asset differences), and more likely to rely on out-of-pocket expenditures to supplement Medicare.[64,65] These differences in insurance status are associated with delaying seeking care, lacking an ongoing relationship with a primary-care provider, or receiving primary care in less appropriate and/or underresourced settings. For example, approximately twice as many older African Americans as whites reported delaying care because of cost.[66] As a result, elders of color are less likely to receive prevention services.[67,68] A report by Christensen and Shinogle[69] demonstrates that having a regular source of care can double the likelihood of physician-provided prevention advice on diet, tobacco cessation, and physical activity. Similarly, Gentry et al.[70] report that patients in Missouri were more likely to disclose behavioral risks for disease if they had a usual source of care. Rather than a focus on developing more educated consumers and more culturally competent professionals, these findings suggest the need to increase equality in access to primary care.

The organization of care has also been implicated in this process of unequal care. For example, in reviewing the causes of racial/ethnic disparities among elders in cancer care, Capitman et al.[14] show that state-of-the-art individually oriented primary prevention programs (smoking cessation, weight loss, physical activity) are primarily sponsored by academic health centers and other settings that serve more affluent and less culturally diverse communities, while settings that serve low-income and minority group elders offer less access to personalized help in behavior change. Focus groups found that, unlike affluent white elders, elders of color generally reported difficulty finding information and support for lifestyle changes or preventive care. This evidence review also found that cancer detection and treatment often require elders to make multiple visits to providers in disparate settings, overcome complex barriers to information sharing among providers, and overcome practical barriers such as lack of transportation or housing. Effective programs to address these barriers do not focus exclusively on patient and provider education but, rather, on ensuring continuity of care and patient empowerment. For example, the Harlem Hospital Patient Navigation Program evolved a model, replicated in Kansas City and Boston, of working with patients from the time of referral based on a suspicious screening finding to assist them in overcoming practical barriers to service use (transportation, grandchild care), benefits coordination, and scheduling services in a timely manner. They seek to avoid missed or rescheduled appointments and work to overcome problems in treatment completion. In addition, these treatment management programs provide counseling, cultural and linguistic translation, and cancer education throughout the treatment process to encourage and support patients in advocating for their own care. This model is consistent with an emerging health care–improvement framework in the Health Disparities Collaboratives in the federal quality community health centers that views unequal care as a failure in clinical system design and administration and engages the whole clinical team in articulating, planning, and implementing consistent diagnostic and treatment protocols. From the perspective of security and solidarity, these broadly targeted organizational solutions are stimulated by evidence of unequal care out of a shared sense that we are all better off if we can count on the health system to ensure access to needed interventions.

Like those based on market-based competitive frames, analysis of just elder care based on the security and solidarity perspective would also highlight practitioner behavior as a central factor in understanding and alleviating racial/ethnic health-care disparities. Yet, this account would see more than the need to increase the skills of practitioners in negotiating cultural differences. Two additional themes might be highlighted.

- *Incentives to address heightened needs*: In the context of most current elder-care systems in the United States, most practitioners must balance concern for patients' well-being with their personal and organizational financial motives. Most settings encourage practitioners to maximize the number of patients seen in a given session, and many encourage them to either minimize services offered (as in some managed-care settings) or promote technologically intensive services with dubious efficacy but high financial return on investment. They do not share clear responsibility for life-course patient outcomes; they are held accountable for providing standard-of-care interventions in response to patient demands in individual encounters but not for maximizing the long-term well-being and community engagement of their clients. In this context, there is little room for practitioners to accommodate the heightened needs for comprehensive patient-centered care associated with the accumulated health consequences of societal racism and other dimensions of social inequality. Only by realigning the incentives of health practitioners and health-care organizations with goals such as maximizing within resource constraints the quality of life and community engagement of each elder during the disablement process can they be expected to act in ways that respond to the health consequences of social inequalities.
- *Cultural humility*: Encouraging practitioners to recognize the importance of relationship building in cross-cultural encounters is a recurrent theme in cultural competence initiatives.[63] Yet, as privileged members of elite professions, most practitioners have few ongoing personal or communal ties to patients in general and elder patients from traditionally excluded racial/ethnic groups in particular. Health-care professional education further distances practitioners from most patients by emphasizing scientific knowledge and technical skills over interpersonal warmth and vulnerability. Tervalon and Murray-Garcia[71] suggest that improved care and outcomes for elders of color may be more readily obtained by teaching practitioners and care systems cultural humility. For Tervalon and Murray-Garcia, cultural competence is becoming expert in the diverse cultures that we serve by acquiring an identified body of knowledge and skill in the application and building of systems of care that support these learnings and behavior. Cultural humility is embarking on lifelong learning about culture and becoming a builder of mutually respectful and dynamic partnerships for health with clients and their families. Focusing elder-care policies on security and solidarity instead of competition and profit would not be expected to diminish the prestige or power of medical professionals, but it would redefine this status in terms of maximizing public health and meeting community needs through relationships based on bidirectional learning and respect.

Implications for Policy and Interdisciplinary Practice

In reviewing the facts and analyses related to the inequities produced by current U.S. elder-care policies, it is difficult to avoid feelings of frustration and impotence. Elders face reduced quality of life and civic engagement because our programs fail to ensure reliable access to chronic disease prevention, self-management, and health-related supportive services during disablement. These challenges are further exacerbated for elders of color and other targets of oppression: Racial/ethnic and gender disparities in health care are prevalent and pernicious. They are created and sustained by care financing and organization approaches that discourage access and leave some settings with inadequate resources. Health systems also fail to interrupt typically unintended discrimination by practitioners. Proposals have been articulated for wholesale reorientation of health-care systems and elder-care policies modeled on the approaches of other advanced knowledge-economy nations that are also grappling with the epidemiological transition. Such proposals call for comprehensive single-payer, universal-access models that eliminate profit motives. These models establish priorities through communal decision making and establish budgets through informed national democratic processes.

But serious debate of these proposals has not occurred in a decade and may be delayed by 2003 Medicare decisions.[36] In the short run, 2007 legislative initiatives to broaden health care access for children first hit the hard reality of wartime budget discipline. Current and emergent approaches already exceed the limits of public taste for health-care expenditures given the range of competing national priorities. Corporate and professional health-care interests and their political elite allies remain staunchly committed to competitive market solutions. They have successfully circumscribed public debate to technical solutions within the existing ethical framework and resource limits. It appears that market-based competition ideology is at the root of elder-care inequities and the elder-care policy impasse. Only by engaging a new kind of national conversation about how values such as justice and beneficence are best reflected in elder-care programming can we expect to break the power of this ideology.

Tesh[72] warns that analyses that identify first causes of public health problems and base proposed solutions on addressing root causes typically present a frightening challenge to powerful economic interests. They provide the solace of understanding but little of the satisfaction associated with alleviating present negative consequences. From her perspective, a useful analysis must also point the way toward short-term solutions. In the case of elder-care inequities, less sweeping proposals inspired by the security and solidarity perspective that leave the U.S. competitive health-care market intact may nonetheless bring important changes. The dual challenges of care for disablement-related needs of all elders and the heightened needs for coordinated primary and preventive care of elders of color can both be addressed through modest expansions of Medicare. Two broad elder-care policy strategies that hold promise for addressing both issues have been proposed in many forms and forums. These proposals call for expanding access for traditional Medicare fee-for-service clients to coordinated patterns of health and health-related services that have been shown to be efficacious in not-for-profit managed-care contexts, partial capitation reimbursement models that extend accountability beyond a single episode of care while establishing clear fiscal constraints, specific attention to respecting individual and cultural diversity, and program evaluation based more on equity than cost-effectiveness goals.

- *Coordinated primary and preventive care*: Currently, neither Medicare nor Medicaid provides specific reimbursement for preventive care or health maintenance medical encounters. The settings that serve low-income and racial/ethnic minority elders are those least likely to have significant streams of private funding to support uncompensated health-promotion and care-coordination efforts. Health-care settings that serve low-income elders and elders of color, such as neighborhood health centers, safety net hospitals, and physician practices in medically underserved communities, and dual-eligible managed-care plans could be eligible for Medicare reimbursement of coordinated primary and preventive care programs. Reimbursement would be on a partial capitation basis, with incentive payments linked to meeting explicit process and outcome standards. Among the process and outcomes standards would be maintaining high levels of patient satisfaction with the individual and cultural responsiveness of services. Eligible providers would implement health-risk appraisals, ensure timely provision of all currently covered preventive health services (cardiovascular and cancer screening, vaccinations, diabetes management, etc.), provide (or purchase) health-promotion and chronic disease self-management programs, and facilitate patient navigation through acute-care systems. By serving elders throughout the disablement process, such programs could reduce the impacts of chronic disease on quality of life and civic participation. Although coordinated primary- and preventive-care programs might prove cost-effective by reducing demand for higher-cost services, they would be evaluated on the basis of reducing socioeconomic and racial/ethnic disparities in health outcomes.
- *Managed community long-term care*: Currently, Medicare provides modest expansions of access to case-managed community-oriented care for physical and cognitive disability–related needs for persons who participate in selected managed-care organizations hosting time-limited demonstration projects,

while Medicaid programs in many states offer diverse versions of these benefits to extremely low-income elders who meet state nursing home–care admissions requirements. A modest managed community long-term care benefit could be offered to participants in traditional fee-for-service Medicare through existing health-care settings that serve low-income elders and elders of color, such as neighborhood health centers, safety net hospitals, and physician practices in medically underserved communities. Community-based social service settings (e.g., adult day centers, senior centers, assisted living/supportive housing sites, etc.) could also be selected as providers of this benefit. Providers would receive partial capitation reimbursement for eligibility determination, care management, and quality-assurance services and would be responsible for assisting elders in spending a dollar-limited individual budget on services to meet disablement-related needs. The individual budget amount would vary based on health and functional status, availability of informal care, and capacity to privately purchase comparable service. Care managers would assist clients in making spending decisions, and participants could decide how much responsibility they wish to shoulder for self-directed and informally provided care. But individual budget amounts would not be contingent on participant decisions with respect to agency-directed or self-directed individual plans. While it is possible that managed community long-term care benefits could show overall cost-effectiveness through substitution of community care for institutional care or less frequent acute exacerbations of chronic conditions, evaluations would focus on reducing rates of unmet disablement-related needs with predetermined budgets.

Proposals such as these for reforming U.S. elder-care policies based on a security and solidarity ethical frame may eventually generate sufficient popular support to gain inclusion in U.S. elder-care programming. But even these modest proposals will need enthusiastic support from a range of elder-care practitioners and other advocates for the aged. Other implications of the security and solidarity framework for interdisciplinary geriatric practice are worth noting. New practitioners in particular may wish to consider the following implications of our shared professional value on just elder care:

- *Consider practice setting incentives*: No matter how committed we are as individual practitioners to meeting the chronic disease and disablement-related needs of older patients, the health-care organizations in which we work create incentives to practice in certain ways that may be sometimes inconsistent with this ethical stance. In selecting the organizational setting in which to practice and as contributors to policy making in these settings, practitioners can seek the alignment of practice incentives (payment and other reward structures, data collected for performance feedback, organizational linkages to support referrals, etc.) with their personal commitments. Just having the awareness that personal values on fairness and kindness in elder care may be short-circuited by excessive pressures to maximize reimbursement or minimize resource use can help practitioners provide responsive and respectful care.

- *Support patient and professional engagement in local policy making*: Increasingly, practitioners are encouraged to engage patients in shared decision making by helping individuals and their loved ones understand the range of treatment and disease management options from the perspectives of benefits, risks, and burdens. Yet, as practitioners, we also can recognize the ways in which broader policy and resource allocation decisions may influence the range of choices that can be offered to patients.[73] If an adult day center with a comprehensive stroke rehabilitation program is available only to private pay patients because of local (and national) resource allocation choices, the opportunities available to individual patients seeking a higher quality of life in the context of disablement have been limited. Two Robert Wood Johnson Foundation initiatives, the Access Project and Community Partnerships for Older Adults, despite different missions and strategies, share the goal of engaging more community members in solving health-care financing and organizational problems at the local level. As practitioners and community members, we can become active participants in similar initiatives that increase public understanding of elder-care policy challenges, create communitywide engagement in addressing these challenges, and hold public officials and private institutional leaders accountable for provision of equitable care.

- *Practice professional and cultural humility*: The hardest lessons for health-care practitioners are reminders of how little they can control outcomes. Those who spend their lives caring for the aged learn and relearn that life chances often trump health care in determining quality of life. If we open our eyes and hearts, we are continually reminded that attention to small human details is at the basis of quality caregiving. For most elders, creating sustainable ties to family and friends, achieving a comfortable and pleasing home life, finding opportunities for lifelong learning and spiritual development, and feeling secure about basic financial needs often have more to do with the health, quality of life, and civic participation than what we can do as health-care practitioners. A complex mix of cultural, socioeconomic, and personal factors shapes the specific meanings and measures of each of these dimensions. Yet, macroindividual forces shape the likelihood that individual elders actually obtain what they sought: Oppression shapes life chances. As practitioners, we cannot know which life experiences and challenges are most salient for each individual we serve or how they interact with the health factors we have been taught to observe and treat. We cannot know in advance which detail of how we present ourselves or what we do in response to apparent patient needs will be perceived as valuable. Assuming that we know puts us at enormous risk for acts of cultural and individual disrespect. By adopting the stance that we can always learn more about how life chances have influenced the health and health-care needs of the people we serve, we can learn to approach each individual as part of a community and view our work as supportive of a larger community.

Many goals have been articulated for elder-care policies in the United States and other countries grappling with the epidemiological transition. Perhaps the most broadly shared of these goals is the creation of a fair approach to meeting the needs of an aging population among whom many face daunting co-occurrence of chronic disease and socioeconomic challenges. The task of meeting this goal is all the more complex in this country because of our competitive market framing of ethical questions in elder-care policy. In this chapter, I have highlighted two of the most notable inequities associated with our patchwork of public and private policies and the associated tendency to multiply limitations and exclusions from care: failure to meet disablement-related needs and racial/ethnic disparities in health care and outcomes. By reframing the goal of just elder care in a context of public desires for security and solidarity, I have pointed out the need for fundamental policy reorientation and new, more inclusive decision-making processes. A focus on security and solidarity in health care also inspires consideration of a short-term reform agenda focused on coordinated primary and preventive services and managed community long-term care. Practitioners engaged by this ethical frame might evaluate their own efforts from the perspectives of practice setting incentives, participation in local elder-care policy formation, and practicing professional and cultural humility.

Application to the Case Study: The Older Adult Care, Training, Research, and Planning Program

The security and solidarity ethical frame for community-oriented elder-care policy and practice can be informative in thinking about the Older Adult Care, Training, Research and Planning Program (OACTRPP). Perhaps most centrally, this framing points to a central task for the OACTRPP researchers and clinicians: developing clinical services that assist elders in self-management of multiple chronic-care problems. Multispecialty clinical care can create opportunities to empower elders to be active partners along with practitioners in promoting their own well-being through engagement in specific disease-prevention and -management activities (adherence to clinical guidelines for Medicare-reimbursed screenings, adherence to medication regimens, etc.) and engagement in health-promoting behaviors (nutrition, physical activity, relaxation, and social participation). At the same time, the OACTRPP may examine its potential roles in providing comprehensive, affordable, managed, community-oriented long-term care services. This might entail development of new service options, such as adult day health care and personal care services, development of partnership arrangements with existing providers of these services to ensure their coordination with health-care interventions, or seeking funding to support a care management program. Given the absence of adequate public or private funding mechanisms for community-oriented supportive services, the OATCRPP may need to consider more difficult new programming that creates ways for elders, other community members, and public or philanthropic funders to work together in financing access to such services.

Whether in the mode of enrolling elders in chronic condition self-management and wellness programs or developing partnerships for new and more consistently coordinated community care, engaging elders in these activities requires understanding and helping to activate individual motivations for obtaining and retaining the best health possible given their health and social resources. At its core, such engagement comes from culturally appropriate, respectful, and individualized interactions with patients and their families. In this context, OACTRPP leaders need to recognize the host of health-care financing, organization, and delivery factors that serve as barriers for patients to accessing needed care. Along with such recognition comes the need for the development of meaningful mechanisms for elder participation in shaping program design and implementation on an ongoing basis. Program leaders will need to struggle with sharing power over program decisions with not only the university medical center managers and multiple funders but also with the community to whom the program is directed.

The case study highlights the mixed "ethnic character" of the OACTRPP catchment area. In light of growing recognition of the challenges faced by communities across the United States in addressing health and health-care equity, the program's leadership and clinical decision makers may need to specifically examine racial and ethnic disparities in health status, health-care access, and health-care quality: seeking racial and ethnic diversity as a complement to the program's interdisciplinary staffing, engaging staff in learning opportunities around their own attitudes toward diversity and how these impact their behavior with clients, and examining the operations of the OACTRPP from the perspective of creating a welcoming environment for all participants. An even greater challenge for the OACTRPP clinicians and other staff may be engaging the university medical center and other community institutions in examining their current and potential roles in contributing to and alleviating physical and social environmental factors in the community that promote health inequities. As individuals and as organizational leaders, health-care providers may have an ethical responsibility that extends beyond professional standards to participating in efforts to create a just and supportive environment for all elders.

References

1. Seow, W., Cowart, M. Epidemiological transition theory and aging: Hispanic populations of North America and the Caribbean. Journal of Health and Human Services Administration 1998;20(3):333–347.
2. Murray, C., Lopez, A. Global mortality, disability and contribution of risk factors: Global Burden of Disease Study. Lancet 1999;349(9063):1436–1442.
3. Marin, P., Wallace, S. Health care for the elderly in Chile: a country in transition. Aging Clinical and Experimental Research 2002;14(4):271–278.
4. Moon, M. 1999. Will the care be there? Vulnerable beneficiaries and Medicare reform. Health Affairs 1999;18(1):107–117.
5. Paccaud, F. Rejuvenating health systems for aging communities. Aging Clinical and Experimental Research 2002;14(4):314–318.
6. Cuellar, A.E., Weiner, J.M. Can social insurance for long-term care work? The experience of Germany. Health Affairs 2000;19(3):8–25.
7. Ikegami, N., Campbell, J.C. Japan's health care system: containing costs and attempting reform. Health Affairs 2004;23(3):26–36.
8. Fuchs, V.R. Economics, values, and health care reform. American Economic Review 1999;86(1):1–24.
9. Cassel, C.K., Besdine, R.W., Siegel, L.C. 1999. Restructuring Medicare for the next century: what will beneficiaries really need? Health Affairs 1999;18(1): 118–131.
10. Daniels, N., Kennedy, B., Kawachi, I. Is Inequality Bad for Our Health? Boston: Beacon Press, 2000.
11. Hofrichter, R. The politics of health inequities: contested terrain. In: Hofrichter, R. (ed.) Health and Social Justice: Politics, Ideology, and Inequity in the Distribution of Disease. San Francisco: Jossey-Bass, 2003.
12. Department of Health and Human Services/Agency for Healthcare Research and Quality (DHHS/AHRQ). 2005 National Healthcare Disparities Report. Publication 06-0017. Rockville, MD: AHRQ, 2005.
13. Smedley, B.D., Stith, A.Y., Nelson, A.R. Unequal Treatment: Confronting Racial and Ethnic Disparities in Health Care. Washington, DC: Institute of Medicine, National Academy Press, 2002.
14. Capitman, J., Bahlotra, S., Ruwe, M. Cancer and Elders of Color: Opportunities for Reducing Health Disparities. Aldershot, UK: Ashgate, 2005.
15. Wong, M., et al. Contribution of major diseases to disparities in mortality. New England Journal of Medicine 2002;347:1585–1592.
16. Yee, D., Capitman, J. Healthcare access and health promotion and older women of color. Journal of Health Care for the Poor and Underserved 1996;7(3):252–272.
17. Wray, L., Blaum, C. Explaining the role of sex on disability: a population-based study. The Gerontologist 2001;41(4):499–510.

18. Leveille, S., et al. Sex differences in prevalence of mobility disability in old age: the dynamics of incidence, recovery, and mortality. Journal of Gerontology Series B Psychological Sciences and Social Sciences 2000;55B(1):S41–S50.
19. Capitman, J. Effective coordination of medical and supportive services. Journal of Health and Aging 2003;15(1):124–164.
20. Stone, R.I. Long-term care for the elderly with disabilities: current policy, emerging trends, and implications for the twenty-first century. Milbank Memorial Fund. Available at: www.milbank.org/0008stone. 2000.
21. Woolhandler, S., Campbell, T., Himmelstein, D.U. Costs of health care administration in the United States and Canada. New England Journal of Medicine 2003;349(8):768–775.
22. Woolhandler, S., Himmelstein, D.U., Angell, M., Young, Q.D. Group single payer national health insurance. Journal of the American Medical Association 2003;290(6):798–805.
23. Williams, J., Lyons, B., Rowland, D. Unmet long-term care needs of elderly people in the community: a review of the literature. Home Health Care Services Quarterly 1997;16(1–2):93–119.
24. Capitman, J., Ritter, G., Abrahams, R. Measuring the adequacy of home care for frail elders. The Gerontologist 1997;37(3):303–313.
25. Lima, J.C., Allen, S.M. Targeting risk for unmet need: not enough help versus no help at all. Journal of Gerontology Series B Psychological Sciences and Social Sciences 2001;56(5):S302–S310.
26. Allen, S.M., Mor, V. The prevalence and consequences of unmet need. Contrasts between older and younger adults with disability. Medical Care 1997;35(11):1132–1148.
27. Leveille, S.G., Wagner, E.H., Davis, C., Grothaus, L., Wallace, J., LeGerfo, M., Kent, D. Preventing disability and managing chronic illness in frail older adults: a randomized trial of a community-based partnership with primary care. Journal of the American Geriatric Society 1998;46(10):1191–1198.
28. Lorig, K., Sobel, D., Stewart, A., et al. Evidence suggesting that a chronic disease self-management program can improve health status while reducing hospitalization. Medical Care 1999;37(11):5–14.
29. Yee, D., Capitman, J., Leutz, W., Sciegaj, M. Resident-centered care in assisted living. Journal of Aging and Social Policy 1999;10(3):7–27.
30. Goldman, D.P., Zissimopoulos, J.M. High out-of-pocket health care spending by the elderly. Health Affairs 2003;22(3):194–202.
31. Gold, M., Achman, L. Average out-of-pocket costs for Medicare choice enrollees increase 10 percent in 2003. Issue Brief Commonwealth Fund 2003;(Aug 667):1–9.
32. Stewart, S.T. Do out-of-pocket health expenditures rise with age among older Americans? The Gerontologist 2004;44(1):48–57.
33. Patel, U.D., Davis, M.M. Falling into the doughnut hole: drug spending among beneficiaries with end-stage renal disease under Medicare Part D plans. Journal of the American Society of Nephrology 2006;17(9):2546–2553.
34. Tija, J., Schwartz, J.S. Will Medicare prescription drug benefits eliminate cost barriers for older adults with diabetes mellitus? Journal of the American Geriatrics Society 2006;54(4):606–612.
35. Stevens, R.A. Health care in the early 1960s. Health Care Financing Review 1996;18(2):11–22.
36. Altman, D. The new Medicare prescription-drug legislation. Journal of the American Medical Association 2004;350(1):9–10.

37. Schlesinger, M. On values and democratic policy making: the deceptively fragile consensus around market-oriented medical care. Journal of Health Politics, Policy and Law 2002;27(6):889–925.

38. Moynihan, D.P. On the commodification of medicine. Academic Medicine 1998;73(5):453–459.

39. Churchill, L.R. Self-Interest and Universal Health Care: Why Well-Insured Americans Should Support Coverage for Everyone. Boston: Harvard University Press, 1994.

40. Silverman, E., Skinners, J., Fisher, E. The association between for-profit hospital ownership and increased Medicare spending. New England Journal of Medicine 1999;341(3):420–426.

41. Stark, F. History versus ideology: the Medicare reform debate. Health Affairs 1999;18(3):265–267.

42. Capitman, J. Defining diversity: a primer and review. Generations 2002; (Fall): 8–15.

43. Verbrugge, L., Leprowski, J., Imanaka, Y. Comorbidity and its impact on disability. Milbank Quarterly 1989;67(3–4):450–484.

44. Verbrugge, L., Jette, A. The disablement process. Social Science and Medicine 1994;38(1):1–14.

45. Verbrugge, L., Patrick, D. Seven chronic conditions: their impact on US adults' activity levels and use of medical services. American Journal of Public Health 1995;5(2):173–182.

46. Wolinsky, F., Armbrecht, E., Wyrwich, K. Rethinking functional limitation pathways. The Gerontologist 2000;40(2):137–146.

47. Weissert, W.G., Hirth, R.A., Chemew, M.E., Diwan, S., Kim, J. Case management: effects of improved risk and value information. The Gerontologist 2003; 43(6):797–805.

48. Leutz, W., Capitman, J., Green, C. A limited entitlement for community care: how members use services. Journal of Aging and Social Policy 2001;12(3):43–64.

49. Green, C., Capitman, J., Leutz, W. Expanded care and quality of life among elderly social HMO members. Journal of Applied Gerontology 2002;21(3):333–351.

50. Leutz, W., Capitman, J., Ruwe, M., et al. Caregiver education and support: results of a multi-site pilot in an HMO. Home Health Care Services Quarterly 2002;21(2):49–72.

51. Kingston, R.S., Smith, J.P. Socioeconomic status and racial ethnic differences in functional status associated with chronic diseases. American Journal of Public Health 1997;87(5):805–810.

52. Krieger, N. Theories for social epidemiology in the twenty-first century: an ecosocial perspective. In: Hofrichter, R. (ed.) Health and Social Justice: Politics, Ideology, and Inequity in the Distribution of Disease. San Francisco: Jossey-Bass, 2003, pp. 428–450.

53. Krieger, N. Does racism harm health? Did child abuse exist before 1962? On explicit questions, critical science, and current controversies: an ecosocial perspective. American Journal of Public Health 2003;93(2):194–199.

54. Bouleware, L.E., Cooper, L.A., Ratner, L.E., LaVeist, T.A., Powe, N.R. Race and trust in the healthcare system. Public Health Reports 2003;118(4):358–365.

55. Brandon, D.T., Isaac, L.A., LaVeist, T.A. The legacy of the Tuskegee and trust in medical care: is Tuskegee responsible for race differences in mistrust of medical care? Journal of the National Medical Association 2005;97(7):951–956.

56. Hannan, E.L., van Ryn, M., Burke, J., Stone, D., Kumar, D., Arani, D., Pierce, W., Rafii, S., Sanborn, T.A., Sharma, S., Slater, J., DeBuono, B.A. Access to coronary artery bypass surgery by race/ethnicity and gender among patients who are appropriate for surgery. Medical Care 1999;37(1):68–77.

57. Horner, R.D., et al. Theories explaining racial differences in the utilization of diagnostic and therapeutic procedures for cerebrovascular disease. Milbank Quarterly 1995;73(3):443–462.

58. Kressin, N.T., Petersen, L.A. The radical differences in the use of invasive cardiovascular procedures: review of the literature and prescription for future research. Annals of Internal Medicine 2001;135(5):352–366.

59. van Ryn, M., Burke, J. The effect patient race and socio-economic status on physicians' perceptions of patients. Social Science and Medicine 2000;50: 813–828.

60. van Ryn, M., Su, S. Paved with good intentions: do public health and human services providers contribute to racial/ethnic disparities in health? American Journal of Public Health 2003;93(2):248–255.

61. van Ryn, M. Research on the provider contribution to race/ethnicity disparities in medical care. Medical Care 2002;40(1 Suppl.):1140–1151.

62. Bogart, L.M. Relationship of stereotypic beliefs about physicians to health care–relevant behaviors and cognitions among African American women. Journal of Behavioral Medicine 2001;24(6):573–586.

63. Betancourt, J.R., Green, A.R., Carrillo, J.E., et al. Defining cultural competence: a practical framework for addressing racial/ethnic disparities in health and health care. Public Health Reports 2003;118(4):293–302.

64. Dunlop, D.D., Manheim, L.M., Song, J., Chang, R.W. Gender and ethnic/racial disparities in health care utilization among older adults. Journal of Gerontology Series B Psychological Sciences and Social Sciences 2002;57(4):S221–S233.

65. Pezzin, L., Kasper, J. Medicaid enrollment among elderly Medicare beneficiaries: individual determinants, effects of state policy, and impact on service use. Health Services Research 2002;37(4):827–847.

66. Janes, G.R., Blackman, D.K., Bolen, J.C., Kamimoto, L.A., Rhodes, L., Caplan, L.S., Nadel, M.R., Tomar, S.L., Lando, J.F., Greby, S.M., Singleton, J.A., Strikas, R.A., Wooten, K.G. Surveillance for use of preventive health care services by older adults, 1995–1997. MMWR Morbidity and Mortality Weekly Report 1999;48(Suppl. 8): 51–88.

67. Potosky, A.L., Breen, N., Graubard, B.I., Parsons, P.E. The association between health care coverage and the use of cancer screening tests. Results from the 1992 National Health Interview Survey. Medical Care 1998;36(3):257–270.

68. Carrasquillo, O., Lantigua, R.A., Shea, S. Preventive services among Medicare beneficiaries with supplemental coverage versus HMO enrollees, Medicaid recipients, and elders with no additional coverage. Medical Care 2001;39(6):616–626.

69. Christensen, S., Shinogle, J. Effects of supplemental coverage on use of services by Medicare enrollees. Health Care Financing Review 1997;19(1):5–17.

70. Gentry, D., Longo, D.R., Housemann, R.A., Loiterstein, D., Brownson, R.C. Prevalence and correlates of physician advice for prevention: impact of type of insurance and regular source of care. Journal of Health Care Finance 1999; 26(1):78–97.

71. Tervalon, M., Murray-Garcia, J. Cultural humility versus cultural competence: a critical distinction in defining physician training outcomes in multicultural

education. Journal of Health Care for the Poor and Underserved 1998;9(2): 117–125.

72. Tesh, S. Hidden Arguments. New Brunswick, NJ: Rutgers University Press, 1988.

73. Capitman, J., Sciegaj, M. A contextual approach for understanding individual autonomy in managed community long-term care. The Gerontologist 1995;34(4):533–540.

8

Health Law for Older Adults

ELLEN A. BRUCE

Developing an interdisciplinary approach to the care of older adults' health may require interaction with attorneys, either as consultants to the team or, in some cases, as part of the team. Lawyers will be particularly helpful when a patient is suffering from diminished capacity and therefore possibly in need of a conservator or guardian and when avenues of treatment seem to be blocked by legal considerations. These considerations may be specific to the patient, such as denial of health-care coverage for a specific procedure, or broader, such as whether a clinic is licensed to provide a particular type of care.

The law, as it is found in statutes, regulations, and case decisions, has a significant impact on the practice of medicine and the care of all patients, including older adults. A lawyer's job is to interpret the law as it applies to a situation and to advise the client on the range of appropriate actions within the confines of the law. Therefore, when working with a lawyer or (heaven forbid) a group of lawyers, it is useful to understand the legal framework within which the lawyer is considering different options and the perspective from which the lawyer is proceeding.

Lawyers are taught to not make value judgments but provide options and advice to a client. The advice will be influenced by the goals of the client. Therefore, the first thing to determine when working with lawyers is who the client is. An attorney will usually be representing some party—for example, the patient, the patient's family, the hospital, the provider, or the state. The job of the attorney is to represent the interests of his or her client, as expressed by the client. Therefore, an attorney will act to protect the wishes of the client, regardless of how foolish those wishes may be. Consider the case of an elderly gentleman who lives alone and is being evicted because his landlord feels he is a danger to himself and other residents. The tenant has forgotten on at least two occasions to turn off the stove, and the fire department has been called due to excessive smoke in his apartment. The elderly man does not want to move. The attorney's job, if he or she takes the case, is to defend the man against the eviction. The attorney may suggest other living arrangements or in-home supports so that the man does not have to cook, but it is up to the client, not the attorney, to make these decisions.

Similarly, an attorney representing an unsympathetic client cannot lecture the client as to what he or she thinks the client should do but must advise within the limits of the law about what the client can do. So, for instance, if an attorney is representing the daughter of an elderly patient whose competency has been questioned and the daughter wants to know how she can take over her mother's affairs, the attorney must advise the daughter of the legal proceedings available. It is not up to the attorney to judge whether the daughter is the best person to make decisions for her mother or whether or not the mother is competent. The attorney, if he or she takes the case, must advocate for the daughter, not the mother. Of course, an attorney should not take a case for which there is no basis to proceed or that he or she knows is based on false information. But it is the attorney's knowledge of the facts and the law that determines whether there is a basis upon which to proceed, not what the attorney thinks would be the best outcome.

With this perspective, a background understanding of the laws that affect the provision of health care to the elderly is useful in providing care to elderly patients and working with lawyers.

Medicare

Medicare is the federal insurance program that covers most people 65 years of age and over as well as severely disabled individuals in the United States. Seniors receiving Social Security or Railroad Retirement benefits either on their own work histories or on their spouses' work history are eligible for Medicare when they reach 65. Some individuals who have never worked in Social Security–covered jobs, such as certain public employees, are not covered. Medicare's history and policy issues are discussed extensively in Chapter 4. Of importance to lawyers and advocates are the rights a patient has if the patient is denied benefits.

Eligibility for Medicare is rarely the reason a person is denied benefits. Eligibility depends on age and work history, and the determination is not complicated. A beneficiary's income and assets do not have to be documented as they are not relevant to the determination. However, Medicare's coverage of services may be an issue. For example, if a patient is denied coverage for home health services because he or she is not deemed homebound, the client may require the services of a lawyer to challenge that determination.

Medicare also will cover only services that are deemed "medically necessary." If the provider determines that Medicare would consider the services medically unnecessary or otherwise not covered because they do not fall within the definition of covered services,[1] the provider will issue a notice of noncoverage to the patient. This notice is not a decision by Medicare that the service is not covered but a determination by the provider. The provider is financially liable for services rendered that Medicare[2] determines are not covered and that the beneficiary had no way of knowing would not be covered. Therefore, providers have a financial incentive to deny services they think Medicare may not cover. After receiving a notice of noncoverage, the patient has the right to insist that the provider submit a bill to Medicare for the services that the patient thinks might be covered. If Medicare denies coverage of the service, the patient may appeal the denial.[3]

The appeal process in Medicare depends on whether you are in "traditional Medicare" or in Medicare Advantage, formerly referred to as Medicare + Choice or Part C. In traditional Medicare you must get a denial notice from the peer review organization (PRO), the intermediary, or the carrier. Once the patient receives the denial notice or initial determination letter, he or she may request a "reconsideration" of that denial. If the coverage is still denied after the reconsideration, the patient may request a hearing before an administrative law judge, then before the Appeals Board, and finally in a court if the amount of money at stake is large enough. During the appeal process the patient must either pay for the services in the interim or go without the services. The exception is for hospital services, which will be covered for 3 days during the appeal to the PRO.

Beneficiaries in Medicare Advantage plans have their initial decisions and reconsideration decisions made by the managed-care organization. If a patient wishes to contest the reconsideration decision, he or she may appeal to the Center for Health Dispute Resolution, an independent agency hired by the Center for Medicare and Medicaid Services to hear these appeals. Medicare Advantage organizations also must have internal grievance procedures and an expedited appeal process for emergency care.[4]

Denial of coverage is not an uncommon problem for Medicare beneficiaries. Because it is usually couched in terms of the patient no longer "needing" therapy or the patient no longer fitting the criteria of a skilled nursing facility, patients don't realize that they have been denied coverage. Instead, they think they don't need the care being requested. Thus, the denial is not often seen as a legal problem. However, a lawyer can be helpful in these situations to identify a patient's rights and explain the appeal process. Providers are required to give written notice to beneficiaries when denying services. In both traditional Medicare and Medicare Advantage appeals, the key to a beneficiary's success is the support of the treating physician.[5] Documentation of the medical necessity of the denied treatment is most persuasive when coming from the patient's treating physician. Ensuring that Medicare pays for all services that are necessary for an individual patient is an area where it is important for treating professionals and lawyers to work together.

In 2003, Congress passed the Medicare Prescription Drug Improvement and Modernization Act, which created many changes in the Medicare program, most notably a voluntary prescription drug program. The prescription drug program, or Part D, began in 2006 and is administered through private drug plans. Part D has been very confusing for elders and their families because of the lack of standardization between plans and because of many administrative complications, which have resulted in some seniors not being able to get drugs or to prove they are covered. Despite the many problems in the administration of the program, it is too soon to tell if the complicated structure of the program will prove beneficial for the majority of seniors or will remain confusing and costly.

Advocates for elders have recommended many changes in the Part D program, including standardizing the formulary, repealing the doughnut hole, and replacing it with a drug benefit run through the traditional Medicare fee-for-service program.[6] Lawyers can be very helpful to advocates trying to change a law such as the Medicare law in that they can explain what needs to be changed and help write the language for bills to be submitted to Congress. Also, the interpretation of a new law often leads to different conclusions, which ultimately must be resolved by the courts. Therefore, lawyers can help elders and their representatives challenge interpretations that are unfavorable to them.

Medicaid

Medicaid is a federal–state program that provides health insurance coverage to certain low-income seniors as well as eligible younger people. To be eligible under the elderly benefit, a person must be 65 years old or over and have limited income and assets. The income level varies widely from state to state, but the assets allowed are only $2000 for an individual ($3000 for a couple) in most states. Other assets that are not counted include the house the recipient lives in, a car, and some other specific assets.[7] Retirement savings are counted toward the $2000 limit, making people who save for retirement ineligible until they have used almost all their savings. This restrictive asset requirement has not changed since 1989 and is one reason that so many low-income elders are not eligible for Medicaid.[8]

"Spend-down" is an often-discussed method of qualifying for Medicaid. There are two forms of spend-down: asset spend-down and income spend-down. Every state requires that countable assets be below the asset eligibility level, but applicants cannot transfer assets for less than the fair market value in order to meet the asset requirement.[9] For example, an elder with $12,000 cannot give her child $10,000 and then apply for Medicaid claiming she has only $2000 in assets. Federal law requires that a state look back 5 years from the time of application for benefits to determine if any assets were transferred for less than fair market value. If they were, the applicant is denied Medicaid eligibility.

Transfer of assets for below market value or the giving away of one's money and property is considered by some to be a serious problem for Medicaid.[10] It is particularly a problem in the long-term care context because long-term care is very costly, few seniors have long-term care insurance, and Medicare pays for very little long-term care. The result is that most people going into nursing homes or needing extensive home-based care must pay for that care out of their own pocket or rely on Medicaid to pay for it. The high cost of long-term care can quickly drain a family's savings, creating a powerful incentive for families to qualify the member needing long-term care for Medicaid. Growing state Medicaid budgets and states' fiscal crises create a powerful incentive for states to restrict access to Medicaid eligibility. The amendments in the Deficit Reduction Act of 2005 restricted eligibility by requiring the 5-year look-back period and making the look-back period start at the date of Medicaid application instead of the date of nursing home application. These more restrictive requirements make transferring assets more difficult, presumably limiting the incidents of false impoverishment.

The second form of spend-down is the income spend-down, in which an individual may have income above the Medicaid eligibility level but medical expenses that, if subtracted from the person's monthly income, leave the individual with disposable income below the income guidelines. For example, an elderly gentleman who has a monthly income of $1500 but is in a nursing home that is costing $2200/month does not have enough income to pay for the nursing home care. If the income eligibility level were $800/month in his state, he would be ineligible because his income is too high. States that allow an income spend-down, however, would find him eligible for Medicaid and pay for the cost of the nursing home that exceeds his income. In these cases, the recipient is allowed to keep a small amount of money for personal expenses, which is referred to as the "personal needs allowance."

Normally, a couple's assets and income are considered together. However, when one member of the couple is institutionalized, Medicaid has special provisions that allow the community spouse to retain some of the couple's income and assets above the Medicaid eligibility limits and still have the institutionalized spouse receive Medicaid benefits.

Medicaid eligibility rules are very complicated and vary from state to state. Also, within a state there are different ways to become eligible for Medicaid depending on the elder's circumstances. For an in-depth explanation of eligibility rules, see Bruen, Wiener, and Thomas, "Medicaid Eligibility Policy for Aged, Blind, and Disabled Beneficiaries.[11]" Medicaid's income and asset tests make the eligibility process complicated, and an attorney may be needed to understand the requirements and to appeal if the applicant is denied eligibility. Like Medicare, applicants are entitled to appeal the denial of an application as well as the denial of coverage once eligibility is determined.

Private Insurance

Since Medicare has many gaps in its coverage, there is a significant market for private supplemental insurance coverage. Many elders receive supplemental coverage through retiree health benefits provided by former employers, although companies have been eliminating this benefit in recent years.[12] Other elders purchase Medigap plans that fill in some of the gaps in coverage. In 1999, 8.4 million beneficiaries were enrolled in Medigap policies.[13] The federal government regulates the benefit packages of individual supplemental insurance plans, limiting the choice of plans offered to 10. In this way individual plans are standardized so that individuals can compare plans. State governments also regulate individual plans.

Retiree health benefits are provided to the company as a group plan and therefore are often less costly than what individual elders could purchase on their own. Privately purchased plans are expensive compared to group plans because their marketing and sales costs are higher. Companies, however, have been cutting back or eliminating entirely retiree health benefits in recent years in an attempt to control company expenses. Findings from a 2003 survey of employers offering retiree health benefits found that employers were capping their contributions to retiree health benefits and that in the previous year retirees' costs for the coverage had increased 18%.[14] Unlike pension benefits that can be vested and therefore become a right of the worker in retirement, retiree health-care benefits do not vest. There is no guarantee that the retiree health benefits offered when you are a worker will be given to you when you retire. There is not even a guarantee that the health benefits you receive when you retire will continue throughout your retirement.

While some retirees from companies that promised in writing lifelong health-care coverage may have a legal claim to continued supplemental coverage for life, very few companies did that. Even if there is an enforceable right on the part of retirees, if a company goes bankrupt, the retirees will have no corporation to enforce their right against. Thus, the loss of retiree supplemental health-care coverage is a very real possibility for many retired workers.

Access to Care

Insuring access to care is a complicated policy problem. The policy issues of equity in financing and access are discussed in depth in Chapter 7. However great is the failure of the American health-care system in providing equal access to care, there are some laws and principles that protect individuals from being denied care. A combination of state and federal laws exists that protects patients' access to health care. Discrimination on the basis of race, type of payment, or illness is generally prohibited in most settings. Under *common law* (practice that has become law because courts have enforced the principles), a physician has a duty to continue to treat a patient under his or her care until the patient has been transferred to another physician, the patient terminates the relationship, or the reason for the treatment ceases to exist.[15] Physicians are under no duty to initiate treatment of a person who is not their patient, but they cannot abandon a patient they are treating without giving the patient adequate time to secure another physician.

Emergency room care is the one situation where federal law has carved out a requirement for a hospital to undertake treatment of a patient regardless of the patient's ability to pay. The Emergency Medical Treatment and Active Labor Act (EMTALA)[16] requires all hospitals that receive Medicare money and have an emergency room to stabilize and arrange for a transfer of any patient who comes to the emergency room with an emergency condition. This requirement is not limited to Medicare patients. Although the requirement is expansive in that it provides no payment for the care it requires, it does not require care past the stage of stabilizing the patient nor does it specify the level of screening required. Therefore, EMTALA protects people in need of emergency care but does not solve the problem of access to care in other situations.

Two other federal laws prohibit discrimination in the provision of health care: the Civil Rights Act of 1964[17] and the Americans with Disabilities Act (ADA).[18] The Civil Rights Act prohibits discrimination on the basis of race, color, or national origin in any program receiving federal aid. This statute has rarely been used to enforce access to care; however, it could conceivably be used if a person is being turned away because of race. The ADA prohibits discrimination by health-care providers on the basis of disability. In the land-mark U.S. Supreme Court case *Bragdon v. Abbott*, a person infected with human immunodeficiency virus (HIV) was found to have a claim under the ADA against a dentist who refused to treat her in his office because of her HIV status.[19] The dentist insisted that the only way he would treat her would be in a hospital setting at a much greater cost to the patient. The court found that HIV infection was a disability protected by the statute and that the dentist did not show that treating the patient in his office posed a danger to him, his employees, or other patients.

The ADA has also been used in the long-term care setting to require the state to provide care to individuals on Medicaid in the least restrictive setting appropriate to their care. In the U.S. Supreme Court case of Olmstead v. L.C.[20] two women with mental disabilities sued the state, claiming that their placement in an institution constituted discrimination on the basis of their disabilities, when they could be treated in the community. The court found that the state Medicaid program had an obligation to provide placement in the least restrictive setting when the state treating professionals said that the person could be treated in the community, the person did not oppose the transfer, and the state could reasonably accommodate the request considering its obligation to other mentally disabled people and the resources available.

The impact of this decision has been to increase pressure for long-term care in the community for both disabled young people and elders. Many states have planning processes in place to increase community-based services for the physically and mentally disabled recipients of Medicaid. The extent to which states must provide community-care services to keep elderly Medicaid recipients out of nursing homes has not been thoroughly tested. The most contentious issues are whether new financial resources are required and how a transition period can be financed. Shifting resources from institutional care to community care can actually increase costs to the state because of the need to maintain institutions that are not fully occupied during the transition period. It can also mean having to move people who still must be cared for in an institution from one institution to another, possibly to their detriment. The transition to community care, however, has been painfully slow even with the ADA and the threat of lawsuits.

Patient Self-Determination and Assisted Suicide

The law starts with the premise that a patient may not be treated without his or her "informed consent." The doctrine of informed consent is based on the concept that a competent adult has the right to determine what shall be done with his or her body.[21] The consent must be voluntary, competent, and informed.[22] The "informed" requirement is somewhat tricky for treating professionals. For consent to be "informed" the patient has to be given information about the treatment, the alternative treatments, and the risks and benefits of each treatment. In this context, not doing anything should also be considered an option. In cases of emergency, a patient who is unable to give consent is deemed to give consent to reasonably necessary treatment.[23] When treating elderly patients, competency to give informed consent may not be clear, as discussed later in this chapter. If a patient is not competent to give consent, someone else with legal authority to give consent must be found for the treatment to proceed.

The corollary to the requirement that the patient must give informed consent is that the patient may withhold consent, that is, refuse treatment. The issue of refusing treatment or terminating life-saving treatment is very controversial and has been the subject of many "end-of-life" cases. The issue arises when, for whatever reason, the patient or someone acting on the patient's behalf refuses further treatment or requests that ongoing treatment be terminated. The U.S. Supreme Court has addressed these issues on several occasions.

In 1990, in the case of *Cruzan v. Director, Missouri Department of Health*,[24] the highest court decided that a state could require clear and convincing evidence of a patient's wishes before terminating treatment of a comatose patient. The patient, Nancy Cruzan, had been in a car accident that left her in a persistent vegetative state. After it became clear that their daughter would not recover consciousness, her parents requested that the court direct the hospital to discontinue artificial hydration and nutrition. All agreed that doing so would result in the patient's death. Although the court did not order the discontinuation of treatment, it did recognize that artificial feeding and hydration was treatment and, therefore, could be requested by a patient to be terminated, even if it resulted in the death of the patient. Justice O'Connor also suggested in her concurring opinion that a competent individual could exercise the right to terminate treatment after he or she became incompetent by completing a health-care proxy or other advance directive. This case settled the question of how far the right to refuse treatment extended. A second important end-of-life case decided by the U.S. Supreme Court was *Washington v. Glucksberg*.[25] This case tested the right of a terminally ill patient to have the assistance of a physician in committing suicide. The plaintiffs claimed that patients have a constitutional right to decide the time and manner of their death. The court decided that there was no such constitutional right and that the right to liberty did not extend to being allowed to have a doctor assist you in ending your life. At the same time the court decided *Glucksberg*, it decided *Vacco v. Quill*,[26] which also claimed a constitutional right (equal protection right) to assisted suicide. The court held in that case as well that there was no constitutional right to assisted suicide.

Although *Glucksberg* found no constitutional right to assisted suicide, it did not foreclose the possibility that a state may give a legislative right to assisted suicide. Oregon has done just that. In 1994 the Oregon voters passed an initiative that allowed a terminally ill, competent adult resident of Oregon the right to request assistance of a physician in ending his or her life.[27] After court challenges to the law, it became operational in 1998. Between 1998 and 2003, 171 patients exercised the right to assistance in committing suicide.[28] The overall number of patients taking advantage of the law is relatively few compared to the number of deaths in Oregon.

The issue of assisted suicide and control at the end of life not only is a legal one but has strong religious, ethical, and philosophical dimensions as well. Physicians and family members report that the loss of autonomy is one of the most prevalent factors for patients choosing to end their life through physician-assisted suicide.[29] Developing a conceptual framework to understand autonomy in the treatment decisions of older adults is discussed in Chapter 5.

A major concern regarding allowing assisted suicide has been the potential for abuse. Specifically, there is a concern that those who are old, poor, or severely disabled may be encouraged to commit suicide or request assistance in committing suicide because they feel guilty about the amount of resources that are being expended to keep them alive. Also, allowing assisted suicide may result in deaths due to depression or undue pain that could have been treated. Interestingly, the sixth Annual Report on Oregon's Death with Dignity Act notes some evidence that the Death with Dignity Law may have increased the medical community's attention to pain management and to recognizing depression in terminally ill patients.[30] As of 2004, only one state has adopted a law allowing assisted suicide. In what is considered the wisdom of a federal system, this policy is being tried and tested in one state. The lessons learned from the experience of Oregon will inform future discussions about the problems and advantages of such a policy.

Patient Confidentiality

Questions about access to medical information arise in many contexts. A patient may want his or her medical records to seek a second opinion or to switch doctors. A family member may want to discuss a patient's condition with the doctor. An insurance company may want to know what treatment a patient has received. Since the uses of medical information vary widely and since the impact of releasing information that is commonly considered private can be devastating, a provider must understand his or her legal obligations with respect to medical information.

The privacy of a patient's medical information is protected in a number of ways. Each state has common law, licensing laws, and/or privacy laws that limit what providers may disclose and to whom they may disclose it. However, the extent of privacy protection by states varies widely, with some states offering very little protection. In 1996, a comprehensive federal statute was passed called the Health Insurance Portability and Accountability Act (HIPAA),[31] which set out privacy requirements for health-care providers and insurance companies. According to the U.S. Department of Health and Human Services' Office of Civil Rights, "A major goal of the Privacy Rule is to assure that individuals' health information is properly protected while allowing the flow of health information needed to provide and promote high quality health care and to protect the public's health and well being."[32]

Information covered by HIPAA (Pub. Law 104–191, 1996) is "individually identifiable health information," and it is protected from being conveyed inappropriately in any way, including orally. Under HIPAA, a provider may continue to disclose medical information for the purpose of treatment and payment of health-care bills. A provider may also share information if the patient authorizes in writing that information may be disclosed. For all patients, but particularly elderly patients, it may be important that they indicate what family members may have access to their health information in circumstances such as an acute hospitalization. If this isn't done, an adult child may not be able to get any information on a hospitalized parent.

Where state laws are different from the federal requirements, the general rule is that the federal law will prevail. However, in some cases where state laws provide more protection than the federal law, providers must follow the state law. Disclosure of health information under state mandatory reporting laws such as elder abuse laws is also allowed.

Also, HIPAA ensures that patients have a right to their personal medical records on request. If an individual is unable to exercise that right, the right may be exercised by "a personal representative." A *personal representative* is someone with legal authority to act on behalf of the patient, such as a legal guardian or holder of a health-care proxy that is in force. In this way, patients' right to their records and their ability to protect their privacy is protected whether or not they are competent.

The act was passed as a response to growing concern over the disclosure of health information. The ease of access to information through electronic databases and the variations between state law left loopholes in the protection of health-care records. The law tries to balance the competing concerns of privacy and need for information to care for patients, protect the public health and welfare, and pay for care.

Competency

Probably one of the most difficult challenges in working with elderly patients arises when a patient's competency is questioned. As a health-care provider, a social worker, or an attorney, the professional takes direction from the patient or client. If the patient is not competent to give that direction, the professional must seek direction from another source. Thus, the question of whether the patient is competent or not becomes crucial. The law assumes that every adult is competent unless proven not to be.[33] Or to put it another way, unless a court has appointed a guardian for an adult, it is assumed that the person can make his or her own decisions.

Courts have used various definitions of "competency." In an often-cited New Jersey case, *In re Quackenbush* (1978),[34] the court looked at whether the patient had the mental capacity to understand the nature and extent of his physical condition and to understand the risks involved in not amputating a gangrenous leg. Although the 72-year-old man was exhibiting some psychotic symptoms and refusal of the operation would result in his death, the court found him competent to refuse the operation because he understood the consequences of his decision.

Courts have not, as a rule, set up clear guidelines to decide whether someone is competent or not but, instead, rely on physicians to make that determination. Obviously, there can be great variation between physicians in the judgment of whether or not a patient is competent and in the standards used to determine competency. In addition to this variation, most courts now recognize that people may be competent for some purposes and not for others. A patient may be able to express a clear desire not to move from his or her house but not to make more complicated decisions such as a choice between two treatments, each of which carries risks and benefits that need to be weighed. Courts in most jurisdictions have the authority to appoint limited guardianships that allow individuals to retain some decision-making authority.

For many years there was no provision in the law for individuals to appoint others to act for them in medical situations when they became incompetent. As advances in medicine enabled doctors to keep patients alive even after the heart or lungs could no longer function on their own, it became not uncommon for individuals to survive with no cognitive functioning. These patients were clearly incompetent. Also, incidences of elderly patients experiencing periods of incompetence due to illness or medical procedures led to the search for ways to make decisions for patients when they could not clearly speak for themselves. After the U.S. Supreme Court decided the *Cruzan* case where Justice O'Connor suggested states could authorize individuals to appoint a friend or family member to act on their behalf when they were incompetent, many states passed laws allowing the appointment of health-care proxies. A *health-care proxy* is an agent who, upon the incompetence of the person who executes the proxy, is empowered to make medical decisions for the incompetent individual. Unlike living wills, which outline specific actions to be taken in certain situations, a health-care proxy turns over the decision to another person who can make the decision based on what the agent feels the patient would have wanted under the circumstances.

The forms of advance directives that are allowed vary from state to state. Under the federal Patient Self-Determination Act passed in 1990, health-care institutions such as hospitals, nursing homes, and home health agencies that receive Medicare or Medicaid must provide each patient with information on the state law on advance directives. The institution must also note in the patient's record whether or not the patient has an advance directive. Although there was great anticipation that the legalization of advance directives would result in most adults executing them, this has not been the case. For example, a study of nursing home residents found that only 32% had advance directives and only 29% had discussed life-sustaining treatments.[35] There is also question about the effectiveness of advance directives in situations where they have been executed.

The Role of the Professional as Advocate

A professional care provider is likely to encounter many situations where an understanding of the law will be useful. In some situations, the provider may be called upon to be an advocate for the elderly patient. In these cases, the provider must decide if he or she can help the patient or if the best help would be to get the patient an attorney. At a minimum, the provider may want to consult an attorney him- or herself to understand the patient's rights and alternatives.

Individual advocacy, however, may be of little use if the law is settled in a situation and it is being followed—for example, when a professional is trying to get health care for an uninsured patient but there is no free care available or the patient does not fit the guidelines for governmental programs such as Medicare or Medicaid. Or it might be that the program the patient is in does not cover the service needed or the required copayment may be more than the patient can afford. These situations highlight the limits of individual advocacy.

Changes in the systems that allow for the provision of care require more than individual advocacy. They require a concerted effort over a long period of time by groups of people determined to see a change. Most system changes during the last 15 years in health care have been driven by the goal of keeping health-care costs down. Questions of quality and access have either taken a back seat to issues of cost or they have been combined with the issue of cost. For instance, the move toward managed care has been advocated as a method of both reducing costs and increasing quality by increasing preventive care.

The continued effort to control costs has fueled the movement to more self-directed care. Like many ideas, it contains both opportunities and concerns for elderly patients. Self-directed care encompasses the concepts of autonomy and choice in the place and method of care. It is likely to result in more home and community-based care for the elderly to the degree that such care can be provided for the same or less cost as care currently being provided in institutions. However, it also is being used as a justification to put more responsibility on patients for choosing health insurance and paying for more of their care out of their own pockets.[36] The argument is that if patients must pay for more of their care directly, they will be wiser consumers of health care and will use only those services that they feel are really necessary, thus reducing unnecessary care. Whether or not self-directed care will result in reducing unnecessary care, and therefore overall costs, is in the exploration stage; but it is clear that it poses problems for both poor patients and patients who are not well enough or competent to manage their own health care.

Providers are in a particular position to influence a number of issues that the health-care system is facing. Protecting quality of care is clearly an issue that providers must be actively involved in as they are in the best position to identify poor care and recommend ways to improve care. However, especially when dealing with elderly patients, the quality of life may be as important as, if not more important than, the quality of care. When does too much care interfere with the quality of life? What is the best balance between the quality of care and quality of life? Who should make these decisions? How should quality of life be measured?

Issues of access and the structure of the delivery system are also in the forefront of policy discussions. Providers have an important perspective to offer in these discussions. They are the ones who will work in whatever system evolves, and they will be seeing the individuals who are either well or poorly served by the health-care system. Can we afford to provide care to all those who need it? Who should decide what care is needed? Is the medical model of care the best model for patients in long-term care? These are just some of the many policy questions that providers must work with elder advocates and policy makers to answer as the health-care system for elders evolves. In these discussions providers will be challenged to represent not only their own interests but also the interests of their patients, many of whom cannot advocate for themselves.

Application to the Case Study: The Older Adult Care, Training, Research, and Planning Program—An Attorney's Place in the Development

The Older Adult Care, Training, Research, and Planning Program (OACTRPP) is a very ambitious project both in its scope and in its timetable. It will be primarily a mammoth administrative undertaking, but there are a number of areas where an attorney will be needed to put it together and administer it, as well as other areas where an attorney could be helpful.

The starting point will be to determine the relationship between the medical school and the OACTRPP. Is the OACTRPP independent of the medical school, or is it a part of the school? If it is independent, it will need some formal legal structure to be set up. A lawyer will be helpful in providing the different options and deciding which one is most appropriate for the situation.

Setting up the OACTRPP will require that a number of entities work together, including the medical school, the OACTRPP planning committee, providers, insurance companies, and government payers. Contracts will be needed with each of these entities to formalize the terms of their working relationships. An attorney for the OACTRPP would be needed, at minimum, to review any contract negotiated. The program will have to be certified for Medicaid and Medicare purposes in order to seek reimbursement. An attorney's contribution when working with a group trying to set up a new program is to insure that it complies with all the applicable legal regulations. Although it may sound as though that simply requires knowing the regulations, the application of regulations to new situations can be complex. There is often much room for interpretation. An attorney who understands and supports the goals of the project will be in a much better position to help the planners accomplish their goals than an attorney who is called in for one technical question. In any evolving project, participants want an attorney who will tell them how they legally can accomplish what they want to do, not list all the reasons they can't do it. Of course, some things will be prohibited, and it is the lawyer's duty to make the planners aware when they cross that line.

A second important aspect of the OACTRRP is that it is intended to be a research project. The project must set up the appropriate protocols and safeguards for client confidentiality under HIPAA and human subject compliance requirements of any grants. The project should also protect against any conflict of interest among researchers, funders, and providers. Knowledge of the applicable state and federal laws will be helpful in creating these protocols.

An aspect of this project that has the potential for conflict is the interface with the community. If handled well and the community is supportive of the project, there should be no need for any attorney involvement. However, if the community opposes the project, an attorney may be needed. In that case, as in all situations when working with attorneys, it is important to clarify whom the attorney represents. In the case scenario, the attorney could represent the medical school or the planning committee. It is very possible that the planning committee and the medical school could have different interests when dealing with the community; therefore, the attorney's role would be different depending on who engaged him or her.

A final consideration for the project is the establishment of appeal procedures for its patients. These procedures will differ according to the payer, and the project must be ready to provide all the appropriate information and the appropriate process.

As noted at the beginning, this project is an ambitious and complex undertaking. Attorneys will be indispensable in sorting out legal requirements, establishing procedures, and generally keeping the project on track. The most important aspect for a project such as this is to have an attorney who understands and supports its goals.

Bibliography

Bruen, B.K., Wiener, J.M., Thomas, S. Medicaid eligibility policy for aged, blind, and disabled beneficiaries. AARP Public Policy Institute, Paper 2003-14. Washington, DC: AARP, 2003.

Bunce, V.C. Medical savings accounts: problems and progress under HIPPA. Cato Policy Analysis 411, Cato Institute. Available at: http://www.cato.org/pubs/pas/pa-411es.html. 2001.

Center for Medicare Advocacy. An introduction to Medicare coverage and appeals. 2003. Willimantic, CT: Center for Medicare Advocacy, Inc.

Center for Medicare Advocacy, Inc. Medicare Part D progress report: six months later headaches persist. Available at: http://www.medicareadvocacy.org/PartD_6MonthReport072006.pdf. 2006. Accessed January 24, 2007.

General Accounting Office. Medicaid: Divestiture of Assets to Qualify for Long-term Care Services. GAO/HEHS-97-185R. Washington, DC: U.S. General Accounting Office, 1997.

Hewitt Associates, Henry J. Kaiser Family Foundation. Retiree Health Benefits Now and in the Future: Findings from the Kaiser/Hewitt 2003 Survey on Retiree Health Benefits. Available at http://www.kff.org/medicare/6105.cfm (last accessed 10/3/08).

Laschober, M.A., et al. Trends in Medicare supplemental insurance and prescription drug coverage, 1996–1999. Health Affairs 2002. Available at: http://content.healthaffairs.org/cgi/content/full/hlthaff.w2.127v1/DC1.

Levin, J.R., Wenger, N.S., Ouslander, J.G., et al. Life-sustaining treatment decisions for nursing home residents: who discusses, who decides and what is decided? Journal of the American Geriatrics Society 1999:47(1):82–87.

McCormack, L.A., et al. Retiree health insurance: recent trends and tomorrow's prospects. Health Care Financing Review 2002;23(3):17–34.

Moon, M., Friedland, R., Shirey, L. Medicare beneficiaries and their assets: implications for low-income programs. The Henry J. Kaiser Family Foundation. Available at: www.kff.org. 2002.

Oregon Department of Human Services. Sixth annual report on Oregon's Death with Dignity Act. Available at: http://www.ohd.hr.state.or.us/chs/pas/ar-disc.cfm. 2004. Accessed March 10, 2004.

U.S. Department of Health and Human Services, Office for Civil Rights. HIPAA compliance assistance. OCR Privacy rule summary, p. 1. Available at: http://www.hhs.gov/ocr/hipaa. May 2003.

Wing, K.R. The Law and the Public's Health. Chicago: Health Administration Press, 2003.

Legal References

Americans with Disabilities Act, 42 U.S.C. sec 12101 et seq. (1990).

Bragdon v. Abbott, 524 U.S. 624 (1998).

Civil Rights Act, 42 U.S.C. sec. 2000d et seq. (1964).

Cruzan v. Director, Missouri Department of Health, 497 U.S. 261, (1990).

Emergency Medical Treatment and Active Labor Act, 42 U.S.C.A. sec. 1395dd, et seq. (1986).

Health Insurance Portability and Accountability Act (HIPAA), Public Law 104–191 (1996).

Lane v. Candura, 6 Mass. App. Ct. 377 (1978).

Medicare Prescription Drug Improvement and Modernization Act, Public Law 108–173 (2003).

Olmstead v. L.C., 527 U.S. 581 (1999).

Oregon Death with Dignity Act, Or. Rev. Stat. sec. 127.800-897 (1994).

Oregon Department of Health and Human Services, Sixth Annual Report on Oregon's Death with Dignity Act.

Patient Self Determination Act, 42 U.S.C. sec. 1395cc(f)(1)(A) (1990).

In Re Quackenbush, 156 N.J. Super. 282 (1978).

Ricks v. Budge, 64 P.2d 208 (Sup. Ct. Utah 1937).

Scholendorff v. Society of New York Hospital, 211 N.Y. 125 (1914).

Vacco v. Quill, 521 U.S. 793 (1997).

Washington v. Glucksberg, 521 U.S. 702 (1997).

Notes

1. For example, Medicare will cover home health care services only if the patient is "homebound" and in need of "intermittent skilled-nursing care." A provider may determine that the patient is no longer considered homebound under Medicare's definition and is therefore no longer eligible for Medicare coverage.
2. The Medicare program is administered by the federal agency, the Center for Medicare and Medicaid Services. For the sake of simplicity, both the program and the administrative agency are referred to generally as "Medicare."
3. Center for Medicare Advocacy, Inc. "An introduction to Medicare coverage and appeals." July 2003: p. 24.

4. Ibid, p. 30.
5. Ibid, p. 33.
6. Center for Medicare Advocacy, Inc. Medicare Part D Progress Report: Six Months later Headaches Persist. Available at: http://www.medicareadvocacy.org/PartD_6MonthReport072006.pdf. 2006. Accessed January 24, 2007.
7. Bruen, B. K., J. M. Wiener, & S. Thomas. Medicaid Eligibility Policy for Aged, Blind, and Disabled Beneficiaries. Washington, D.C.: AARP Public Policy Institute, 2003: p. 3.
8. Moon, M., R. Friedland, & L. Shirey. Medicare Beneficiaries and Their Assets: Implications for Low-Income Programs. The Henry J. Kaiser Family Foundation. www.kff.org. 2002.
9. Bruen, Wiener, & Thomas, op. cit., p. 30.
10. GAO. Medicaid: Divestiture of Assets to Qualify for Long-term Care Services (GAO/HEHS-97-185R). Washington, D.C.: U.S. General Accounting Office, 1997.
11. Bruen, Wiener & Thomas, op. cit.
12. McCormack, L. A. et al. Retiree health insurance: recent trends and tomorrow's prospects. Health Care Finance Review 2002:23(3) pp. 17–34.
13. Laschober, M. A., et al. Trends in Medicare supplemental insurance and prescription drug coverage, 1996–1999. Health Affairs. 2002. Available at: http://content.healthaffairs.org/cgi/content/full/hlthaff.w2.127v1/DC1.
14. Retiree Health benefits now and in the future; Findings from the Kaiser/Hewitt 2003 Survey on Retiree Health Benefits. Available at: http://www.kff.org/medicare/6105.cfm (last accessed 10/3/08).
15. For example, *Ricks v. Budge*, 64 P.2d 208 (Sup. Ct. of Utah, 1937).
16. Emergency Medical Treatment and Active Labor Act, 42 U.S.C.A. sec. 1395dd, et seq. (1986).
17. Civil Rights Act, 42 U.S.C. sec. 2000d, et seq. (1964).
18. Americans with Disabilities Act, 42 U.S. C. sec 12101, et seq (1990).
19. *Bragdon v. Abbott*, 524 U.S. 624 (1998).
20. *Olmstead v. L.C.*, 527 U.S. 581 (1999).
21. *Scholendorff v. Society of New York Hospital*, 211 N.Y. 125 (1914).
22. Wing, K. R. The Law and the Public's Health, Chicago: Health Administration Press, 2003: p. 320.
23. Ibid.
24. 497 U.S. 261 (1990).
25. 521 U.S. 702 (1997).
26. 521 U.S. 793 (1997).
27. *Oregon Death with Dignity Act*, Or. Rev. Stat. secs. 127.800–897 (1994).
28. ODHS. Sixth Annual Report on Oregon's Death with Dignity Act, Oregon Department of Human Services. Available at: http://www.ohd.hr.state.or.us/chs/pas/ar-disc.cfm. 2004. Accessed on March 10, 2004.
29. Ibid.
30. Ibid.
31. *Health Insurance Portability and Accountability Act of 1996,* (HIPAA), Public Law 104–191 (1996).
32. U.S. Dept. of HHS. Office for Civil Rights, HIPAA Compliance Assistance, OCR Privacy Rule Summary. p. 1. Available at: http://www.hhs.gov/ocr/hipaa. May 2003.

33. For example, *Lane v. Candura*, 6 Mass. App. Ct. 377 (1978).
34. *In Re Quackenbush*, 156 N.J. Super. 282 (1978).
35. Levin, J.R., et al. Life-sustaining treatment decisions for Nursing home residents: Who discusses, who decides and what is decided? Journal of the American Geriatrics Society, 1999:47(1):82–87.
36. Victoria B.C. Medical Savings Accounts: Problems and Progress under HIPPA. Cato Policy Analysis No. 411, Cato Institute. Available at: http://www.cato.org/pubs/pas/pa-411es.html. 2001.

9

Acute Care

Access To Health Care

MARTIN P. SOLOMON
EDITOR   DAVID G. SATIN

Our health-care system for the elderly is like an old overcoat. It looked good when first purchased many years ago, trim and well-fitted to our youthful shape, with stylish features that were appealing to the eye. As our nation grew and our population aged, the increasing size and complexity of our elderly population have stretched the fabric to its limits, leading to inadequate coverage and exposing the elderly to the harsh, cold realities of illness, confusion, and shame. At the same time, the sense of responsibility to insure that our elderly are cared for appears to have lost much of the moral and political imperative that brought us as a nation to confront this issue. Any discussion of this wretched garment that constitutes health care in America, now a patchwork of different efforts to hold together some form of cover, must be retrospective. Attempting to piece together each of the threads of the system into an understandable whole can only lead to frustration and disappointment. (Chapter 4 gives more detail about the development and structure of the U.S. health-care system.)

For the elderly living in the community rather than in chronic care or organized care facilities, the critical problem areas in accessing health care can be broken down into demographic and cultural issues, financial and economic issues, and changes in the medical profession. Each of these issues weaves through the other in a continuum. In spite of this, they can be viewed separately in order to understand the dangers and to help to consider new options for styling a better system.

Demographics and Cultural Changes

In developing countries a crisis looms, with the population of those under 30 growing exponentially. In contrast, here in the United States as well as in other developed countries birth rates have slowed dramatically in the past 20 years. The elderly, those over 65 and particularly those over 85, have been growing steadily in both numbers and age (see Fig. 9.1).

To make matters worse—or better, depending on your point of view—we have succeeded in prolonging the life span of our elderly to the point where their needs have escalated and the demands on our society to support them have become a major moral, financial, and political issue.

As evidence confirming the rule that says the older you are, the older you get—or to paraphrase further, survivors survive—Figure 9.2 illustrates how those who are 65 today, an increasingly larger proportion, can expect to live to 85.

We have done such a great job of immunizing against influenza, pneumonia, tetanus, and diphtheria; maintaining a safe water supply; and, to a large though occasionally violated degree, facilitating a safe and protected food chain that people are living longer with fewer disabilities. My elderly patients are not dying of influenza, infectious hepatitis, or infectious diarrhea. They

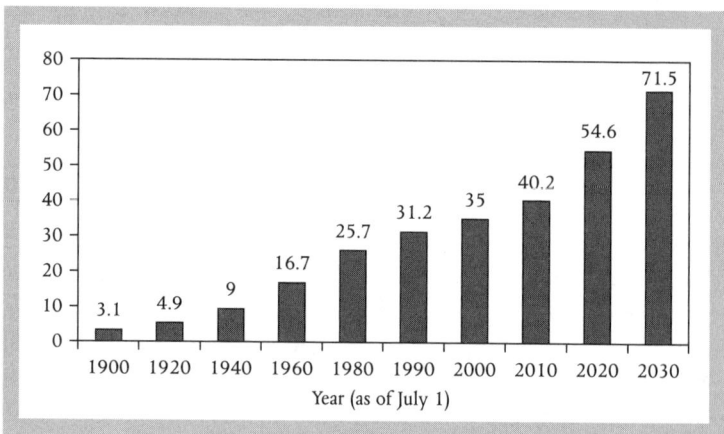

FIGURE 9.1 Number of persons 65+ (1900–2030).
SOURCE: Adapted from Current Population Reports, Special Studies. Available at: http://www.elderweb.com/home/.

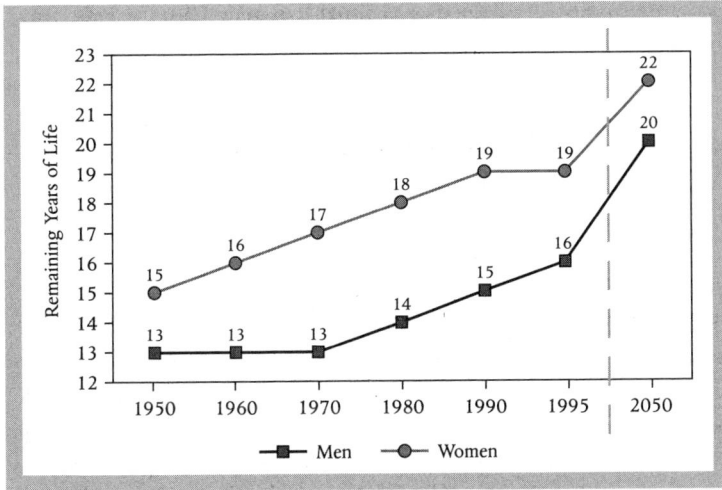

FIGURE 9.2 Remaining life expectancy at age 65.
Source: Copyright 1999, ElderWeb. Available at: http://elderweb.com.
ElderWeb, accessed 7/28/08.

are not, with a few notable exceptions, subjected to dangers of war and violence like much of the rest of the world. While we have many children who go to bed hungry, this is a rare occurrence in the elderly, who are able to avail themselves of home cooking, institution-based nutrition, or community programs such as Meals on Wheels.

What the elderly are suffering from today are the natural consequences of outliving the previously normal bounds of survival. They experience failure of the systems that are crucial to sustain a functionally viable human being. Like an aging building with a rotting foundation, corroded and clogged boilers, cracked ventilation ducts, and clouded and broken windows and doors, age has given way to a wearing out of the systems that keep us alive, such as kidney failure, heart failure, other circulatory failure such as stroke or heart attack, bone marrow failure, cancer (a failure of immune surveillance or earlier habits), degenerative disorders, and mental illnesses. While the ultimate mode of death is often infectious in the form of pneumonia or urinary tract infections, the predisposing factor is usually one of the above-mentioned. These catastrophic processes put enormous emotional and physical strain on families and caregivers, who remain the primary source of care for the elderly. Nearly two-thirds of the disabled elderly living in the community rely exclusively on family or volunteers for their care and sustenance. (Chapter 6 addresses prevention as a way of dealing with chronic and degenerative diseases.)

From my perspective as a primary-care physician, I remain impressed with the numbers of elderly patients I see who continue to live alone or with families and outside of institutions. And yet we know that ever increasing numbers of the elderly are without this support as families continue to fragment, with children moving out of town, state, or region in search of education, job opportunities, careers, or just a new life. I often receive calls from desperate children or other relatives living in distant parts of the globe wondering what can be done to help an aging parent, aunt or uncle, or friend.

In this setting, physicians in the community typically turn to the Visiting Nurse Association, hospital-based home nursing care services, as well as private organizations that will provide some form of home evaluation and management of care. These are usually financed to a limited degree by Medicare for care immediately after hospitalization, Medicaid for some community services in qualified patients, and, to a more limited extent, charitable organizations. Gone are the days when church or synagogue groups would rally around the needs of the home-based elderly, bringing meals, companionship, and home support. Our social structure has become too fragmented, and the younger generations have long ago forgotten the human service aspect of civic life. (Chapter 11 describes community care institutions and their struggle to function effectively.)

These home-care agencies are able to provide medical supervision on an intermittent basis to monitor health-care issues such as vital sign monitoring, medication oversight, or assessment for changes in clinical conditions such as diabetes, heart failure, and asthma. They can recognize when counseling or nutritional intervention is required. However, not everybody is eligible for this service, and there are limits to the duration of service that insurance will cover. Once an elderly patient becomes stable, the nursing care groups must terminate their care or be liable to punitive action from the funding government agency for billing for care deemed not covered. In essence, this means that once a patient has achieved the targeted goals for nursing intervention, care must be stopped.

Illustration

Mrs. Davis is an 89-year-old widow living alone in Brookline, Massachusetts, outside of Boston, in a small apartment since her husband died 20 years earlier. When she moved into this third-floor unit 45 years earlier, there was no elevator; but a small three-person elevator was adapted to the stairwell around the time of her husband's death. It was barely large enough for a wheelchair and not for the stretcher on which his body was removed to the funeral parlor. Now, at her advanced age, she finds it difficult arranging to get out with her walker and bags. Since her recent hospitalization for congestive heart failure, she has had to add a portable oxygen tank to the paraphernalia she needs to drag along whenever she leaves the apartment. In order to monitor her lungs, blood pressure, weight, ankle swelling, medications, and blood tests on a weekly basis to adjust her warfarin (a blood anticoagulant she needs because of the development of atrial fibrillation in the hospital), a visiting nurse comes in once a week and spends about 30 minutes with her and a homemaker is provided for her for 2 hours 3 days a week to help with cleaning and cooking.

This all worked well for a period of time, until the nurse, with the agreement of the supervising physician, found that Mrs. Davis had become stable and was no longer in need of the weekly services to recover from her illness. It may be true that without supervision she will slip back into trouble in a matter of weeks. Regardless, since that is not a certainty, she will lose her weekly nursing visits and most of her homemaker care. Given her advancing age and difficulty with mobility and egress from her apartment, she is once again isolated and likely to again develop difficulties. If she is lucky enough to have a physician who can come to her home to assess her once a month or a practice with a nurse-practitioner who can do the same, she may escape the need for medical attention in between these visits. However, the effects of age being what they are, we can anticipate some acute illness occurring in the future when there will probably be nobody to help, ultimately leading to an ambulance trip to the hospital or worse.

In the best of worlds, homebound elderly like Mrs. Davis would have family or friends checking on them regularly and somewhat trained to recognize problems when they arise, perhaps even able to check vital signs, monitor medications, and transmit this information either electronically or by phone to a receptive and waiting medical provider. In our real world, the homebound elderly are usually isolated and at risk.

In addition to the simple isolation of being old and alone in our polyglot society, many of our elderly are confronted with the more complex issues created by differences in language, beliefs, and values. Older members of minority populations in this country have a significantly higher rate of chronic illness (see Fig. 9.3).

The language barrier contributes not only to difficulty accessing good and regular medical care but also to problems with medications and treatments. In one study, Spanish-speaking Hispanic patients were significantly less likely than non-Hispanic white patients to have had a physician visit (relative risk [RR] = 0.77, 95% confidence interval [CI] 0.72–0.83), mental health visit (RR = 0.50, 95% CI 0.32–0.76), or influenza vaccination (RR = 0.30, 95% CI 0.15–0.52). After adjustment for predisposition, need, and enabling factors, Spanish-speaking Hispanic patients showed significantly lower use than non-Hispanic white patients across all four measures. Black patients had a significantly lower crude relative risk of having received an influenza vaccination (RR = 0.73, 95% CI 0.58–0.87). Adjustment for additional factors had little impact on this effect but resulted in black patients being significantly

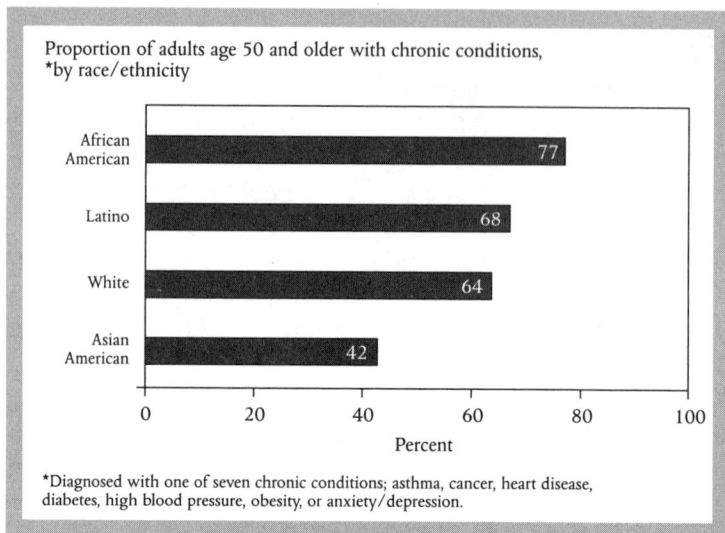

Proportion of adults age 50 and older with chronic conditions,
*by race/ethnicity

*Diagnosed with one of seven chronic conditions; asthma, cancer, heart disease,
diabetes, high blood pressure, obesity, or anxiety/depression.

FIGURE 9.3 Older African Americans and Latinos are more likely to have chronic conditions.
SOURCE: Collins, K.S., Hughes, D.L., Doty, M.M., Ives, B.L., Edwards, J.M., Tenney, K. Diverse communities, common concerns: assessing health care quality for minority Americans. New York: Commonwealth Fund, 2002.

less likely than non-Hispanic white patients to have had a visit with a mental health professional (RR = 0.46, 95% CI 0.37–0.55).[1] (Chapter 7 addresses the maldistribution of health services to subpopulations in society.)

As Figure 9.4 indicates, racial and ethnic minorities are less likely to have a regular doctor and effective health insurance, further compromising their care. This kind of data is even more serious in the isolated elderly in the community, though it is notable that recent studies suggest our minority and immigrant communities appear to do a far better job of caring for their elderly in the family unit than do traditional Caucasian families. While the addition of interpreter services helps to bridge this gap, there are real limits to the availability of professional interpretive services in the community. In my private outpatient experience, most of the interpretation occurs via friends or family. One study has pointed out that patients who have professional interpreters for their visits are far more satisfied with the care they receive than are those who have a family member or friend. Because minority elderly are often brought to clinic by children, it is rare that this issue is met satisfactorily.[2]

Given the shift in populations in our country with the increasing numbers and proportion of the elderly, the widening geographic gaps between aged family members and those who traditionally provided support in the past, the increasing ethnic and social diversity of our communities, obtaining medical

Proportion of the nonelderly population who do not have a usual source of care, by race/ethnicity

Proportion of the nonelderly population who are uninsured, by race/ethnicity

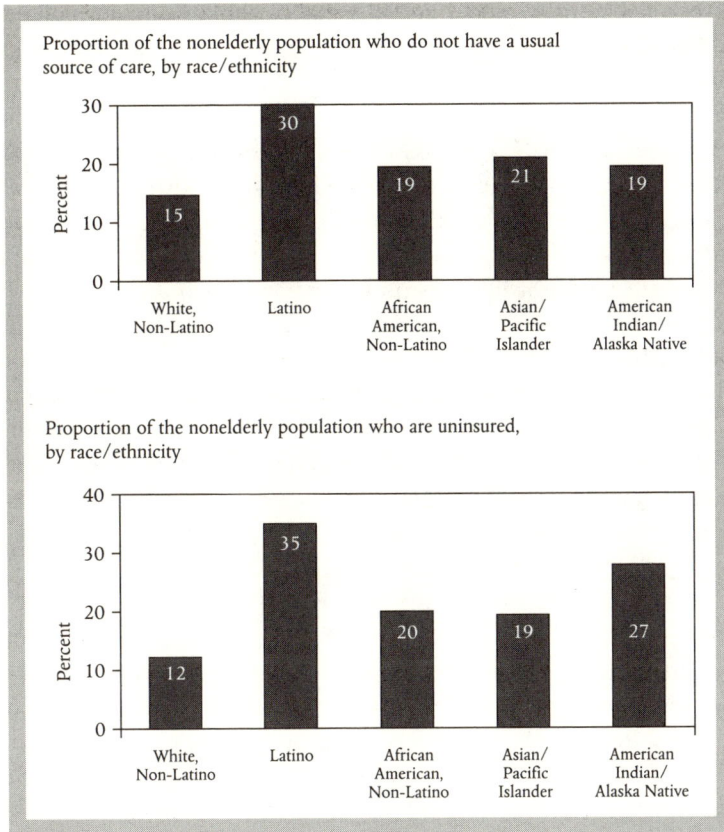

FIGURE 9.4 Racial and ethnic minorities are less likely to have a regular doctor and health insurance.
SOURCE: Lillie Barton, M., Rushing, O.E., Ruiz, S. Key Facts: Race, Ethnicity and Medical Care. Washington, DC: Kaiser Family Foundation, 2003.

care through our old-fashioned and rapidly wearing system has become an increasing challenge. And yet that would all be surmountable if it wasn't for the worsening crisis in the cost of health care for the elderly.

Financial Considerations

Even if we could solve all the cultural and social issues surrounding health-care access for the elderly, the financial and political aspects of the problem confound every effort to find solutions. As our population ages and our national mix of workers and retirees shifts, we face a diminution in the size of the taxable population available to support health care for the elderly at the same time as the numbers and needs of those who are aging are increasing rapidly. Since, as noted, we are not set up to care for large numbers of elderly in the community, we face a shift to progressively more care from institutional settings.

Not only do we have more people in the category of needy or dependent elderly but the nature of those who we describe as elderly has changed. Since much of the data previously available in this category are based on the over-65 population, we have to change our definition of the elderly. As a result of medical technology, public health measures, and advances in treatment and drug therapy, we have more functional and independent elderly but more dependent and disabled extreme elderly.

Figure 9.5 illustrates the accelerated rise in the numbers of those living longer and thus needing more health care longer.

Not only are more people remaining in the work force beyond age 65 but they remain functional and independent longer. This means, however, that, as they reach retirement or are disabled from working because of illness, our elderly are older and sicker than in the past. In fact, the sad truth is that, because they are working longer (21.6% of those over 65 are employed compared to 13% only 5 years ago) and living longer, by the time the elderly get sick they are older and sicker than we ever experienced in the past and often have less income and savings left to pay for their needs.

By the time they reach the point of needing assets to pay for their medical care, many of our elderly are now running out of money to pay. Often, their illnesses are more debilitating and they are forced to rely on others for their care.

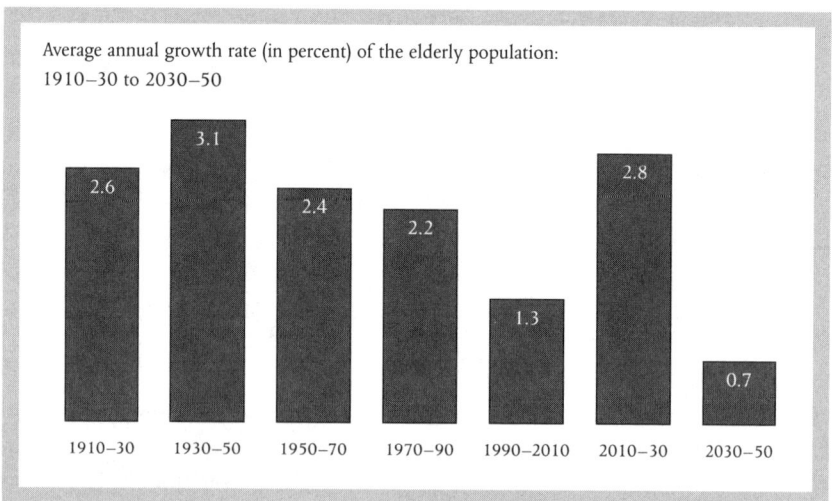

Average annual growth rate (in percent) of the elderly population:
1910–30 to 2030–50

1910–30	1930–50	1950–70	1970–90	1990–2010	2010–30	2030–50
2.6	3.1	2.4	2.2	1.3	2.8	0.7

FIGURE 9.5 Fifteen years from now, elderly population growth will explode.

If residency ratios remain unchanged, the number of persons residing in nursing homes will double or triple by 2030. The number could rise by over 300% for those aged 85 and over.[3]

From 1997 to 2030 individuals aged 85 and older, the group most likely to require long-term care, will more than double from 3.9 million to 8.5 million and by 2050 will more than double again to 18 million (to as high as 27 million).[4] (Chapter 10 reviews the range of resources for older adults needing long-term care.)

Health-care costs for the over-65 and over-85 population groups are substantially higher than those for younger people and are rising at a faster rate. For the community-based population, the average cost of health care per year is close to $15,000, more than four times that of those younger than 65.[5]

As the insurance industry and government attempt to reduce costs by limiting coverage for services, medications, nursing care, and medical treatment, the costs are transferred or, to use the more appropriate parlance, "shifted" to patients and providers of care. The elderly, living on progressively less income, find themselves paying out-of-pocket for more costly medical care, prescriptions, and treatments. We know that many are choosing to forgo needed drugs and medical visits because of issues of cost. I, like many other medical care providers, have seen elderly patients skip pills, reduce the frequency of dosing, postpone treatments, and miss visits due to the costs as well as the sometimes misplaced fear of added costs associated with each visit.

I know patients with pneumonia who delay getting their medications because they can't afford a cab to go out and buy them and are unable to find a pharmacy willing to deliver to their homes, either because of location in perceived unsafe communities or due to an inability to deliver the medication at a cost that would justify the effort. I vividly recall my elderly patient with asthma who recently spent 2 days in the hospital because she couldn't afford her asthma medication and allowed herself to get progressively more short of breath, revealing to me in a tearful state the sorry condition of her financial affairs.

Going back to our Mrs. Davis in Brookline, using her social security check of about $1000 per month along with small savings left over from her husband's life insurance and money they had put aside, she pays her rent, Medicare fees, Medicare D cost for prescription drugs, groceries, and the daily newspaper. She has a small amount left over for taxi fares for her doctors' visits and the rare trip to a friend's house. When she is fortunate, her niece, who lives in Denver, comes once every 6 weeks or so to take her shopping, on errands, and for any professional visits she is able to arrange. Nothing is left for emergencies. Unfortunately, because of the cost of her multiple medicines for heart failure, diabetes, hypertension, and thyroid problems, she has no cash left over. Then she hits the "doughnut hole" of Medicare D, when she must pay out-of-pocket for the next $2300 cost of prescription drugs. At this point, she starts asking if I can eliminate any medication but with the excuse of side effects and fear of drugs, rather than admitting to her desperate financial straits. Or she simply lies and says she is taking the medication as her blood pressure control and heart failure slowly deteriorate.

This is a real scenario that happens every day. The tragedy of it is that those who should be protecting the frail elderly and poor are busy passing legislation which protects the pharmaceutical and insurance industries at the expense of these more vulnerable people. Medicare D has benefited the companies that administer Medicare D and the pharmaceutical manufacturers that make the drugs preferred by these plans. The problem was painfully easy to push past Congress and should be even easier to fix: Simply eliminate the lapse in coverage, insist that the insurers negotiate the lowest price possible with the pharmaceutical companies, and push the Food and Drug Administration to process the currently delayed backlog of generic drug applications that are sitting on hold as the expensive brand-name drugs are pushed through. (See Chapter 8 on the legal and governmental process for developing the health care system and policies, and Chapter 15 for policy making and changing.)

Lurking in the background is the potential fear of the failure of Social Security, with catastrophic consequences for the elderly of the next generation. At that point, the key issues for maintaining the health of our elderly will shift from medication and technology to housing and food. Clearly, financially the elderly are in an increasingly painful bind.

Figures for 2003 show that overall the elderly spent an average of $537 a person on prescription drugs compared to $192 by those under 65, a difference of $345. About 63% of the elderly's drug spending came out of pocket compared to 56% for younger adults. The sums represented 3.55% of family income for the elderly but only 1.25% for the under-65 group.[6]

Now add the increasing costs of health care for the elderly to the burden of finding somebody to reliably provide the health care they so desperately need. I mean, of course, the primary-care doctors and nurses who have been the traditional first-line source of medical care and the people responsible in the past for managing and directing this care. We are in the downward spiral of a crisis in primary care that will threaten the very roots of health care in the United States, endangering, first and foremost, the elderly, poor, and poor elderly.

There are good data supporting the contention that primary-care physicians (general internists and family physicians) provide more cost-effective, high-quality care than general practitioners and non-primary-care internists. And yet the number of new doctors entering primary care is dropping at an accelerating rate.[7]

As this trend continues, more and more of the physicians who flocked to primary care a generation ago are reaching retirement age, switching to other

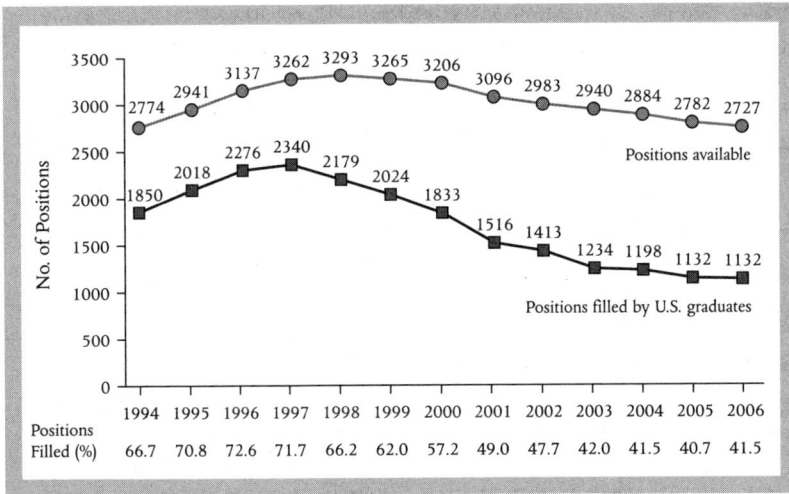

FIGURE 9.6 Filling primary-care physician positions.

specialties, going into concierge-type practices for the wealthy, or just calling it quits. Of those who remain in practice, increasing numbers are refusing to accept Medicare patients. Even if the elderly could overcome the steep and rising costs of health care, they will be in desperate straits to find physicians or nurses interested in and available to care for them.

These considerations apply to the interdisciplinary health-care team that is needed by older adults with complex health-management problems. Medicare, Medicaid, and other health insurance funding for rehabilitation therapies, social work, and other disciplines are grossly inadequate for effective care and maintenance of function. There is no funding for the hallmarks of interdisciplinary care: meetings, travel, communication, team treatment sessions, etc. Government funding for professional training in all areas has been slashed to an inadequate level. Health-care professionals' reimbursement for the care of older adults, with their complex, chronic, and bio-psycho-socio-spiritual needs, has been substandard enough to discourage professionals from caring for older adults and certainly from specializing in this population. Thus, while the interdisciplinary approach is needed, policy and economic forces discourage it.

Summary

The crisis in health care for the elderly in our country is no longer a semantic tool used by health-care academics to bludgeon each other in intellectual arguments. For our increasing numbers of elderly, it is a painful reality today. We neglect addressing the issues outlined in this chapter at the risk of putting the lives and security of our elders and ourselves in peril. (Chapter 2 gives a vivid example of the needs and suggestions of older adults in this health-care system.)

Application to the Case Study: The Older Adult Care, Training, Research, and Planning Program

DAVID G. SATIN, BASED ON CONCEPTS BY MARTIN P. SOLOMON

Two of the Older Adult Care, Training, Research, and Planning Program's (OACTRPP's) missions are to study factors affecting health and functional status and to develop and test theories about the development of heath care in a community setting. The target community is ideal for this purpose, being mixed in class, ethnicity, and culture. The project can test our observations of inadequate funding and resources for health care for the old, poor, and ethnic minorities and their effect on health status. It can then develop pilot programs for funding and staffing adequate and equitable health care for these subpopulations in the experimental catchment area. The fact that funding is fragmented and limited and that politicoeconomic factors block support from Medicaid, for instance, does not make this research and experimentation unfeasible but only more realistic. If it can be done by the OACTRPP, then there is a good chance that it can be exported to the real world.

Training for students in the various health professions must include learning to appreciate and deal with the delivery of health care and the programmatic and financial factors that affect it. This is an opportunity to prepare a cadre of health professionals who will not be ignorant of or callous to the health-care system that is such a powerful influence on their patients' health and their own professional practices. Part of this education should be not only to know but to influence these forces in their own practices, in their professions, and in the political arena. This is an opportunity to learn that "no man is an island." When such an educational program is developed, it can be implemented in other settings.

Another part of the professional education process should be to consider the disciplines and specialties that are needed for the health of the community and to work toward making them available. We have written about the lack of primary-care health professionals in medicine and in other disciplines. The OACTRPP should select students for training in its program who are committed to primary care and specialty care in the proportions needed by the community. Beyond this, it should advocate with the professional education programs in the parent medical center and beyond to prepare professionals in specialty proportions that are responsive to community health needs.

Finally, the clinical care programs for the study community should be informed by the community's health, economic, and cultural needs. The planners, administrators, and caregivers should plan, administer, and care according to these needs. This will probably be a wrenching endeavor because it diverges from usual patterns in several ways: It differs from traditional professional education and practice and will discomfort those committed to traditions. It may also strain the university medical center's self-interest in terms of patient referrals, income, professional advancement of influential staff members, and the reaction of staff to unfamiliar and uncomfortable new values and practices. Finally, it must be remembered that funding sources have their conscious or unconscious agendas. HealthCo, Inc., may not see the expected profit from the values and practices developed by the OACTRPP. City, state, and federal agencies which fund and oversee the project have to deal with the ideas and self-interest of their constituencies. Thus, one of the major tasks and achievements of the OACTRPP may be negotiating social change with social forces invested in other outcomes. If this is not recognized, addressed, and resolved, the whole experiment may be, to use an appropriate term, academic—a self-serving job for those who are employed by it. This, too, would be a significant research finding.

Bibliography

Center for American Progress. Better benefits, lower costs: three steps to improving Medicare. Available at: http://www.americanprogress.org/site/pp.asp?c=biJRJ80VF&b=368873.

Center for American Progress. Privatization threatens Medicare and Social Security. Available at: http://www.americanprogress.org/site/pp.asp?c=biJRJ80VF&b=40071.

Collins, K.S., Hughes, D.L., Doty, M.M., Ives, B.L., Edwards, J.M., Tenney, K. Diverse Communities, Common Concerns: Assessing Health Care Quality for Minority Americans. New York: Commonwealth Fund, 2002.

Current Population Reports. Special studies. Available at: http://www.elderweb.com/home/.

DeLew, N., Weinick, R. An overview: eliminating racial, ethnic, and SES disparities in health care. Health Care Financing Review 2000;21(4):1–7.

Federal Interagency Forum on Aging-Related Statistics. Older Americans 2000: Key Indicators of Well-Being. Washington, DC: U.S. Government Printing Office, 2000.

Federal Interagency Forum on Aging-Related Statistics. Older Americans 2008: Key Indicators of Well-Being. Available at: www.agingstats.gov.

Henry J. Kaiser Family Foundation. The Faces of Medicare and Minority Americans. Menlo Park, CA: Henry J. Kaiser Family Foundation, 1999.

Intercultural Cancer Council. Elderly & cancer. Available at: iccnetwork.org/cancerfacts.

Koh, L.T., Corrigan, J.M., Donaldson, M., et al. To Err is Human: Building A Safer Health System. Washington, DC: Institute of Medicine, 1999.

Ku, L. Shift in costs from Medicare to Medicaid is a principal reason for rising state Medicaid expenditures. Center on Budget and Policy Priorities. Available at: http://www.cbpp.org/3-3-03health.htm.

Lillie Barton, M., Rushing, O.E., Ruiz, S. Key Facts: Race, Ethnicity and Medical Care. Washington, DC: Kaiser Family Foundation, 2003.

Liu, H., Sharma, R. National Healthcare Disparities Report. Health and Health Care of the Medicare Population: Data from the 1998 Medicare Current Beneficiary Survey. Rockville, MD: Westat, 2002.

McWilliams, J.M., Zaslavsky, A.M., Meara, E., Ayanian, J.Z. Health insurance coverage and mortality among the near-elderly. Health Affairs 2004;23(4):223.

Wray, L. Health policy and ethnic diversity in older Americans: dissonance or harmony? Western Journal of Medicine 1992;157(3):357–361.

References

1. Fiscella, K., Franks, P., Doescher, M.P., Saver, B.G. Disparities in health care by race, ethnicity, and language among the insured: findings from a national sample. Medical Care 2002;40(1):52–59.

2. Carrasquillo, O., et al. Impact of language barriers on patient satisfaction in an emergency room department. Journal of General Internal Medicine 1999;17:641–646.

3. U.S. Bureau of the Census, 1996. United States Bureau of the Census, found at http://www.census.gov/main/www/cen1996.html

4. U.S. Bureau of the Census, 1996. United States Bureaur of the Census, found at http://www.census.gov/main/www/cen1996.html

5. Administration on Aging, U.S. Department of Health and Human Services, to be found at http://www.aoa.gov/prof/Statistics/statistics.aspx (July 2008).

6. Levin, A. Low-income elderly hardest hit by prescription costs. Health Behavior News Service, September 9, 2003.

7. Bodenheimer, T., Grumbach, K. Understanding health policy: a clinical approach. New York: Lange Medical Books/McGraw-Hill, 2002.

10

Long-Term Care

LEN FISHMAN with DAVID G. SATIN

Immediately before coming to Boston I was president of the American Association of Homes and Services for the Aging, which is the national organization that represents about 6000 nonprofit senior counseling and health-care organizations around the country. Its headquarters are in Washington, D.C. And that's where I first got to know the Hebrew Rehabilitation Center of Boston.

I'm going to give you a bit of an introduction. I'll talk about our situation in the year 2000. I'm going to give you a kind of environmental scan of the demographics and trends as they looked to us around the year 2000. (Chapter 4 goes into the history and broad organization of health care for older adults.) And then I'm going to talk about what we did to accommodate to these conditions and what happened during the intervening period.

Figure 10.1 is one way of conceptualizing some of the different options along the continuum of care for seniors in terms of different kinds of facilities. Starting on the left side are people who are fully independent and progressing toward the right side are people who are increasingly dependent. Lasell Village in Newton and Orchard Cove in Canton, Massachusetts, is an example of a continuing care retirement community (CCRC). You pay refundable entrance fee on going in. Initially you are independent, and generally on that campus there are assisted living and long-term care facilities for people who

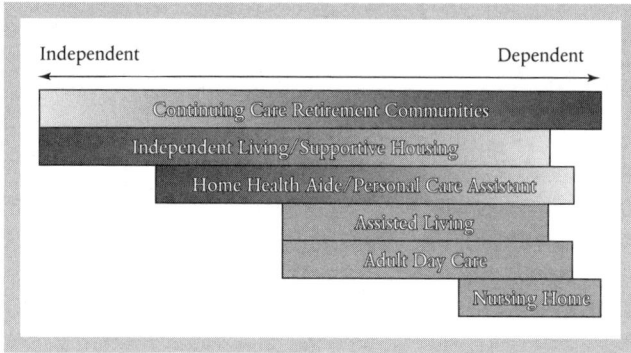

FIGURE 10.1 The continuum of care and services for seniors.

come to need them. The idea is to provide the complete continuum of care right on one site. Independent living or supportive housing is obviously for people who are independent. But nowadays people who are quite frail can be maintained in independent living environments.

Home health services are generally for people who need some assistance—personal care, for example assisted living is for people who are in need of more help. Adult day care is similar. And then the most intensive care is delivered in a nursing home. The most important thing to note about this continuum is that there are not highly specific positions on the continuum—there's a lot of overlap. And that overlapping is, if anything, occurring more and more. Another way to think about this is to consider the elements that go into different settings. There's the housing resource. There's what I call convenience services—meals, activities programming. There's assisted living or personal care. And then there is the health-care component. And these building blocks can be put together in an almost infinite number of ways.

In the old days the package was very rigid. If you think about a nursing home, it is comprised of housing; it's obviously a place where people live. It has meals and programs. It's got personal care—getting people up in the morning, helping to bathe them and get them to meals. And then it has health care—the nursing component and the medical component. But if you think about a nursing home, which one of these building blocks really stands out in your mind? What's driving the whole engine there? It's health care. We don't really think about meals in nursing homes as being a primary activity in the same way we do in independent living. We don't think about the programming that's driving the day. It's really built around the delivery of health care and, generally, in a way that's most convenient for the institution. The reason I dwell on that is that it's very easy for people to fall into a particular frame of mind, myself included when I started in this field some 25 years ago. The nursing home package appeared to make sense; I figured people must have put the thing together in that way because it was a logical way to do it. It's a minihospital, much different in physical appearance from assisted living facilities. But then you step back and ask yourself, "Why would you design an environment for frail elders, who may be living there for 2 or 3 years, that resembles a hospital?" This frankly isn't a great place to stay for 5 or 6 days. A lightbulb goes off, and you realize those who put that package together made a mistake. Unfortunately, there are 17,000 of them around the country now, and it's not going to be that easy to change. But it's a lesson. The people who did it weren't dumb. They just had a particular worldview. And they elevated this component above all the others. But that's not really the way people want to live their lives. And that's one of the reasons that there has been quite a lot of ferment in this field in recent years.

When I started in this field in the early 1980s, if you were old and frail and you weren't capable of living alone anymore, the chances were that you would end up in a nursing home, whether you really needed that level of care or not. It was basically a "one-size-fits-all" system. And there were a lot of people living in nursing homes who did not really require that level of care. But there just weren't alternatives. There was no such thing as assisted living in this country. There was in Sweden and in other countries in northern Europe but not in the United States. Independent housing—the kind subsidized by the Department of Housing and Urban Development housing, for example—was basically for independent seniors. And aging in place back then was considered one of the features of senior housing that was a problem. It wasn't a goal to be aspired to. People who ran senior housing facilities used to sit around and talk about strategies for getting people out if they weren't fully independent anymore. The idea of bringing services into that setting so they could age in place was really pretty radical.

So if I step back and ask myself what are the really big things in the field that have happened over the last 20 years, I would distill them into these three bullets.

- The first is the blurring of the line between housing and personal health care. As I was suggesting earlier, it used to be that housing was over here and health care was over there, and they weren't supposed to mix. That's really changed, and a good example of that is assisted living or some of the facilities that we and Jewish Community Housing for the Elderly in Boston and other good providers in the city have developed: housing where a lot of personal care and health care is being delivered. This is really a radical change from what was going on a couple of decades ago.
- A second is that consumers are basically saying, "We insist upon having choices. One size fits all is unacceptable." And the single greatest example of that is assisted living. That's gone from zero to practically a million residents over the last 10 years. Consumers are saying they want a different

environment, and they've really been insisting on it. (Chapter 5 discusses freedom of choice and influence on care by older adults.)

- The third big difference is that this field historically has been a backwater. It has not attracted the best talent or the most creative thinkers, and at a cocktail party somebody in acute care was probably going to have an easier time opening a conversation than somebody in long-term care. I don't think that's true anymore. There have really been big changes. You can't go anywhere without somebody talking about what's going on with their mom (or with a sister, depending on the age), and very often it involves some element of long-term care.

So I think that our field is coming front and center, and this is the most exciting time by far to be in this field. There are a lot of problems with regulations, with reimbursement—all the stuff that I'm going to talk about that characterizes our difficult state currently. But notwithstanding that, I think that we are on the threshold of the most transformative years in the history of our field. And that's really something to be excited about.

I remember when an issue of *Time* magazine came out about 6 or 7 years ago. It was the first time that *Time* or any national publication had a cover story on our field. It was really interesting. It had a guy who was supposed to be frail—he looked pretty good to me—with a cane in his hand. But it was not directed at seniors; it addressed taking care of our parents. So they're talking to the boomer generation. And the subtitle is "The New Alternatives to Nursing Homes" because assisted living and other alternatives were really heating up. So this is a wonderful little snapshot of where the country was 6 or 7 years ago. It really distilled a lot in very few words. And then you have *Modern Maturity* deciding that they ought to have great-looking women on the cover. Look how sexy they are: Susan Sarandon was, I think, 55 years old when they put her on the cover. I can't believe she ever looked better than that when she was younger. Most recently, two issues ago, they moved up to age 60: Goldie Hawn is sexy. And you can predict in 5 years there'll be a 65-year-old on the cover who will be sexy and sultry.

Another thing that's worth noting is a public television documentary that aired in Boston on station WGBH, the first time there's been a nationally telecast documentary on this field. And it was nuanced and sympathetic and serious. It was not an exposé on nursing homes, which is what has appeared in the national press or on TV in the past. It was a wonderful piece about couples aging unevenly in a continuing care retirement community and what it means when one of the spouses has to go into the long-term care facility. The other plot is that this nursing facility is trying to implement really radical culture change, which is something that we are also in the process of doing. So it tells two stories. Again, I think this is an example of how this field is gaining greater prominence.

Now, I'm going to describe the situation of my organization, which used to be called Hebrew Rehabilitation Center for Aged. You can probably figure out already why we changed our name. We were preparing to celebrate our centennial year. We were founded in the year 1903 as the Moshav Zekeinem, which is Hebrew for "old age home." It opened, caring for 15 elderly men and women. It was located on Queen Street in Dorchester, part of Boston. In the last 100 years we've become a seven-site system of senior housing and health care serving 5000 seniors in the greater Boston area. We're the largest non-profit senior housing and health-care provider in the state. We have a terrific staff of geriatricians, 16 of them in fact, which is more than 12 states have. It may be the largest concentration of geriatricians in the country. Those of you who know something about long-term care know that it's hard to find a doctor in a nursing home and if you find one, he or she is probably not a terrific doctor. All but two of our physicians are faculty members of the Harvard Medical School. We're also, by far, the largest geriatric teaching site in the state. Every year we train over 500 medical students, nursing students, and other students in the health-care professions; and we're headquarters for Harvard Medical School's Geriatric Fellowship program.

We also are home to the largest provider-based geriatric research facility in the country. The Institute for Aging Research is divided into two parts: what we call the social gerontological part does research on issues like designing the assessment tool the Minimum Data Set, which assesses functional status of frail elders—quality indicators, work we do for the federal government—and then the clinical component, which looks at things like exercise, hip fractures, falls, osteoporosis, and dementia. And these folks talk to each other. Most of our research is interdisciplinary, which is a very exciting aspect of the institute. So you've got social researchers and clinical researchers existing within an environment where caregivers are delivering care and seniors are actually living. All of this calls upon us to take an interdisciplinary approach to all aspects of our work.

We also take seriously our role as a citizen of the Commonwealth of Massachusetts. We are home to the Harvard Cooperative Program on Aging, which serves the greater research community in the Boston area. Basically, what the program does is to recruit subjects of color to make sure that when research is done panels are not just comprised of white males or even white males and females but also have a racial and ethnic mix. We sponsor the Multicultural Coalition on Aging, which is comprised of 80 different governmental and nongovernmental organizations representing every racial and ethnic group in the state. And we're also active in the Boston Partnership for

Older Adults, which is trying to figure out ways to make Boston neighborhoods more senior-friendly. (Chapter 7 addresses the degree to which the needs of these various populations are met by our health-care system.)

A review of the Hebrew SeniorLife facilities starts with the Roslindale campus. This campus opened in 1963 and was the successor to the original Jewish Home for the Aged. The first building that opened, the Berenson Building, houses 475 residents. It is 400 feet long and 60 feet wide. It's like a cigar box standing on its side. It was designed in the late 1950s, and it was really conceived of as a dormitory because in the late 1950s some of the people who were living on this campus were actually still driving cars and many of them spent their winters in Florida. Since then, the population has aged very considerably.

Ten years later we built the Burger Building. This building houses 250 residents. Rooms were a little bit larger because by then the architects were realizing that, because of increasing frailty, more people were staying in their rooms and on their floors. In this building the expectation was that people would get up in the morning, go down to the main dining room, take their meals, and spend the rest of the day roaming around the campus. Well, today that's much less true because the population in 2004 was much older. How much older? Well when the Red Sox won the World Series and we brought the World Series trophy to our campus, we discovered that 388 of our residents were alive the last time the Red Sox won the World Series (in 1918).

The average age on this campus in Roslindale is a few months shy of 90, which is almost 3 years older than that in the average long-term care facility in Massachusetts. We offer long-term care there in 640 of our beds. We have an adult day health program, both here and on the premises of Jewish Community Housing for the Elderly, which is an all-Russian adult day health program. And this slide shows you some of the problems that we are dealing with in Roslindale. I mentioned that it was conceived of as a dormitory, where people would get up in the morning, leave their rooms, and go downstairs. The dining areas were very small on the floors because the expectation was that people would go to the main dining room. But today, with people so frail, we're running out of space in our small dining rooms. Back then the double-bed room in Berenson measured 182 square feet; that's smaller than the single-bed rooms that we're designing now. And you see the bane of all long-term care administrators, which is the lineup of wheelchairs in the hallway because there's not enough activity space on the floors. We offer great quality of care, fabulous staff, but a very obsolete building.

Figure 10.2 shows the problem of a growing gap between what our costs were per day and what Medicaid was paying us per day. So by the year 2000 we were losing about $25 a day on each of our Medicaid residents. And with 200,000 plus Medicaid days, that means that every budget year started with a

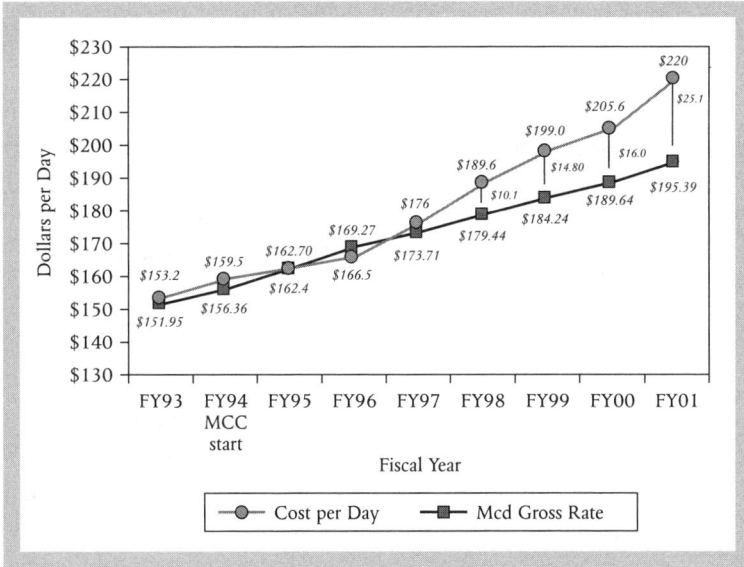

FIGURE 10.2 Cost-per-day vs. Medicaid gross daily rate.

structural deficit of over $4 million. Within a year of building the Roslindale campus in 1963, we had a waiting list of 500 and a building that housed 475. It was clear that we were not going to get around to caring for most of the people on that waiting list because they wouldn't be living by the time we had a bed for them.

Our first researcher, Dr. Silvia Sherwood, had this idea that maybe some of the people on our waiting list didn't need to be in an institutional setting. She applied for a grant from the federal Department of Health, Education, and Welfare, the predecessor of the Department of Health and Human Services. With that grant she did research on people on our waiting list and other long-term care facilities' waiting lists and discovered that 50% of them could be sustained in the community in a housing setting if they had the right supportive services. (Chapter 6 addresses the preventive approaches that can maintain older adults in independent living.) The result of that was Jack Satter House in Revere, which is a low- and moderate-income facility. It is home to 300 seniors. This, in its time, was really radical. It was a congregate housing facility, one of the first in the country. People here get meals, transportation, social services, and personal care. The average age in this building is 85. People here are quite frail, but we're able to sustain them because of all the supportive services they have. This is an amazing building because of the age group: Franklin Roosevelt is still president; these are basically New Deal Democrats who are living in this building. And they're very grateful for the support they get from the federal government because they know that without it they would never be able to live in accommodations like these. We think it's the only affordable housing site in the country where every apartment has a view of the ocean—it faces Revere Beach. The residents refer to it as "A cruise ship that hasn't left the docks." It was so successful that we then built a facility for about 200 low- and moderate-income seniors in Randolph, a more suburban environment but basically the same idea.

And then, 12 years ago, we built Orchard Cove, which is a continuing care retirement community. A total of 375 seniors live there, all at market rate. They are independent living seniors when they move in, with assisted living and long-term care for the very small portion of people who come to need it.

So this is a summary of our situation in the year 2000. The Roslindale physical plant, especially the Berenson Building, is terribly obsolete. We had no post-acute-care unit; we only offered long-term care on the campus. Our census was down; we actually had empty beds, probably for the first time in our history. The acuity level of our residents was up, which is one of the reasons that we had this big gap between our costs and what we were being paid because we were being paid as if our residents were still lighter care, when in fact we needed more staff to care for them. Our Medicaid census was 90%; when 90% of your residents are Medicaid and you're losing $25 a day, it's kind of difficult to cost-shift to your remaining payers because they make up only 10% of your census. Reimbursement was relatively flat. As you remember from that graph, deficits were up. Liquidity was good: We had very little debt, so we had a lot of cash on hand. Our fund-raising was a plus: We were doing a pretty good job of raising money. Orchard Cove, our market-rate facility, was a plus. It was contributing over $1 million a year to the corporation as a whole, and it had raised our image. It was the first time the organization said, "You know what? If we can do a great job of providing care to low- and moderate-income seniors, how about doing it for people who can afford to pay their own way?" In addition, it was making a contribution to the organization. Jack Satter House and Simon C. Fireman Community were marginally profitable; I mean, they would basically break even, which back then was a plus. Research was both a plus and a minus: It was certainly something that added to our image and distinction but also cost us money because we had dedicated funds to support our research mission. Likewise, our academic teaching program made us different from our competitors, but it was also something that was costly to us because we weren't reimbursed our additional costs.

So now that I've told you about us in the year 2000, let me give you a quick run-through of the environment in which we were operating and that hasn't changed all that much. I start with the obligatory chart that shows the growth in the number of people 65 and older, an elevenfold increase in the last century.

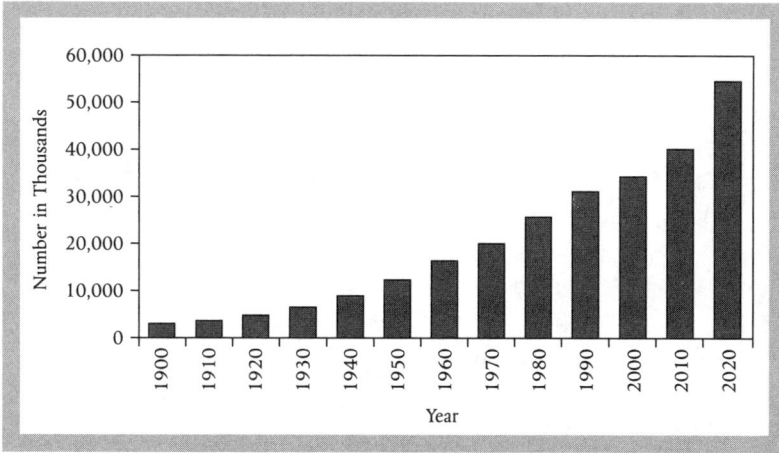

FIGURE 10.3 Growth in the number of adults 65+.

But what I think is really more important is that we added more years to the human life span in the last century than in all of recorded history until the year 1900. And most importantly, the country has really begun to age in the last 40 years. So we are really pioneers in an experience no other generation in humanity has ever had. It's not just that people are living longer; it's that for the first time people are expecting to live longer and are beginning to plan for it. My parents retired in their late 70s, and they figured they'd live another 5 or 10 years. In fact, 20 years later they were still going strong. They had outspent their assets because they didn't think they'd be alive that long. But that's not true now. People retiring in their late 60s are expecting to live to their 80s or maybe even longer. So the expectations have changed dramatically. And, of course, the demographics are going to become even more dramatic in the next 20 years because between now and the year 2020 the 85 and over population is going to increase by 128%. And by the year 2030, the 65 and over population will have doubled. That means that in the year 2020 Massachusetts will look demographically exactly the way Florida does today, and we will be one of the younger states in the country.

So we are on the cusp of what will be the most dramatic change, demographically, in all of human history. And I sometimes feel like Noah building an ark, trying to get ready for that reality, because God knows there aren't a lot of other people, especially the federal government, who are really preparing for that reality. (Chapter 15 discusses the making and changing of health-care policy.) If you realize that one out of four people aged 65 and over today is going to live to 90 or more and that in a few years it'll be two out of four people 65 and over who will live to age 90, how do you justify Social Security beginning at age 65 or even age 62? It shouldn't; it's crazy! I mean, that's a system that was designed for people who would be dead within 5–10 years, but it's now serving a population that will be alive for 15 or 25 years after payments kick in. That's one small example of how radically our reality has changed and how impoverished the conversation is on the federal level among policy makers for this new reality that we're about to enter. And right now we're in a trough that's going to last another 8 or 9 years, and then there's really going to be a rapid uptake because the boomers are going to start to age into that population.

It's also important to note that successive generations are going to be better-educated (see Fig. 10.4). Most of the people we're caring for are high school graduates. In the future, a much higher proportion will be college graduates. The elder poverty rate is at its lowest since we began measuring it after the Second World War; it's actually at its lowest in U.S. history (see Fig. 10.5). One out of 10 elders is impoverished. I should note that a large proportion, 40%, have incomes under 200% of the federal poverty level. The fact is there's a lot of disposable income among elders, more than has ever been true before.

The elder population is becoming more diverse (see Fig. 10.6). It lags behind the rest of the country because when you're looking at people who live in senior communities, it's sort of like a little archeological dig. You're looking at what the country looked like 60 years ago. So the diversity of the elder population lags behind the diversity of the younger population for obvious reasons.

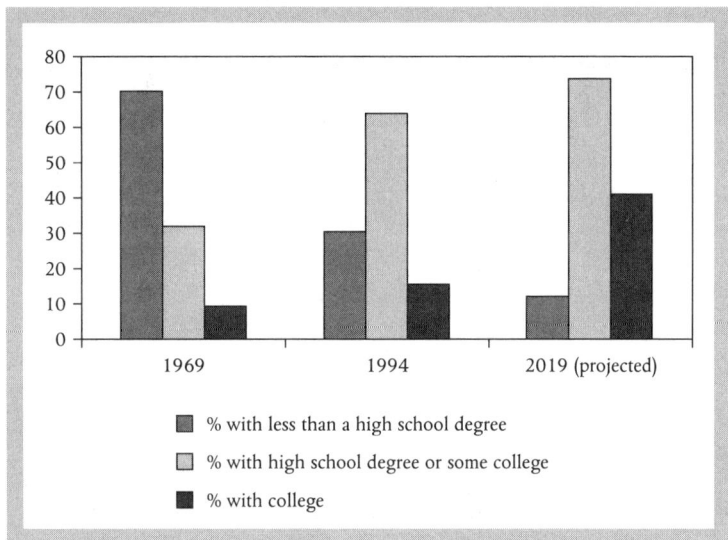

FIGURE 10.4 Successive generations of elders in the United States better educated than the last.
SOURCE: Hadley, J. Analysis of Data from the 1969 and 1994 Health Interview Surveys. Washington, DC: Institute for Health Care Research and Policy, Georgetown University, 1998.

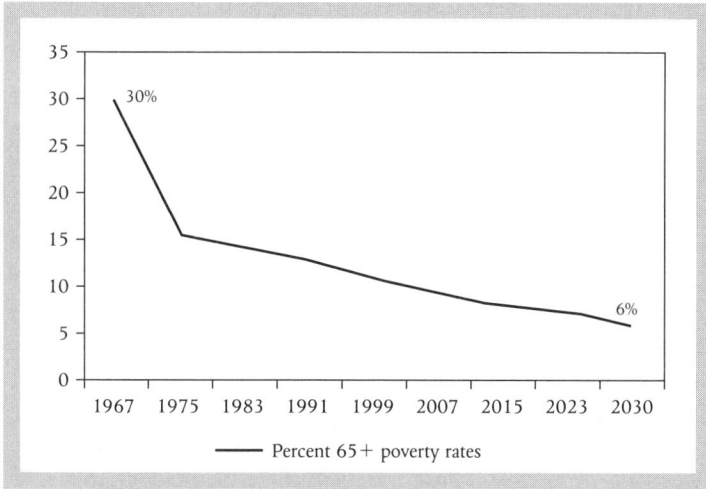

FIGURE 10.5 Decline in elder poverty in the United States, 1967–2030.
SOURCE: Current Population Survey, March 1998 data file and U.S. Census Bureau poverty tables. Access via http://www.census.gov/hhes/www/poverty/poverty.html, accessed 7/28/08

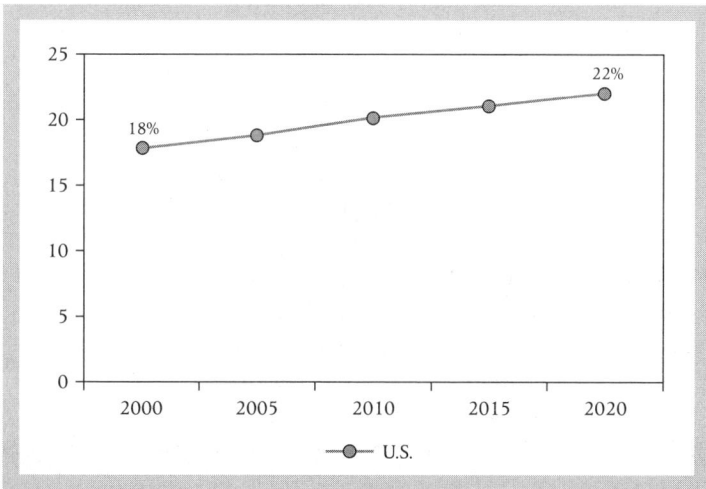

FIGURE 10.6 Growth in diversity of elders in the United States, 2000–2020.
SOURCE: U.S. Census Bureau, 65+ in the United States. P23–190, Table 2-1, 1996. Access via http://search.census.gov/search, accessed 7/28/08

There's also been a big decline in elder disability rates (see Fig. 10.7). Every year since 1985 there has been a decline in the disability of elders. It's not clear that that's going to continue because the middle-aged population is not as healthy in some respects as the population it's replacing. And those of you who are in public health know you can go back to the 1964 Surgeon General's

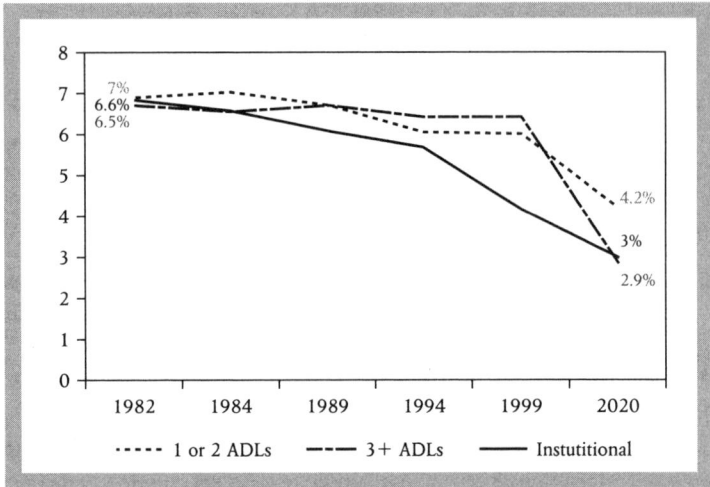

FIGURE 10.7 Decline in elder disability rates in the United States, 1982–2020. ADLs, activities of daily living.

report on smoking and see the results of that campaign really playing out here in the declining disability rates and the decline in mortality. These public health campaigns really make a difference: stop smoking, exercise, better diet. But it's also important to remember that most frail elders are not living in places like the Roslindale facility that I showed you; they're living in their own homes, being provided care informally by family and friends.

Long-term care is 35% of Medicaid spending, even though it's only about 10% of Medicaid beneficiaries (see Fig. 10.8). And Figure 10.9 shows the projection for institutional long-term care spending, according to the Congressional Budget Office. That's just not a sustainable rate of increase. (Chapter 6 discusses some of the changing characteristics of the older adult population.)

A quick reminder—not all seniors are alike. We tend to think that there's one big homogeneous group that we call "seniors." In fact, there are three pretty distinct groups: the New Dealers; people we sometimes call the "GI Generation," or the "Greatest Generation," born between 1901 and 1924; and then there's the "Silent Generation." New Dealers are those whose political icon is Franklin Delano Roosevelt. The big events in their lives are the Depression and World War II. This generation is politically very Democratic. They're dying out at a rate of about 4000 a day. The Silent Generation's icon is Dwight D. Eisenhower. This generation is a lot more Republican, and it's one of the reasons that Congress is Republican. Boomers (1946–1964) are going to be better-educated, they're going to be wealthier, they're going to be more demanding, they're accustomed to having things their own way. This is the most narcissistic, self-centered generation in human history. And just like us.

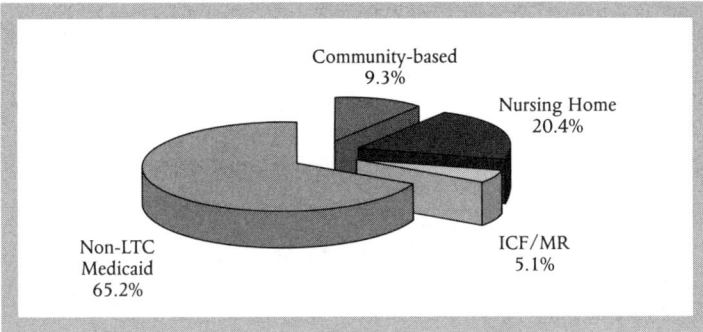

FIGURE 10.8 Long-term care is 35% of Medicaid spending. LTC, long-term care; ICF/MR, intermediate care facility for the mentally retarded.
SOURCE: Medstat HSBC. Available via http://www.hcbs.org/browse.php/sby/ Date/source/150/Thomson%20Reuters%20(formerly%20Medstat); accessed 7/28/08.

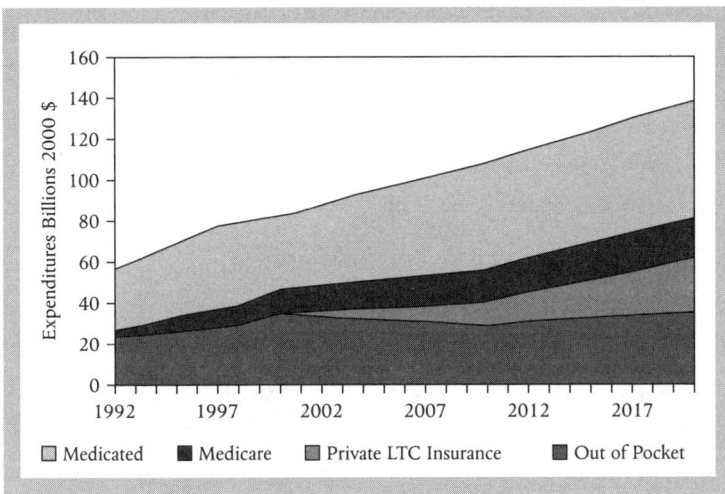

FIGURE 10.9 Institutional long-term care (LTC) spending—Congressional Budget Office projections. Accessable via http://www.cbo.gov/; accessed 7/28/08.

We (the Boomers) are going to be the generation from hell when you're trying to provide services.

Finally, I want to talk a little bit about cultural change and the fact that, at least in the progressive organizations, we are in the midst of figuring out how to change the way we provide long-term care and senior care. An editorial appeared in the *New York Times* in 1999 citing a number of nonprofit organizations that were leading the way. One of them is called the Wellspring Model. What links all of these cultural change models together is rethinking the physical environment to make housing and meals and programming more prominent and thinking about how to empower frontline caregivers and change what has been a very hierarchical organization into one with a little more parity among the nurses, the nurses' aides, the doctor, the social worker, the dietitian, etc.

Putting all of this together, we're really at a moment of very radical transformation in this organization and in our field. The social safety net is fraying and is demographically flawed. One example is that the age of retirement is very out of sync with what we know is the actual health and capacity of people who are attaining the age of 65. This seismic shift of longevity is reverberating throughout society. Seniors are demanding autonomy and choice. And providers like us, I think, had better throw their old models out the window or they're going to become obsolete. (See Chapter 5.)

So now we come to the part where we have to decide how to tackle these problems.

It's amazing how resistant organizations are to the obvious things that are going on outside. If you've done things in a particular way, and particularly if you've been successful at it for decades, and things suddenly aren't going right, the natural human reaction is to assume that everybody else is crazy and eventually they're going to figure out that what you're doing makes perfect sense. And that's why sometimes you just have to look out the window and see what's happening and try to suspend denial. This is what I'm trying to do with my organization.

Around the year 2000, the Board of the Hebrew Rehabilitation Center for Aged decided to bring in Abt Associates, a consulting firm, to ask them to help take a look at where the future was going. The question was, How can we come up with a strategic vision for moving the organization in a direction that would allow it to thrive for the next 100 years? That requires two things, both taking a broad view: First, what are the big things that the organization needs to do differently, and what's the thread that runs through the changes that need to be made? Second, what are some of the more specific things that you would do to implement that plan?

When I was commissioner of Health and Senior Services in New Jersey, we used to go through the appropriations process every year, which is kind of a hazing process for public officials because you're going up there to defend your budget. But the legislators, when they're questioning you, aren't really interested in your budget. They're interested in the issues that they care about, the controversial issues: whether you're giving out condoms at parties of transsexuals, let's say. And that may be a very tiny line item in the budget as compared to something else they ignore entirely. And it's always a process you've spent weeks preparing for; I would have mock appropriations hearings where my own staff would drag me over the coals. But the good thing is that at the end of the day you were handed a bag of money by the legislature and you didn't have to raise it. All you had to worry about was how you were going to spend it. It's a little different when you're out in the private sector because you have to worry not only about expenses but also how to raise this money. And when you have a shortfall you can't make it up the way the government does by printing more money. You have to actually get close to breaking even.

I'm going to run through some of the things that we actually did. I want to stress that we have not solved this problem; unfortunately, it's still a work in progress. But we've set a strategic vision, and we've come up with some ways of implementing it. We're still struggling a little financially, but I think we're headed in the right direction.

What the organization did is a self-assessment, an environmental scan, a kind of vision about where it wanted to go and then put together a strategic plan to implement that. Figure 10.10 summarizes the strategic plan that we came up with.

The first decision was to serve a broader community in terms of age, socio-economic status, and levels of need. This was an important change for an organization that historically had really focused on the oldest, the poorest, and the frailest people in the community, mainly the Jewish community.

The second decision was to expand and balance the continuum of care, balancing it meaning not being entirely focused on long-term care with a little bit of subsidized housing as we had been.

The third decision was to diversify the revenue streams and reduce our reliance on government subsidies, particularly in the Medicaid program.

The fourth decision was to develop a more flexible and entrepreneurial culture.

The fifth decision was to expand our research agenda.

The CEO's job is to take what the board of directors decided, develop plans for implementing it, send it back to them, and make sure that all are in agreement.

When I was younger, I used to scoff at strategic planning as a waste of time: "Why talk about it? Let's do it." Since I've gotten older I've learned

⊗ Serve a broader community – in terms of age, socio-economic status and levels of need

⊗ Expand and balance continuum of care

⊗ Diversify revenue streams and reduce reliance on government subsidy

⊗ Develop flexible and entrepreneurial culture

⊗ Expand research agenda

FIGURE 10.10 Strategic plan (2001).

that strategic planning is really, really important because whenever I discuss an innovation with the board, I go right back to this slide and I talk about the strategic plan. I remind them that these are the things that they said the organization ought to do, and it's a very powerful springboard to be able to go back to this so that it doesn't look like something pulled out of left field but an implementation of the board's own thought. Now, ultimately, the board has to decide whether they think that's true or not, but it's very powerful to come up with a few ideas and be able to keep going back to a strategic plan as a touchstone. Otherwise, when you're proposing a new project, you're starting from scratch all over again, and the same controversies that you had to push through at the beginning rise up again. Now, that may happen anyway, but I think having a strategic plan to refer to is very important, and it's something that has taken me longer than it should have to recognize.

I'm not a big fan of management gurus, and when we went through this strategic planning I hadn't read *From Good to Great* by Jim Collins, the same guy who wrote *Built to Last*. I think this is the best book I've read that deals with effective management. Following are three of the book's big ideas.

The first is, "who, then what?" The concept is you have to get the right people on the bus. Collins looked at the country's 11 most successful Fortune 500 companies and interviewed the CEOs. Most of them said what one expressed as "I didn't really know where the company should be going. But I knew if I got the right people on the bus they would figure out where the bus ought to go." It was very interesting to Collins because he was expecting that the CEOs of the most successful companies would be people who were visionaries who came out and announced to their senior staff and to everybody else, "This is where the organization is going." In fact, they turned out to be people who built very strong teams of independent-minded people, who really liked to mix it up. Out of that process came a plan that senior managers bought into and could support.

The second thing is to confront the brutal facts. It's very hard for an organization to really look at what's going wrong. There are a million reasons why it's really not going wrong or if it really is going wrong, it's going to go away. Or if it's really going wrong and it's not going to go away, that's too bad because we're not going to sacrifice our principles in the interest of continuing to thrive financially. Confronting the brutal facts but never losing faith is something that most people can't do. Holding both of those things in mind is a very difficult exercise. People talk about only seeing dollar signs. On the one hand, you must keep your mission in mind; but on the other hand, you want to make sure that it's a mission that is financially sustainable. And this, I think, is a terrific piece of advice.

The third thing is what he calls "simplicity within the three circles" (see Fig. 10.11). He says that organizations should do those things that fall within

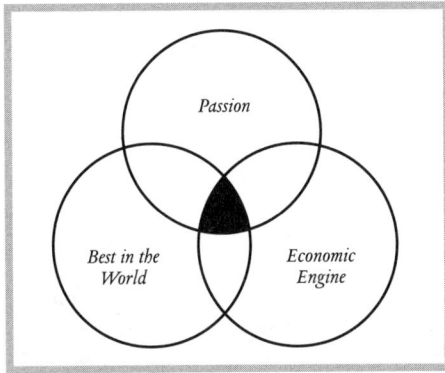

FIGURE 10.11 Simplicity within the three circles.

the middle of these three circles. What do you have a real passion for? What can you be the best in the world at doing? And what drives your economic engine? If you can find areas of activity that fall within these three circles, that's the best thing for your organization to be doing. To develop skills in management, I don't think time would be better rewarded than picking up this book. In hindsight, I think it framed a lot of my own and our organization's own thinking as we went through this process.

The pyramid in Figure 10.12 represents where the system was in the year 2000. Most of what we were doing was long-term care, some supportive housing, and a little bit of community-based services. What we decided was that we had to turn that pyramid upside down and have something that looked more like the second figure—much more community-based services like adult day health, outpatient care, assisted living, and others. Chapter 11 explores such service further. Of course, we think of research and teaching as the things that we do that reach the widest audience.

We decided that we wanted more supportive housing because when we looked at Jack Satter House and Simon C. Fireman Community, we saw that these were great platforms for delivering services to seniors, even when they were really frail. If we had the right supportive services there, instead of building more long-term care facilities that were 90% Medicaid-supported, we could provide pretty extensive care in a supportive housing environment. We decided that we wanted to shrink long-term care, although it would remain a very important component of what we did. Then we decided that we wanted to increase the part of our system that was more acute, namely, post-acute care, which is rehabilitation, typically with a 2–4 week stay. You fracture a hip or you have a stroke, and you get rehabilitation; then, after two to four weeks or more, you go home. Finally, we decided to develop long-term acute care— really an acute level of care for very complex patients who typically require

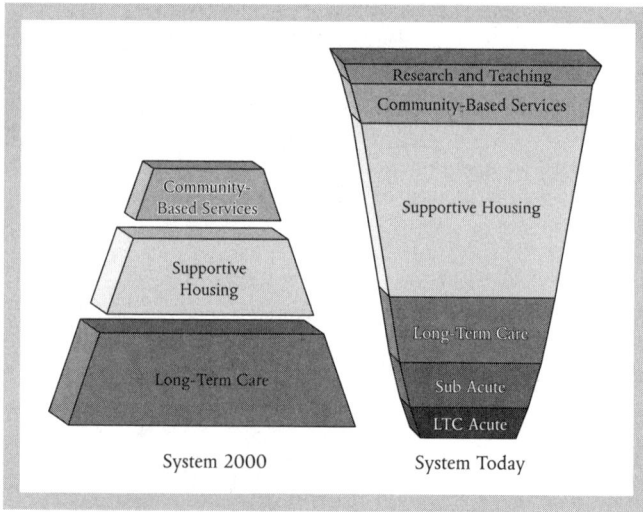

FIGURE 10.12 A new paradigm of senior care. LTC, long-term care.

about a month or more of rehabilitation. So we wanted to increase the continuum on both ends: more community-based services and more acute care.

We also redefined our mission. We defined it in terms of our roots: We talked about our mission starting with the Fifth Commandment, described as honoring our elders by respecting and promoting their independence, their spiritual vigor, their dignity and choice. (This is discussed in more detail in Chapter 5.) We talked about this special responsibility for a long time at the board level because some of our members insisted that we have specific language addressing caring for the frailest, neediest members of our community, which we did. We described our duty as reflecting *tikkun olam*, which is Hebrew for "to repair or heal the world," because while we take very seriously the responsibility to provide care for the seniors under our direct care, we think of our mission as serving seniors everywhere. We were specific about providing a high quality of health care and housing, conducting research, teaching, being advocates, being leaders, and raising standards in the field.

All of this tended to create a platform from which we could innovate. I describe this as a system that rests on four pillars: health care, housing, research, and teaching. This was the first time that we had elevated housing, research, and teaching to the same level as health care. Earlier, if you would ask people "What's Hebrew Rehabilitation for Aged about?" they would have said, "Long-term care." We made a conscious effort to say that we are an academic teaching hospital, but we are also a research facility and a senior housing organization; each of these pillars is equal.

Then we went about implementing this vision and strategic plan. The first thing we did was to implement post-acute care. We opened a subacute unit, converting 46 of our long-term care beds into a skilled nursing facility. Many people called on us to do that, and it has been a tremendously successful service for us. Whereas 5 years ago we were admitting about 250 people a year, we're now admitting 1700 people a year because many of them are coming for short stays and then going home. I run into people all the time now who have experience with the organization because they've come for a couple of weeks and then gone home. How great it is to get rehabilitation and then to go home! We also are interested in ethnic units: We expanded our Russian service. One out of every six residents in our place today is Russian-speaking. When we opened a post-acute unit, we ended up serving a much broader population—well over half the population we serve is non-Jewish, which is also a first for us. (Chapter 7 speaks to the needs of minority populations.) This 46-bed unit is the largest in the state. It runs an average occupancy of 43, which is almost impossible; and we're thinking seriously of expanding it. One of the great assets is our location: We're just a couple miles from the Harvard Medical School campus and surrounding teaching hospitals, so we're well located for admissions from the medical school–affiliated hospitals.

We then opened a long-term acute-care unit, which is 31 beds now and has a very high rate of reimbursement. We're providing 4–5 weeks of treatment there. So we took 85 long-term care beds that had been 90% Medicaid-reimbursed and converted them to beds that are now almost entirely Medicare-reimbursed at a much better rate.

So we improved out financial situation, we expanded our continuum of care, we are serving a broader community, we're diversifying our revenue stream, and it has helped bolster our census, which is now operating at a 99% occupancy level.

We then decided to move more decisively into housing. We doubled our housing portfolio by acquiring three housing facilities in Brookline, Massachusetts. These were so-called expiring use buildings. They were built about 35 years previously by private developers who promised that they would provide affordable housing for 35 years. When they were built, it seemed that 35 years was a long time; but we were now at the end of the term, and the developers who were fortunate enough to build in neighborhoods like Brookline were turning all of their units to market rate. They were about to sell, and with encouragement from Brookline and the state, we stepped in and acquired the buildings and then renovated them. These were like the senior housing facilities that I talked about at the beginning: for independent seniors who would get their mail in the morning and then go upstairs and spend their time in their apartments because there was very little common space. Our goal was to take these buildings and make them more like Jack Satter House and Simon C. Fireman Community. So we spiffed up the exteriors a little bit, but more importantly we took all of the space on one-half of the first floor of the building that had been private apartments, gutted it, and turned it into common space. We created a big community room for live entertainment, movies, and lectures. We have a nurse-practitioner on staff there, so residents can actually see her or him, even without an appointment, as well as medical office hours during the week. There is a beauty salon—that's one of the most popular things that we did. There is also a big fitness room, a coffee shop, a library with computer stations, a livingroom, an outside terrace where people can spend time when the weather is nice, and a big reception area.

So it went from a place that really felt bleak to one which, within the constraints, now really is quite nice. And 60% of the apartments are low- and moderate-income, and 40% are market-rate. The average age of people living in this building is 86 years—and many of these people would be living in assisted living facilities if not for the supportive services here. In fact, some people have moved into this building from assisted living facilities. So you've got independent, very dependent, low-income, moderate-income, and market-rate seniors. What I love about it is that it's taking all the categories that used to be segregated and mixing them all together in a way that really works in a setting that is probably the best neighborhood for seniors in America.

The low-income people are Section 8–supported, and they're paying no more than 30% of their income; and the people who are paying market rate for a two-bedroom apartment are probably paying, with meals, about $2100 a month. But you have to remember that people living in a building like this don't have a lot of excess expense because you're got your meals, transportation, an incredible activities program, and a lot of other stuff that's provided on-site.

When we first bought these buildings, I went to each of them to introduce our organization and myself. After I made my remarks, I asked if there were any comments or questions. In the first building I approached, there were about 200 people in the dining room, and a woman stood up and said, "Mr. Fishman, I'm so glad Hebrew Rehabilitation Center for Aged has taken over this building. What I want to know is, will you care for me at the Center if I can't live here anymore?" ("The Center" refers to our Roslindale long-term care facility.) I was a little taken aback because I was there to talk about housing, not long-term care, and the last thing that I wanted was for the people living in these buildings to think that we were going to try to fill up our long-term care beds with the people living here. So I gave a long-winded, politically correct senior housing answer about supporting her where she lived and making sure that she had everything she needed to spend the rest of her life there.

But then I said, "If you can't live here anymore, then of course we'll care for you at the Center. In fact, we'll make sure that you have preferential admission." And the entire room burst into applause, which was a shock because seniors usually don't clap about getting on a fast track to a long-term care facility. But the lesson that I learned that day, which I knew in my mind but I didn't know in my guts, is that it was a tremendous relief of anxiety. These folks don't want to go to Roslindale, but the fact that they knew that if they needed it, somebody would hold their hands and help them get there and that they wouldn't be strangers when they arrived was incredibly powerful. And it was like taking two plus two and getting 10; it was just extraordinary for them. So this place now functions like a virtual CCRC for people who can't afford the entrance fee, and it's incredibly gratifying to be able to put that together.

We also decided that the Roslindale campus was going to be impossible to renovate to attract a larger private-pay crowd for long-term care. Furthermore, we decided that in order to renovate the Roslindale campus, we had to move beds off-site so that we could have room to decompress. For example, one possibility is to take double-bedded rooms and turn them into single-bedded rooms. But you can't do that without moving people. So we decided we had to find a parcel of land to move 240 beds—frankly, an arbitrary number—off that campus. And then we thought, well, if we're going to have long-term care, we should have the full continuum of care with assisted living and supportive housing. And then we thought, well, if we're going to do all of that, let's not just have it for seniors; let's see if we can do a multigenerational campus. So we approached four day schools that were looking for a permanent location and asked them if they'd like to locate with us. Three of them were Jewish day schools and one was a nonsectarian school. And the result was New Bridge on the Charles, a multigenerational campus, still in the planning stages, to be built on the Dr. Miriam and Sheldon G. Adelson campus. And this really is in some ways the linchpin of our future because it will help serve the community needs by strengthening our financial future, further diversifying our revenue stream, moving Roslindale beds so that we can then renovate the Roslindale facility, expand our geographic coverage, and, we hope, extend our leadership in long-term care in senior facilities and services. It's a beautiful parcel: 162 acres surrounded by the Charles River, right off an exit from a main interstate and state highway. The Rashi School, a k-8 Jewish day school, will serve about 400 kids.

The current campus site plan (see Fig. 10.13) calls for a 270-bed health center with long-term and post-acute care services, as well as a 91-bed assisted living facility with 40 dementia units. There will be 256 units of housing— some apartment-style, some cottages. The Rashi School is being built just 200 feet away from the senior housing; there'll be an early childhood education or day-care center for kids embedded in the long-term care facility. And within

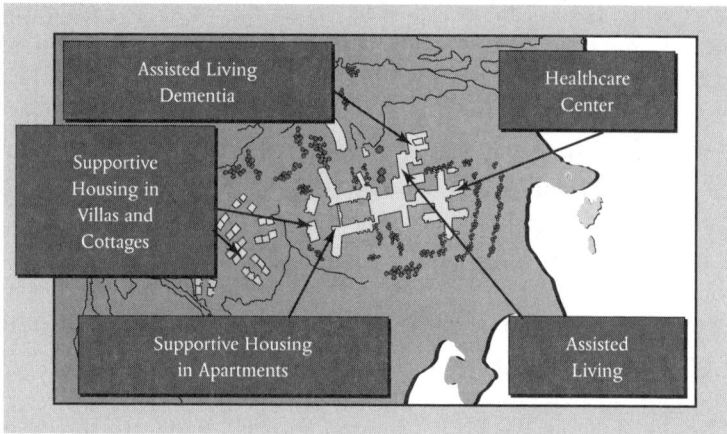

Figure 10.13 Campus organization: five distinct senior programs plus school.

the center will be a village center that will house three restaurants, a kosher deli, a movie theater, a pool, a spa, etc. That will serve the entire community and is intended to be a hub where the seniors and the kids come together. We're expecting 400 kids to come running into that center at around 3:30 p.m. for ice cream, pizza, whatever. And the seniors who don't want it will have cleared out by then and will reappear when the kids go home.

Inspiration for the housing communities we are building comes, in part, from Rotterdam in the Netherlands and other parts of northern Europe. In Rotterdam a renovated hospital has 160 units: some are rental, some are condo; some of the people living there are young, some are old; some are receiving long-term care and some are receiving an assisted living level of care. There's a common space with a supermarket on the bottom. It's right in the middle of downtown Rotterdam, and it's called Apartments for Life because the idea is to design the units so that people can live there for the rest of their lives. The units have a universal design to support people aging in place. And it's cost-effective to bring services in so that people can stay there. And the Apartment for Life concept is being built into all of our apartment units on the new campus.

The new long-term care facility will be comprised of a series of households. Each room will be private, with a private bath and a private shower. These households will come together in neighborhoods of 80 so that we can mount large-scale activities—live music, etc. —for the population that we're serving. In the center will be a country kitchen, where real food is served, not on plastic trays, but family style. Entrees will be brought to the kitchen and put on a steam table so that the meal can be served over a period of time. When you work at a facility like the one that I work in, you learn that the meal program organizes the entire day. It's something I never realized, but when you think about the trays coming up to the dining room, every minute that the meal is sitting on the tray is a minute that the food is less fresh and less hot. And think about what that means for the morning breakfast: When that tray cart comes up, every resident has to have been awakened, groomed, dressed, washed, and zipped out into the dining room so that he or she is ready to eat. That's a ridiculous way to organize your life, but that's how every meal and every day is in a long-term care facility. So if you bring the food up in bulk and put it on a steam table, you now have a 1 hour and 15 minute window of opportunity. If somebody wants to sleep in, that's not only OK but better because now you don't have the dining room full all at one time. You can have that person show up an hour later; the food is still hot and the person can be served in a way that feels much more natural and home-like.

This plan is more expensive—much more expensive—to build, and the only way we can do that is through philanthropy and an expectation that 25% of our beds will be occupied by private-paying patients instead of the 10% occupying our beds on the Roslindale campus. And you can see the difference before and after the new Dedham campus (see Fig. 10.14): Right now 49% of our revenue comes from the Medicaid program, 11% comes from Medicare, and 28% comes from private sources. Post-Dedham, 42% of our revenue will come from private sources, 28% will come from Medicaid, and 21% will come from Medicare. If half your revenue is coming from Medicaid, you're going to be struggling year after year. If it's more like 30%, that model is probably sustainable. Chapter 4 explores more exhaustively the planning and funding of health care for older adults.

Our concepts and programs of senior care have evolved tremendously over recent years, as Figure 10.15 shows. Consequently, we changed our name because we wanted to convey to people that we weren't just about long-term care or rehabilitation anymore. We changed it from "Hebrew Rehabilitation Center for Aged," which was quite a mouthful, to something that we thought reflected our broader focus "Hebrew SeniorLife." We chose the tagline "Care, Community, and Innovation." We kept "Hebrew" because we wanted to hold onto our heritage, we chose "Senior" because I think people prefer that to "Aged," and "Life" was something that we thought captured a vision, a more active vision. We changed our governance system. We expanded the Institute for Aging Services as the strategic plan called on us to do. We also expanded home health care and our outpatient services. And we launched a capital campaign to help us pay for all of these things.

You can see that all these housing, health, recreation, administration, planning, and funding activities will engage a wide range of disciplines. Since the programs and the care are intended to be integrated, it requires that the disciplines integrate their work. This is a prime opportunity for interdisciplinary

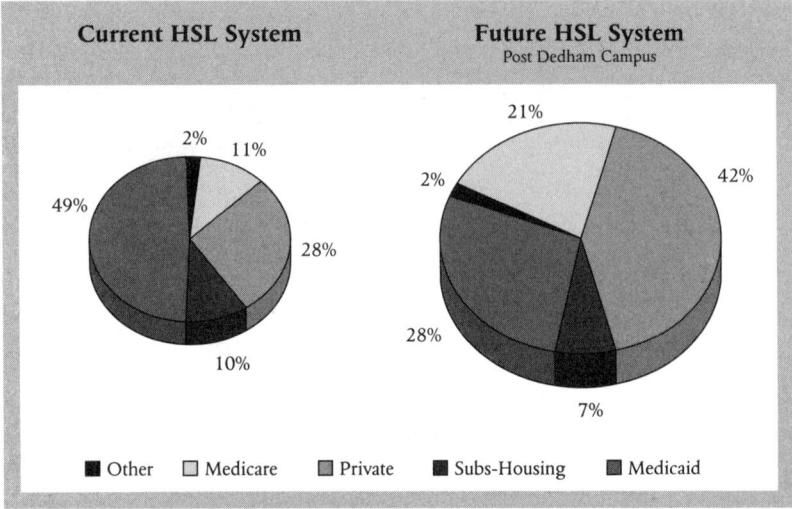

FIGURE 10.14 Current and future Hebrew SeniorLife (HSL) system. Subs, subsidized.

collaboration in the provision of services and care. Hebrew SeniorLife is also a major teaching facility for many disciplines, and research is a major commitment in all aspects. Therefore, an interdisciplinary approach will be called for in care, teaching, and research. The logic in this program to meet the long-term needs of older adults is the logic of all geriatrics: Life is interdisciplinary, so professional education and practice must be interdisciplinary to meet these needs. So Hebrew SeniorLife can be a leader in interdisciplinary collaboration as well. Would it be too much to think that this is also a model for meeting the needs of other age groups too?

I hope this leaves you with at least two conclusions: first, that you can teach an old dog new tricks and, second, that we're really living through a time of amazing innovation. And it if it feels to you like this field is exciting, now you're really going to be in the middle of what's going on in this country in every way—socially, economically, health care-wise—5–10 years from now. So I hope most of you, if not all of you, end up in this field for good.

Application to the Case Study: The Older Adult Care, Training, Research, and Planning Program

The residential environment and long-term care of this diverse population need to be addressed. Our experience with a comprehensive array of living

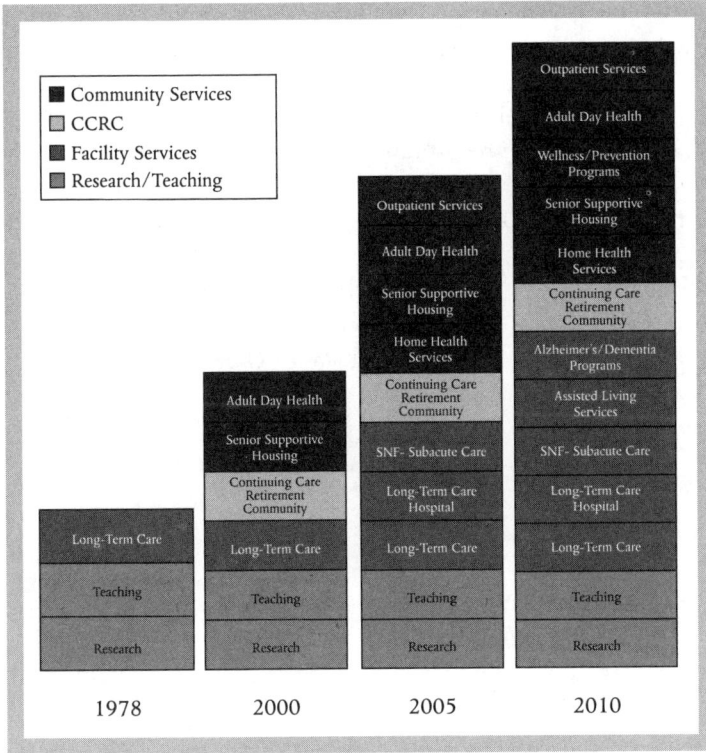

FIGURE 10.15 Evolution of Hebrew SeniorLife (HSL). CCRC, continuing care retirement community; SNF, skilled nursing facility.

environments to match the stages of life needs of older adults should be a part of the planning for health care in a community setting. This community, too, should plan health and social care in the context of older adult lives, rather than the traditional health planning of bringing people to health-care programs. It would contribute valuably to developing and testing theories of funding this approach, as well as integrating professional health care into the lives and dwellings of older adults.

Certainly, long-term residences for older adults in community settings should be developed. The integration of older adults with children, young adults, and those transitioning to old age is an intriguing problem whose many potential approaches can be explored in this project. Involving the community population in this planning and experimentation will give it new perspectives and acceptance.

It is essential that the students from various disciplines learn about the lives, abilities, wishes, and needs of the older adult population. From this enriched knowledge base they should then learn how to contribute their disciplinary expertise to support and enhance the lives of older adults. Health, seen in this life and community context, will be better served than with the usual approach of cure of isolated pathology. Students should learn the place of residence and supportive services in their professional practices. Working in the lives of the older adults gives a more realistic picture of their capacities and needs than does work in health institutions.

Finally, the study of the effect of home and housing on health and functional status would recognize a dimension often forgotten in biological and psychosocial research. As home provides strength and comfort and loss of home causes anxiety and grief, so supportive housing is a factor in maintaining and regaining health and functional status. Our experience in integrating health, social, and recreational care in housing, based on such assumptions, would benefit from careful testing and confirmation.

Bibliography

Collins, J. Good to Great, 1st ed. New York: HarperCollins, 2001.

Collins, J. Level 5 leadership. Harvard Business Review 2001;(January):66–76.

Committee on State and Community Psychiatry Systems, Council on Psychiatric Services. Guidelines for Psychiatric Practice. I: Public Sector Psychiatric Inpatient Facilities. American Journal of Psychiatry 1994;151(5):797–798.

Hadley, J. Analysis of Data from the 1969 and 1994 Health Interview Surveys. Washington, DC: Institute for Health Care Research and Policy, Georgetown University, 1998.

Institute for the Future. Health and Health Care 2010: The Forecast, the Challenge, 2nd ed. San Francisco: Jossey-Bass, 2003, chapter 14. Available at: http://www.iftf. org/system/.../deliverables/SR-794_Health_&_Health_Care_2010.pdf.

Lichtenstein, B. (producer, director). Almost Home. Motion picture. Available from the University of Wisconsin, Center on Age and Community: http://www.uwm.edu/ Dept/ageandcommunity/Resources/products.html. 2006.

National Academy on an Aging Society. Demography is not destiny. Available at: http:// www.agingsociety.org/agingsociety/pdf/destiny1.pdf. 1999.

Taylor, B.E., Chait, R.P., Holland, T.P. The new work of the nonprofit board. Harvard Business Review 1996;74(5):36–46.Figure 10.13 Campus organization: five distinct senior programs plus school.

11

Community-Based Care for the Elderly

SEYMOUR J. FRIEDLAND

Ask most elderly people how they would like to live out their lives and you will typically get a response that indicates a preference for remaining at home. In a recent national study,[1] 64% indicated that in the event of a serious illness they would prefer to live at home, 3% preferred to move to an institution such as a nursing home, and only 15% preferred moving in with family. Yet, 72% of the $98 billion spent in 2000 on long-term care for the elderly was directed toward institutional care.[1] Clearly, then, we continue to have service systems that are geared toward institutional models and are only now beginning to look at community alternatives. The purpose of this chapter is to explore a number of new models of community care, issues involved in developing and sustaining community approaches, and implications for the interdisciplinary model.

Defining Community-Based Care

As more models of community care develop, it becomes more difficult to define what is meant by "community-based care." If we take a purely physical or geographic approach, we would restrict community-based care only to those who live in their own homes. However, a more useful definition is based on a set of dimensions that results in seeing community versus institutional care on more of a continuum.

The first dimension is independence; clearly, settings that foster great independence and self-care are more toward the community-based end of the spectrum. Second, environments that are least restrictive are more representative of the community-based model. When services are brought directly to the elder or in close proximity, there is greater affinity with a community model. Finally, settings that foster normalization are characteristic of the community approach. By "normalization" we mean approaches that encourage elders to be involved in activities and interests that are age-appropriate and that we would expect to be important aspects of human functioning, that is, what we would expect are important characteristics of being a social being—opportunities for social contact, intellectual stimulation, learning, entertainment, and emotional support.

It is important to consider all dimensions. One may be cared for in a truer community model in elderly housing than in one's home if all the conditions are right. Once we consider the multidimensional aspect of community care, a number of situations may fit the model: living at home, elderly housing, assisted living, senior communities, and continuing care facilities. We can suspect that this list will grow in the future and opportunities and models for community care will become more diverse.

Forms of Community-Based Care

There are many forms of community-based care. They all have a goal of keeping people in the community, out of nursing homes, and functioning as independently as possible. We will look first at comprehensive health models that are incentivized for keeping people in the community, then at approaches that focus on where people live, and finally at specific vehicles for delivering services.

Comprehensive Health Approaches

The Program of All-inclusive Care for the Elderly (PACE) is a federal program that serves individuals 55 or older and who are certified as nursing home–eligible. Although it is possible to buy coverage on a private basis, the vast majority of seniors seen in PACE are Medicaid-eligible. The purpose of PACE is to keep frail elders with chronic care needs in the community. Payment to the individual PACE organizations is based on a capitated fee that provides incentives for developing innovative and comprehensive community-based services. Thus, PACE provides all the traditional medical services such as physician care and hospitalization but also adult day care that offers rehab services, meals, nutritional counseling, social work, and personal care. The program differs from most health maintenance organizations (HMOs) in that it provides social services and a high level of case management. The PACE projects began in 1971 in the Chinatown–North Beach area of San Francisco with what later became known as On Lok Senior Health Services. In 1997 PACE became permanently recognized under the Medicaid and Medicare programs. Today, there are 45 PACE programs in 22 states serving more than 13,000 seniors. The typical PACE participant is very similar to the average nursing home resident. On average, she or he is 80 years old, has 7.9 medical conditions, and is limited in approximately three activities of daily living. Forty-nine percent of PACE participants have been diagnosed with dementia. Despite a high level of care needs, more than 90% of PACE participants are able to continue to live in the community.[2]

PACE is impressive in assembling a tightly managed interdisciplinary team that oversees treatment planning and service delivery.

> An interdisciplinary team, consisting of professional and paraprofessional staff, assesses participants' needs, develops care plans, and delivers all services (including acute care services and when necessary, nursing facility services) which are integrated for a seamless provision of total care. PACE programs provide social and medical services primarily in an adult day health center, supplemented by in-home and referral services in accordance with the participant's needs. The PACE service package must include all Medicare and Medicaid covered services, and other services determined necessary by the interdisciplinary team for the care of the PACE participant.[3]

A model similar to PACE has recently been developed in Massachusetts. Senior Care Options (SCO) provides comprehensive health care similar to the PACE model. However, enrollees do not have to be nursing home–eligible. The SCO therefore is operating on a different actuarial model. Again, enrollees must be Medicaid-eligible. However, by reaching out to healthier elders, this effort expands the PACE model. Some of the services provided include[4]

- All health-care services covered by MassHealth (Medicaid) Standard
- Coordination of health care, including a centralized record of medical information
- Specialized geriatric support services
- Adult day care
- Dental care and eye care
- 24-hour access to medical support
- Home-care services
- Family caregiver support

The SCO reimbursement system again provides incentives to keep people healthy and living in the community.

The PACE and SCO programs are significant in that they address both acute and long-term needs of the elderly living in the community. Because they are capitated models, payment is based on the individual's health status rather than an individual service; there is encouragement for using whatever disciplines, methods, and service-delivery models that will keep the person out of more expensive settings such as the hospital or nursing home and keep the individual at the maximum level of health. There are other forms of capitated health care, but they are focused primarily on acute care and do not attend to longer-term needs. These models are less interested in a more comprehensive view of the person and essentially view the elderly person through a medical lens.

Health Maintenance Organizations

Of the 43 million elders and disabled on Medicare, 81% are covered under a traditional fee-for-service model. Only 19% receive care through private health plans funded by Medicare.[5] Since 1970 HMOs have been available to Medicare recipients. However, the Balanced Budget Act of 1997 created a variety of new Medicare plans: Preferred Provider Organizations, Provider Sponsored Organizations, and Private Fee for Service. The Medicare Modernization Act of 2003 further expanded options, creating regional Preferred Provider Organizations and Special Needs Plans for people who were eligible for both Medicare and Medicaid.[5] Medicare pays these private plans a percentage of the average fee-for-service costs in a region. Any savings achieved are passed onto the consumer in the form of additional benefits or reduced premiums. There was a steep decline in membership in private Medicare plans, but enrollment has increased since the 2003 legislation and these plans are now more attractive. However, they are still quite limited in providing the kinds of services needed to keep people in the community. They continue to pursue an office-based model, provide only some preventative services, and do not readily address the needs of the chronically ill. The HMOs may result in some improvement in medical care, but this isn't sufficient to insure quality of life and continued functioning in the community. Because they are under pressure to save money, they provide less case management, less service integration, and less of an interdisciplinary model.

Social Health-Maintenance Organizations

An interesting hybrid that is a better fit with a community-based emphasis is the social HMO (SHMOs). These were mandated by Congress in the Deficit

Reduction Act of 1984. The model emphasizes an "expansion of care" as enrollees get older and more disabled. The SHMO has a greater willingness to deliver care directly to the consumer at home and in the community. The goal was to avoid nursing home placement and costly hospitalizations. The SHMO model has had inconsistent popularity. From 1985 to 1999 there were 157,237 SHMO members. However, by the end of 1999 only 79,785 were participating.[6] The SHMOs did succeed in keeping people out of nursing homes and ensured a more functional life for many highly disabled elderly. The extensive use of personal care assistance and homemakers demonstrated how important the use of paraprofessionals could be in the care of frail elderly. The SHMOs in many ways were precursors of the PACE projects and other comprehensive plans. However, they suffered from a stagnant capitated reimbursement rate that greatly prevented expansion. It is interesting to note that even though expansion of care was made available as a person got frailer, it was not always used. Much of what was used depended on the presence of informal care-givers such as spouses and family members. When such alternative care was available, costs of additional personnel and services decreased.[6]

It should be evident at this point that we don't lack for models that provide comprehensive health care. What we do lack are approaches that are focused on both acute and long-term care, that expand care as the elder gets more frail, and that bring that care directly to where seniors live. These more comprehensive approaches provide better quality of life and delay nursing home admission. Because they don't result in excluding care by spouses or other family members, they can be cost-effective. The best of these models use extensive case management and an integrative approach emphasizing the coordination of various disciplines and paraprofessionals. They offer some of the best examples of an interdisciplinary approach. However, they appear unable to compete with the traditional fee-for-service medical model. Perhaps this comes from American values that center on free enterprise and a focus on short-term costs. Because they engage the elder at home, they may go against the ideal of the person's sense of privacy and supremacy in his or her own home. However, the end result is that the traditional model of care results in greater longer-terms cost and decreased independence as a result of earlier nursing home admission.

Housing Approaches

Over the last couple of decades there has been greater interest in the importance of where a senior lives as related to aging. This would seem to be an obvious consideration, yet it has taken quite a while to recognize how we might impact functioning and longevity through the physical structures in which people live. Peter Townsend in an interesting article about social dependency and the elderly suggests that economic factors cause us to see the elderly as more dependent than they are and provides the rationale for institutional care allowing for greater control and financial efficiency.[7] This may account for our interest in building nursing homes rather than senior communities.

Housing approaches have been motivated by one or more of the following considerations:

- Reducing social isolation
- Increasing the efficiency of service delivery
- Providing a more facilitating physical environment to counter increasing disability and frailty
- Improving quality of life
- Increasing availability of care

The housing approaches we will discuss attempt to maximize one or more of these considerations. They may, however, achieve one goal only to worsen another. We will take a brief look at the more popular approaches to housing the elderly. The first three involve physical housing; the last is a more "virtual" approach:

- Congregate elderly housing
- Assisted living
- Continuing care retirement communities (CCRCs)
- Naturally occurring retirement communities (NORCs)

Congregate elderly housing

This is housing built specifically for the elderly. Funding may be public or private. Frequently, this housing is in part funded by the federal agency for Housing and Urban Development. Therefore, rental costs are usually below market value, and there is the expectation of a minimal level of services. However, services that are provided vary greatly across locations. In some states there may be specific publicly funded services available to these sites, while in other areas services may be almost nonexistent. In addition, some areas may have very mixed elderly housing in terms of income level and disability, while others may be segregated enclaves for poor and disabled elderly. Frequently, there is no mechanism for efficiently coordinating care. This type of housing is a good example of the outcome of inconsistent regulation and criteria for care. However, elderly housing does provide a potential base for helpful services. The economies of scale permit the provision of services at significant savings. The availability of space in such housing also allows for many social activities and increased interaction among residents. However, very much like senior centers, elderly housing suffers from the isolation and segregation of the elderly and the "unnatural" environment this produces.

Assisted living

Assisted living is another form of congregate housing. Here, the population is defined by limitations in activities of daily living. This is typically a population that cannot fully care for itself in terms of housekeeping, bathing, errands, etc. The typical assisted living facility will provide meals, housekeeping, and some personal care assistance. Nursing assistance may also be provided, and medical care is frequently facilitated. Social and cultural events are also promoted. Many assisted living programs are private for-profit and therefore quite expensive for the average senior. Those run by not-for-profits are less costly but may still be beyond the means of many people. There are some instances where an assisted living facility may be required to have a number of Medicaid or reduced-cost units. However, this is relatively rare. Assisted living facilities may provide a comfortable environment and services that ensure some quality of life. However, outside services are not always coordinated, and the assisted living model is not equipped to accommodate more severe levels of disability. For example, those with advancing dementia may find the need to move to a nursing home when functioning decreases significantly. Because there may not be good mechanisms for the coordination and integration of outside care, these sites may not be particularly encouraging of interdisciplinary approaches.

Continuing care retirement communities

A relatively recent entry into community-based housing, these settings provide a continuum of housing from independent living to nursing home care all on the same "campus." They offer continuity of care and some flexibility in services. This is because staffing from the nursing home and assisted living facility can be made available to those elders living in the independent units. People who are independent can also avail themselves of meal services. The CCRC is frequently quite expensive, requiring a large down payment and monthly charge. There are some CCRCs that are run by nonprofits but may still be expensive for the average person. In addition, because they take up a good deal of land, they may be located remotely. Depending on the availability of internal services as compared to external services, they vary in the ability to coordinate and integrate care.

This is a model that provides generally good service, social stimulation, and the opportunity to use services at a pace that tracks changes in the individual's functioning and frailty.

Naturally occurring retirement communities

An NORC is a community with a large proportion of older people residing within a defined geographic area. It is distinguished from other areas that also have high concentrations of older residents, such as assisted living communities or continuing care retirement communities, in that it is "naturally occurring," that is, it was not designed specifically as a community for older people but rather evolved in such a way that a large proportion of its residents are older.[8]

The NORCs are the ultimate method for helping people "age in place." Their goal is to bring services to a particular geographic area in order to lengthen the amount of time a person can live at home. In a sense they create an "elderly housing option" where housing already exists. They may be brought to urban areas within high-rise buildings (vertical NORCs) or created in suburban areas where people live in private homes (horizontal NORCS). It is an approach that at this point has not been extensively applied to more rural areas.

Hunt[9] has described NORCs as centering on three kinds of populations: aged and left behind, aging in place, and in-migration. These three groups may well be associated with different levels of economic and social well-being. Thus, NORCs may be applicable to the poor as well as the relatively well off. This makes them even more interesting because one can have a subscription model in a relatively affluent part of Boston, Beacon Hill, or a subsidized approach in a rather poor industrial city in the same state. Many of the NORCs that exist nationally are a result of activity by the organized Jewish community. These are funded by specific budget amendments and flow through the Administration on Aging. Although initiated by faith-related organizations, they are generally nonsectarian.

Typically, NORC projects begin with a survey of what is wanted and needed by residents. Thus, each NORC may be quite different depending on specific local needs. Most NORCs provide transportation, housekeeping, social activities, and meals.[8] Generally, the goals of the NORC are to reduce social isolation, build community, maintain and encourage wellness, and sustain the fit between the person's health status and the environment in which she or he lives. Thus, resources may range from poetry reading groups to blood pressure clinics to ambulance services to cooking classes. The NORCs frequently encourage volunteer-based activities and promote models where the more able in a site help the less able.

Historically, funding for NORCs frequently came from specific federal budget lines or philanthropic dollars. The recent reauthorization of the Older Americans Act now has an authorization for NORCs. Only a handful of states and cities fund NORCs. In New York, housing owners are required to provide a match for public funds. It is a good indication of the advantage of NORCs to apartment operators: less turnover, better maintenance of physical structures, and more content residents. Also, NORCs are funded by a variety of not-for-profits. There are NORC-like elements in many programs for the elderly.

The NORC concept is exciting because it focuses on client identification of needs, brings services directly to clients, uses existing assets where people live, and reduces the dislocations often associated with aging. This model incorporates many kinds of disciplines: nursing, social work, nutrition, physical therapy, occupational therapy, and psychology. Because coordination is an important component, it fosters an interdisciplinary approach.

Nonhousing Options in the Community

In many housing situations elders can avail themselves of services that can support continued living in the community. There is a long list of these services, and all are not available in every location. Popular services provided in the home include

- Family caregiving
- Home health
- Homemaker and personal care assistance
- Volunteer programs
- Assistive technology

Frequent services provided outside the home include

- Adult day services, respite
- Senior centers

In-Home services

Family caregiving It is important to remember that most of the care provided to elders at home is from family members and spouses. Informal caregiving, unpaid help provided by spouses and children, has long been the most common source of long-term care for older persons with disabilities in the United States.[10] In fact, in the period 1994–1999 the number of spouses and children providing care to older persons with disabilities increased while the use of formal care decreased.[10] This is primarily attributable to federal cuts in programs. Family caregivers are an aging resource as well, and ultimately we will reach a point where the limitations of this kind of care are evident. Much of the time, family caregiving is ineligible for funding. However, in a few states, such as Oregon and Massachusetts, such kinship care may be paid for at nominal rates. Availability of training and support can be quite minimal. Respite services are also rare in many locales or too expensive to be commonly used. The death of a caregiving spouse can therefore be very disruptive and frequently is the cause of nursing home placement.

Home health This is a service typically funded by Medicare or Medicaid but may also be provided by HMOs. Home health offers skilled nursing care;

rehab specialties such as speech therapy, occupational therapy, and physical therapy; social work; and home health aide services. Medicare home health is oriented toward more acute medical problems and requires that the patient be homebound. Medicaid home health is a bit more forgiving and more tolerant of longer-term conditions. These services have become more popular as hospital stays have shortened. In fact, from 1986 to 1998 Medicare home health expenditures went from $3 billion to $18 billion. However, the Balanced Budget Act of 1997 brought with it a prospective payment system that greatly impacted how home health was provided. Within 2 years after passage of the act there was a 52% drop in home health expenditures, the percentage of Medicare beneficiaries receiving home health services declined by 20%, and actual use of services declined by 39%. The biggest drop in specific services was a decline of 59% in services by home health aides.[11] It is clear that use of home health services by people with more chronic conditions was greatly curtailed, and users were considerably more limited in the services they could obtain. Home health continues to be useful for posthospitalization; however, there is little that has replaced it for longer-term conditions. This is a good example of a phenomenon frequently found in community-based services for the elderly. A service designed for a particular population is applied in a wider form because alternatives don't exist. In an attempt to save money, that service is then curtailed but not replaced by another service that will address the issues that are still present.

Homemaker and personal care assistance These are direct care services that are critical if a disabled elder is to remain in the community. Homemaker services focus on the person's physical environment, while personal care assistance consists of services that relate to the person him- or herself, such as bathing, lifting, and assistance with other personal requirements. These services can be purchased privately or may be publicly funded. When publicly funded, they are often through Medicaid waiver dollars. When this is the case, these services are usually available to frail elderly who are at the poverty line or at most 200% or 300% above the poverty level. These services are essential if a person is to remain in the community and has some disabling condition. Recently, these services have become the focus of a controversy about how services should be obtained and paid for. Traditionally, these services are provided and paid for by either not-for-profits or public agencies. Personnel are hired and compensated by formal organizations. However, a new model that has gained popularity in assisting younger individuals with disabilities has now made its way to elderly care. The consumer-directed service model is based on an approach where the elderly person is directly given funds and may hire and pay directly for homemaker and personal care assistance services. There are variations in this model. In some approaches assistance is provided either in screening and hiring or in generating payment.[12] There has been a national demonstration of this approach, Cash and Counseling, that has suggested that it is an effective and efficient model that can be used by a variety of groups. In many instances, family members can be paid through such a model for their caregiving.

Volunteer programs According to the Bureau of Labor Statistics, 61.2 million Americans volunteered in a recent year. Many volunteers work with the elderly, and the elderly volunteer at a high rate, particularly through religious organizations. Many organizations provide volunteer visiting programs for the elderly, frequently called "Friendly Visitor." These may be limited to social contact, but often volunteers do chores and light housekeeping. The value of these services in making it possible for elders to remain in the community should not be underestimated. As government cutbacks continue, volunteer services will become even more important.

Assistive technology Although this is not a service in the traditional sense, assistive technology will eventually become an important component of community-based care. Many people rely on low-tech assistive technology devices such as canes, walkers, and bath benches. Environmental interventions such as ramps, lowering of cabinets and counters, special lighting, and grab handles are also useful and becoming more common.[13] At this point, such devices can be expensive and are not typically reimbursed by third-party payors. However, this is beginning to change. There is now some public assistance for emergency signaling devices such as Lifeline and even more advanced devices such as pill-dispensing machines for those with cognitive impairment. Telemetry devices that can measure weight and blood pressure are becoming cheaper, as are methods that can help a senior check in electronically with a home health nurse. Mann et al.[13] found that assistive devices can slow decline in functioning and are cost-effective. As more evidence accumulates that technology can be effective, it will become more common and available.

Out-of-home services

Adult day services, respite These are community-based group programs with specialized plans of care designed to meet the daytime needs of individuals with functional and/or cognitive impairments.[14] Adult day services (ADS) started in 1974, and as of 2001 there were 3493 centers nationally. Some centers are based on a social model offering transportation, meals, and social activities. Others are based more on a medical model offering basic nursing services, diagnostic screenings, and even rehab specialties. The majority of ADS centers are a combination of the two models. Most ADS centers are not-for-profit. However, for-profit companies are beginning to offer this service. Most of the clients attend on a private-pay basis. Medicaid is the major public funder. However, recently Medicare has made an exception to its homebound criteria and will pay for some centers through the home health benefit. Long-term care insurance policies are now also a more frequent funder of ADS because they have a financial interest in keeping a beneficiary out of a nursing home. The ADS centers that serve individuals with dementia are particularly valuable. They provide social stimulation and respite during the day for family caregivers. They can be invaluable in monitoring more chronic conditions and can improve quality of life for seniors with significant deficits.

As we have seen, many elders survive in the community only because of family caregiving. This makes respite care extremely useful. Even the most devoted family member can become overwhelmed by the stress and fatigue of caring for a disabled elder. In recent years there has been some help in accessing respite services through the National Family Caregiver Support Program, which was passed in 2000 as an amendment to the Older Americans Act. Every state can now provide assistance. However, respite is an expensive service, and it is difficult to find providers. Clearly, ADS are a more economical and more therapeutic solution to providing relief for caregivers.

Senior centers There are 15,000 senior centers nationally, serving more than 10 million adults. The National Institute of Senior Centers defines a senior center as a place where "older adults come together for services and activities that reflect their experience and skills, respond to their diverse needs and interests, enhance their dignity, support their independence, and encourage their involvement in and with the center and the community."[15] Senior centers typically provide nutrition, recreation, social, and educational services. Through informational fairs and meetings they provide comprehensive information about other services and referral. Many centers offer medical screening programs, fitness activities, computer learning, and caregiver support. One does not need to fit financial eligibility or impairment criteria to attend a senior center. They are generally for healthier seniors. Although they serve a very useful purpose, there has been some concern about their tendency to segregate elders. As multigenerational approaches become more popular, as in mixed housing models, the senior center model can be seen as too limiting.

Coordination and Advocacy

Even in this brief review, it is evident that there are many services available in the community. Medicare and Medicaid have a prominent role because they are a major source of funds. Many innovations have arisen over the last few years through Medicaid funds that get used via the Home and Community-based Waiver Programs. Another source of funding, services, initiatives, and coordination is the Older Americans Act.

The Older Americans Act (OAA) was enacted in 1965 to promote the well-being of older persons and help them remain independent in their communities. The OAA distributes federal funds to states, which, in turn, establish centers for information about services available to older persons. Title III of the OAA provides funds to help states organize and pay for meals and a broad range of social services. All persons age 60 and older are eligible to participate, but states are required to target services to persons with the "greatest social or economic need."[16]

The OAA has been reauthorized a number of times since its original passage, mostly recently in 2006. In 2004 total federal funding for the OAA was $1.4 billion. A large part of this funding goes for supportive services and meals for the elderly. Most importantly, the OAA established the Area Agencies on Aging (AAAs) as a conduit for funds and a coordinating mechanism. The AAAs provide services themselves, contract out services, coordinate state and federal programs, and advocate for the elderly. Many of the better-known senior services, such as Meals on Wheels, come out of Title III of the OAA. Although most of the services that stem from the OAA are community-based, it also funds the Nursing Home Ombudsman program, which surveys nursing homes and responds to complaints.

The OAA is an excellent vehicle for stimulating discussion about community-based services and a concrete method for achieving funding and important policy regarding the elderly. The reauthorization of the act provides a means for publicizing the needs of the elderly and promoting new ideas for community care. In this regard, what is most significant in the 2006 reauthorization is a proposal to pilot Choices for Independence. This is a $28 million demonstration project to promote consumer-directed and community-based long-term care options. This program is motivated by an interest in promoting services that better ensure quality of life and dignity for the elderly.

There are numerous organizations that advocate for the elderly on an ongoing basis: the American Association of Retired Persons, the National Council on Aging, and the National Association of Area Agencies on Aging. In addition, professional and gerontological associations are active in promoting community-based models. Most states have a division on aging, and the federal government coordinates aging issues through the Administration on Aging. Many faith-based organizations are also ardent supporters of services for the elderly. Because of the baby-boomer surge, the public has become particularly aware of issues that relate to aging, and this has brought a closer, more personal concern for what happens to people when they get older.

What Must We Focus on in the Coming Years?

There are a number of areas that require a good deal of investigation and action if we are to accommodate the burgeoning number of seniors that will come in the next 20 years with the surge of baby boomers. Here are some key areas that should take on great importance.

Integration and Coordination of Services

Systems of care are quite fragmented and complex at this point. Reimbursement methods, differences between disciplines, and variations among government bodies can make it difficult to bring services together in a meaningful way. It is important that case-management services get funded as a primary service and that payment systems recognize the importance of interdisciplinary approaches.

Quality of Life

Services for the elderly are frequently at the survival level. We need to address issues such as housing, transportation, and social activities if living the last years of one's life in the community is to be meaningful.

Dignity

To be old frequently results in having a lower social status. We need to develop approaches that provide elders with greater control, more choice, and increased flexibility.

Staffing

Even at this time there is an insufficient number of trained individuals to care for the elderly. The need for both professionals and paraprofessionals will grow as the baby-boomer generation takes hold. We will have to not only train more people but also discover ways of caring for the elderly that are less labor-intensive. For example, eventually it will be necessary for home health aides and personal care assistants to do many of the tasks now done by registered nurses. Technology will need to be a major substitute for direct care.

Funding

Society will need to be prepared to expend more. This may well burden the younger generation, but it is a fact that total expenditures will grow at a vastly accelerated rate. For example, by the year 2035 federal spending for Medicaid, Medicare, and Social Security will double as a share of the gross domestic product compared to expenditures at the turn of this century in 2000. By 2040, the number of elderly people living in the United States will double. By 2050 projected long-term care expenditure for the elderly could nearly quadruple.[17] These are sobering numbers.

Implications for the Interdisciplinary Approach

It should be evident at this point that the best care is integrated and coordinated care. Maintaining older people in the community in an efficient and sensitive manner requires many disciplines and systems. A good example is fall prevention. If devastating falls are to be prevented, coordination of physicians, pharmacists, nurses, rehab specialties, and social work is required. It is safe to assume that most outcomes for the elderly are the result of many factors, not just one. This is particularly true for maintaining people in the community. Currently, the reliance on a fee-for-service payment model reduces the attractiveness and affordability of an interdisciplinary approach. Each discipline gets paid separately and many times from a different reimbursement system. Generally, there is no payment for time spent in case consultation and coordination, and rarely is there payment for case management. As capitated approaches become more popular, we will see a greater use of interdisciplinary models. This is not only because of integrated payment systems but also because a capitated model rewards more effective and efficient care. As discussed previously, the interdisciplinary model will have to include paraprofessionals. Demand in the future will require that paraprofessionals take on more responsibility and, therefore, will need to be a part of the core team. Finally, the recognition of the importance of accessibility of service will foster an interdisciplinary approach. With more people living in the community, there will be greater recognition of the value of locating services close to high concentrations of the elderly. The popularity of NORCs, satellite clinics, and mobile medical units is a sign of what is to come.

Application to the Case Study: The Older Adult Care, Training, Research, and Planning Program

The Older Adult Care, Training, Research, and Planning Program (OACTRPP) provides an excellent starting point for an interdisciplinary approach to community-based care. Some of the positives include the following:

- It is situated in the community it plans to serve
- There is early contact with community groups
- Many disciplines are involved
- Not all funds are based on fee-for-service

Therefore, there are opportunities to work with local retail business in developing senior-friendly policies, with tenant groups to consider a NORC, and through public agencies in fostering collaboration with other providers. Because the OACTRPP comes out of a medical center, is funded in part by a drug company, and has a major goal to feed a tertiary-care facility, it will have to be diligent in avoiding focusing on just acute issues and only medical services. In this respect, it is notable that there was mention of problems with traditional Medicaid reimbursement but no indication of trying to participate in a Home and Community-based Medicaid Waiver program. This would have provided more opportunity for flexible programming and service coordination and management.

There are some aspects that, if made prominent, would more readily guide the OACTRPP toward a truer community-based interdisciplinary model. These include

- A multicultural staff and orientation
- Use of supportive services such as homemaker and personal care assistance services
- A mission statement that emphasizes keeping people in that community
- Use of outreach teams within that geographic area
- A reliance on a team approach
- Formation of a community advisory group

There should be concern that without these additional components the OACTRPP may well fall back on the traditional fee-for-service medical model. In fact, the method of supporting training, fees, may well push the training model away from an interdisciplinary approach.

There is a Chinese proverb that tells us, "If we do not change our direction, we are likely to end up where we are headed." This can be read as don't get distracted and keep your destination in mind. It can also mean that if we start in the same way we always do, we will wind up in the same place. The OACTRPP sets out to go in a worthy direction. However, as this chapter has tried to convey, we may at this point need to radically change direction if we are to adequately care for the elderly. For the OACTRPP to be successful and relevant even 5 years from now, it may need to start on a different road and go in a different direction.

Bibliography

AARP. Reimagining America: How America Can Grow Older and Prosper. Washington, DC: AARP Public Policy Institute, 2005.

Butler, R., Grossman, L., Oberlink, M. Life in an Older America. New York: Century Foundation, 1999.

Centers for Disease Control and Prevention, Merck Company Foundation. The State of Aging and Health in America: 2007. Whitehouse Station, NJ: Merck Company Foundation, 2007.

Enguidanos, S. (ed.) Evidence-Based Interventions for Community Dwelling Older Adults. Binghamton, NY: Haworth Press, 2006.

Gist, J., Raetzman, S., Gaberlavage, G., Gibson, M., Kochera, A., Straight, A. Beyond 50: AARP Reports to the Nation. Washington, DC: AARP Public Policy Institute, 2005.

References

1. Slagter, E., Haase, L., Magyera, A. Expanding home and community-based services for the elderly. Issue Brief 3. The Century Foundation. Available at: http://www.tcf.org/publications/healthcare/longtermcare.pdf. 2002. Accessed March 10, 2007.

2. National PACE Association. Who, what and where is PACE? Available at: http://npaonline.org. Accessed June 3, 2007.

3. Centers for Medicare and Medicaid Services. PACE fact sheet. Available at: http://www.cms.hhs.gov/pace/. Accessed June 3, 2007.

4. Massresources.org. Senior care options (SCO). Available at: http://www.massresources.org/pages.cfm?dynamicID=830&subpages=yes&contentID=51&pageID=13. Accessed June 3, 2007.

5. Kaiser Family Foundation (March, 2007). Medicare fact sheet: Medicare advantage. Available at: http://www.kff.org/medicare/upload/2052-09.pdf. Accessed June 19, 2007.

6. Social HMO Consortium. Available at: http://socialhmo.brandeis.edu/home.html. Accessed June 19, 2007.

7. Townsend, P. The structured dependency of the elderly: a creation of social policy in the twentieth century. Aging and Society 1981;1:5–28.

8. Ormond, B., Black, K., Tilly, J., Thomas, S. Supportive services programs in naturally occurring retirement communities. Urban Institute Report for the U.S. Department of Health and Human Services, Asst. Secretary for Planning and Evaluation and the Office of Disability, Aging and Long-term Care Policy. Available at: http://aspe.hhs.gov/search/daltcp/reports/norcssp.pdf. 2004. Accessed March 10, 2007.

9. Hunt, M. (1998) Naturally occurring retirement communities. In: Encyclopedia of American Cities and Suburbs. New York: Garland, 1998, pp. 517–518.

10. Coleman, B., Pandya, S. Family caregiving and long-term care. AARP Public Policy Institute Fact Sheet 91. Available at: http://assets.aarp.org/rgcenter/il/fs91_ltc.pdf. 2002. Accessed June 28, 2007.

11. Fishman, E., Penrod, J., Vladeck, B. Commentary: Medicare home health utilization in context. Health Services Research 2003;38:113–135.

12. Squillance, M., Firman, J. The myths and realities of consumer-directed services for older persons. National Council on Aging. Available at: http://www.ncoa.org/downloads/myths and realities.pdf. 2002. Accessed March 10, 2007.

13. Mann, W., Ottenbacher, K., Fraas, L., Tomita, M., Granger, C. Effectiveness of assistive technology and environmental interventions in maintaining independence and reducing home care costs for the frail elderly. Archives of Family Medicine 1999;8:210–217.

14. Pandya, S. Adult day services. AARP Public Policy Institute Fact Sheet 98. Available at: http://assets.aarp.org/rgcenter/il/fs98_service.pdf. Accessed June 28, 2007.

15. National Council on Aging. Fact sheets. Senior centers. Available at: http://ncoa.org/content.cfm?sectionID=103&detail=1177. Accessed June 27, 2007.

16. Kessner, E. The role of the Older Americans Act in providing long-term care. AARP Public Policy Institute. Available at: http://www.aarp.org/research/longtermcare/trends/aresearch-import-670-FS12R.html. Accessed June 28, 2007.

17. Walker, D. Long-term care: aging baby boom generation will increase demand and burden on federal and state budgets. GAO, Testimony before the Special Committee on Aging, U.S. Senate. Available at: http://www.gao.gov/new.items/d02544t.pdf. 2002. Accessed May 7, 2007.

12

Models of Disciplinary Practice

CLARE E. SAFRAN-NORTON AND SUSAN NEARY

The value of teamwork in providing health care for older adults has been a strongly held tenet of geriatric medicine. In a review of the team concept, Tsukuda[1] dated the first mention of health-care teams to Richard Cabot, who in 1915 mentioned a team involving a physician, an educator, and a social worker. The evolution of teams continued through the twentieth century, with emphasis shifting in the 1970s from public health–oriented teams to those targeting the health-care needs of specific populations. Teamwork in geriatrics is of particular importance, given the growth in numbers of this group and the complex social and health-related needs of this population.[2]

It is generally accepted that interdisciplinary teams offer the most comprehensive model of care for older persons.[2-8] Given changes in health-care financing, the growing number of older Americans, and the reorganization of the health-care system, however, is the interdisciplinary team still a viable and effective method of providing health care to elders? This chapter will consider some of the benefits and challenges of the interdisciplinary team model, with reference to the current literature and application to the Older Adult Care, Training, Research, and Planning Program (OACTRPP) case study. We will start with a review of the models of disciplinary practice, considering the benefits and limitations of each. We will next consider the challenges involved

207

in implementation of the interdisciplinary approach, with an examination of the current context for interdisciplinary practice.

Models of Disciplinary Practice

As noted in Chapter 1, there are varied models of disciplinary working relationships. There is confusion and controversy, however, about the definition of these models, as well as their application in the current health-care system.[7,9] The models most frequently confused include multidisciplinary and interdisciplinary. The following section will define the characteristics of each of these models.

Multidisciplinary Practice

Multidisciplinary working relationships are characterized by Satin[7] as having discipline-defined roles and tasks. Professional education is discipline-specific, and there is little interaction among students during their training. Although team members understand and respect the competencies of other team members, each works within his or her own discipline. The multidisciplinary group meets to discuss the patient's care and goals for health interventions; however, team members continue to practice individually and separately, with little to no overlap of services.[6,10,11] A hierarchical structure is implied, with a physician generally viewed as the head of the multidisciplinary team and ultimately responsible for decision making.[12]

If the OACTRPP project were to choose a multidisciplinary model, for example, a team would be assembled, perhaps including physicians, nurses, nurse-practitioners, physical therapists, and social workers. The physician, by tradition, would be the team leader and other professionals, particularly the nurses and physical therapists, would defer to the physician for "orders" for care. A weekly team meeting would involve presenting individual patients to the team for consultation, but approval would be sought from the physician team leader. Each professional might precept students in their individual practices, but there would be little communication between students across disciplines.

Interdisciplinary Practice

In contrast to the multidisciplinary model, the interdisciplinary team offers a more comprehensive approach to collaborative practice. According to Satin,[7] interdisciplinary practice is characterized by overlap among disciplines. Leadership of the team is determined by competency needed in a specific area, not by hierarchical tradition. Role assignments are flexible and based on the nature of the problem at hand. As team members work together, they learn about the other's discipline and areas of expertise. Students from various disciplines also learn and work together, developing respect for other disciplines at an early point in their careers. Enhanced problem solving as well as resource conservation occur in the interdisciplinary model as aspects of each case are examined from multiple perspectives.[2,3,9] Decisions are made, not in a hierarchical fashion, but by inclusion of input from team members, patients, and families. Decision making does not occur at one point but is continuous as the patient's status evolves.[6,12]

The interdisciplinary team is particularly relevant to managing the continuum of care in geriatrics, given the multiple health and social issues involved in geriatric care.[4,6,7,12,13] Several professional organizations and accreditation bodies, including the Joint Commission on Accreditation for Health Care Organizations,[14] recommend this model for elder care. According to an Institute of Medicine report,[15] two-thirds of all current health care–delivery deals with the complex problems of the elderly. The current primary-care system, where 10- to 15-minute blocks are allotted to each patient, does not adequately address elders' needs.[16,17] In order to better meet these needs, there have been multiple initiatives over the past several years involving comprehensive geriatric inpatient and outpatient (community-based) services. Recognizing that geriatric care extends beyond medical care to address psychological, social, and functional needs, the American Geriatrics Society[2] recommended the interdisciplinary team as one of the seven critical components of community-based health-care services for elders.

The geriatric interdisciplinary team may function in a variety of settings. Inpatient teams range from case management teams consisting of a physician, nurse, and social worker (more multidisciplinary than interdisciplinary) to dedicated geriatric units within hospitals. The latter include units providing acute care, palliative care, and transitional care. Other interdisciplinary programs focus on outpatient management, with provision of care over time in the settings in which patients reside, either in the community or in long-term care. With the shift in emphasis from acute to community care, these programs are particularly suited to meeting the long-term needs of elders. In the OACTRPP example, an interdisciplinary team model would be well-suited to management of geriatric community health care. The goals of the project, including clinical care, professional education of students, and research on factors affecting health, functional status, and health-service utilization, would be enhanced by the interdisciplinary team approach. The following section will consider both the advantages and challenges of the interdisciplinary model, with further application to the case of the OACTRPP. Outcomes of the model will also be discussed, with reference to existing interdisciplinary programs.

Benefits of the Interdisciplinary Model

It is generally assumed that the interdisciplinary model is advantageous to patients, providers, and the health-care system. Outcomes of the interdisciplinary team approach can be viewed in terms of health effects for elders, benefits for providers, and benefits for the health-care system as a whole. Of these three categories, patient outcomes have been studied most extensively and will be considered first. The patient outcomes that have been most comprehensively researched are factors related to hospitalization, including length of stay and rehospitalization rates; mortality; effects on physical, cognitive, and emotional function; and quality of life.

Patient-Related Outcomes

Hospitalization/length of stay

The effects of interdisciplinary teams on decreasing length of hospital stays or preventing rehospitalization have been mixed. Sommers and colleagues,[18] in an evaluation of an interdisciplinary outpatient geriatric practice, found both decreased hospital admissions and readmissions for enrollees compared to a control group receiving traditional physician's office–based geriatric care. Stuck and Siu,[19] in a meta-analysis of outcomes of several types of geriatric assessment teams, including inpatient and home-care models, found an overall reduction in rehospitalization rates of 12% across programs. Rehospitalization rates among programs varied, however, with only two home health programs demonstrating a statistically significant reduction in hospital admissions.

Other studies have found that interdisciplinary teams do not reduce length of stay and hospital readmissions. Palmer et al.,[20] for example, in evaluating the outcomes of two inpatient acute care for elders units, one in a university hospital and one in a city hospital, found no statistically significant differences in length of stay between the elders assigned to the acute-care unit and those assigned to receive usual hospital care. Similar lack of effect on hospitalization and length of stay was found in the evaluation of an outpatient interdisciplinary palliative care program,[21] a Veteran's Administration (VA) outpatient geriatric evaluation and management program,[22] and a long-term home health program for frail elders.[23]

Given these mixed results, rates of hospitalization or length of stay may not be the most relevant outcomes for measuring the effectiveness of either inpatient or outpatient geriatric interdisciplinary team programs. Other variables, such as decreased expected length of stay, reduced outpatient visits, or fewer admissions to long-term care facilities, may be more pertinent. For example, in an analysis of data from the well-known Program of All-Inclusive Care for the Elderly (PACE), Wieland and colleagues[24] reported that the number of hospital days for PACE enrollees was comparable to that of the general Medicare population. This finding is significant as PACE enrollees are generally sicker than the general Medicare population and could be expected to have longer hospital stays. Several studies have reported decreased office visits for older patients managed by interdisciplinary teams. Burns et al.,[22] in an evaluation of the effectiveness of outpatient geriatric evaluation and management teams at the Memphis VA Medical Center, found that the program did not reduce hospitalizations; however, clinic visits were reduced over time, with the control group needing 40% more clinic visits than the intervention group. Reduced clinic visits were also cited as outcomes in other studies.[18,21]

The return of elders to community care after hospitalization and the avoidance of nursing home placement are other important outcomes. In the inpatient transitional care setting, for example, Palmer et al.[20] found that although there were no statistically significant differences in hospital charges or length of stay, fewer patients were discharged to long-term care. Stuck and Siu[19] also demonstrated an impact of some interdisciplinary geriatric assessment programs (hospital geriatric assessment units, home assessment services, and hospital home assessment services) on the likelihood of the elder's living in the community setting, with enrolled elders more likely to be living at home 6 months after evaluation.

Mortality

The impact of interdisciplinary teams on reducing mortality is also controversial. Stuck and Siu,[19] for example, found that although individual programs in the meta-analysis failed to show an outcome of decreased mortality, the hospital geriatric evaluation and management units reduced mortality risk at 6 months by 35% and home assessment programs reduced mortality risk at 36 months by 14%. Other programs, however, showed no effect of interdisciplinary interventions on decreasing mortality.[20,22,25] As above, the PACE program[24] offers a more complex view of this outcome variable. Eight percent of PACE deaths occurred in the hospital, but fewer than one-third of the elders spent time in the hospital during the 6 months prior to death. Perhaps interdisciplinary management of the patients at home prevented more costly hospital admissions and facilitated the patients' remaining in their homes in the months prior to death.

Physical and cognitive functioning

Several controlled trials have indicated that interdisciplinary team management has beneficial effects on physical function, cognitive function, and quality of life. The effects of interdisciplinary practice on these variables are complex, however, in that improvements have been demonstrated in some types of programs but not in others. Comprehensive interdisciplinary programs addressing prevention of falls and delirium, for example, have been effective at reducing morbidity and mortality from these two common geriatric problems.[2] Other studies indicate that improvements have been noted in some, but not all, facets of physical and cognitive function and that effectiveness of interventions varies by setting. In the meta-analysis reported by Stuck and Siu,[19] for example, only the geriatric inpatient units reported improvements in physical function at 6-month and 12-month follow-up evaluations; there was no effect on physical function for the other comprehensive geriatric assessment programs reviewed. Similar mixed results were reported for effects on cognitive function.

Research has demonstrated varied effects on activities of daily living (ADLs) as well. Burns and colleagues,[22] in their evaluation of interdisciplinary outpatient geriatric management at the VA, did not find positive intervention effects on ADLs over 2 years of follow-up but did find significant changes in instrumental ADL (IADL) scores. The intervention group also demonstrated significant improvement in global social activity over 2 years. Palmer and colleagues,[20] in an evaluation of two inpatient geriatric units, found improvement in selected (mobility, bathing, and dressing) ADLs, but these improvements were not consistent across the two intervention sites. Significant improvements in ADLs were also demonstrated by Cohen and colleagues,[25] in patients treated in a VA inpatient interdisciplinary geriatric unit; patients treated in an outpatient geriatric clinic had significantly better scores on the Short Form 36 Health Survey (SF-36) mental health subscale than did patients assigned to usual outpatient care.

Quality of life

Several studies have indicated benefits of interdisciplinary team care on quality of life and measures of emotional well-being. Burns and colleagues,[22] for example, reported greater improvement in general well-being in the intervention group as well as improved scores on the Cantril Life Satisfaction Scale and the Center for Epidemiological Studies Depression Scale. Wieland and others[24] noted improved quality of life in terms of fewer symptoms experienced by PACE enrollees as well as better emotional function and environmental mastery. Similar improvements in symptoms as well as decreased anxiety (but not depression) scores were reported by Rabow and colleagues[21] as outcomes of an interdisciplinary palliative care team.

Provider-Related Outcomes

Participation in interdisciplinary teams offers several benefits for providers, including relief of isolation, exposure to new ideas and practices, and broadened perspectives.[10,26–30] Though these advantages are widely touted, there has been little research on provider-related benefits of interdisciplinary team work. Benefits such as work satisfaction may vary, depending on the provider's professional status and role on the team. In a recent study evaluating team members' assessment of team performance in 26 PACE programs, for example, Temkin-Greener and colleagues[31] found a difference in perceptions of team effectiveness between professional and paraprofessional team members. On all team process domains, professionals rated team functioning better than did paraprofessionals. There were also differences in perceptions of team effectiveness related to age of respondents, with older individuals rating team effectiveness more positively than did younger respondents. Based on these results, it seems that provider perceptions of the benefits of participation in an interdisciplinary team are complex and further research should be conducted on this aspect of teamwork.

Benefits to the Health-Care System

The benefits of geriatric teams to the health-care system are generally expressed in financial terms. According to Tsukuda,[1] the issue of cost-effectiveness, though a recurring concern, has not been sufficiently addressed. Recent research has demonstrated that interdisciplinary care can be beneficial to elders without increasing the overall costs of care.[25,32] There are cost savings, for example, in terms of decreased office visits[18,21,22] and, more significantly, fewer nursing home admissions.[5,20,23,24,33,34] As Capitman notes in Chapter 7, there is evidence from the 115 Medicaid and Medicare waiver demonstration projects that indicates that these projects "reduce unmet needs for disablement-related care, support family and others in their informal caring role, and improve the health-related quality of life of elders within reasonable budgets." The PACE model, developed over 30 years ago, demonstrates the melding of interdisciplinary practice and cost-effectiveness. This Medicare and Medicaid capitated managed-care program provides comprehensive care for frail elders who meet state criteria for nursing home eligibility. According to Gross and colleagues,[33] "the average PACE enrollee is 80 years old, has an average of 7.9 medical conditions and three activities of daily living (ADLs) limitations." PACE providers are able to monitor patients for changes in their conditions, intervene early in acute illnesses, and thus prevent hospitalizations. Using pooled funds, the program is able to offer participant services not normally available under Medicare, e.g., respite care and extended home nursing.[34] The program supports both patients and family caregivers in their efforts to stay at home, avoiding or postponing costly nursing home care. Though PACE programs require backing from funding agencies for start-up, they become financially self-sustaining with time. Gross and colleagues[33] estimated that a program "breaks even" when it has approximately 100 enrollees. Gong and

Greenwood[5] predicted that a PACE program can break even at 38 months and get a return on net revenue within 5 years.

Challenges of the Interdisciplinary Team Model

Despite the many benefits of interdisciplinary practice in geriatrics, there are several challenges to implementation and follow-through of the model. There are the difficulties engendered by melding diverse disciplines into a functioning team and the conflicts inherent in this process. There is the ongoing challenge of measuring outcomes for older patients.[4,19,20] There are also new challenges related to the changes in structure and financing of the health-care system that may pose larger problems for interdisciplinary practice.

Team Structure and Role Conflicts

Of the potential barriers to interdisciplinary health care, team structure and role conflicts among team members have received the most attention. These factors will be considered in more detail in Chapter 14 but will briefly be addressed here. As Satin[7] noted, the effectiveness of the team depends on the willingness of team members to recognize the strengths of others and to extend the boundaries of their role identities. The traditional health-care hierarchical structure leads to turf issues and power struggles that are detrimental to team functioning.[10,35] Leipzig and colleagues,[36] in a survey of 592 interdisciplinary training students—medical residents, nurse-practitioners, and social work students—found disagreement about team leadership and decision making. A majority (80%) of the medical residents felt that they had the right to change care plans and that they had the final legal responsibility for team decisions. There were interprofessional differences in attitudes toward the value of an interdisciplinary team, with significantly higher scores on team value among nurse-practitioner and social work students compared to the medical residents.

Similar conflicts involving physician team roles were noted by Albinsson and Strang[37] in a qualitative study involving staff on a unit caring for patients with dementia. Interestingly, a review of the literature did not reveal discussions about role conflicts in other professions, including nursing, physical therapy, and social work. Leipzig and colleagues[36] noted that medical students, trained in a unidisciplinary hierarchical model, have less educational exposure to interdisciplinary teamwork than do students in nursing and social work. It may also be true that physicians, traditionally the leaders in health care, have more to lose by participation in the more egalitarian interdisciplinary team. Iutcovich and Pratt,[16] for example, in reporting findings from a process evaluation of

10 demonstration geriatric health centers, described resistance of physicians to referring their patients to the geriatric health centers. Physicians viewed the centers as a competitive threat and felt that they could provide similar holistic care in their traditional primary-care practices.

Interdisciplinary professional education has been viewed as a solution to team disharmony and as a powerful contributor to optimal team functioning. Several programs have been implemented within the context of medical education[13] and within other disciplines.[8,27,38–40] These projects demonstrate the importance of introducing interdisciplinary practice early in the curriculum and of following through so that students have the opportunity to apply what they've learned to actual interdisciplinary practice.

One of the most comprehensive initiatives, involving multiple professions, is the Geriatric Interdisciplinary Team Training (GITT) program, funded by the John A. Hartford Foundation. This two-phase project involves 13 sites, training students and health professionals in 17 disciplines, with a focus on primary-care interdisciplinary teams.[4] The project is committed to interdisciplinary team training in managed-care settings, addressing potential barriers such as cost and efficiency of training. Initial evaluation of this program at eight sites revealed difficulties in the team training process.[4,41–43] Differences in length of clinical experience led to conflicts between nurse-practitioner and medical resident trainees, for example. Medical residents, who were less clinically experienced than their nurse-practitioner colleagues, felt that their contributions were valued less.[4] Reuben and colleagues,[43] in citing results of the GITT evaluation, described "disciplinary split" as a factor detrimental to team cohesion and training. These authors reported that physician trainees participated "less enthusiastically" than other trainees. They attributed this decreased commitment to inadequate support from medical faculty and to the fact that medical students had shorter GITT experiences than the other disciplines. Other factors contributing to disciplinary split were requirements of professional accreditation bodies and differences in levels of training of participants. Some settings may be more conducive to team training: Team experiences at home-care sites, for example, better facilitated interdisciplinary teamwork.

Measurement of Outcomes

According to Fulmer,[44] if the interdisciplinary team is to remain a viable geriatric care model, there must be an evidence-based rationale for its existence. The long-term impact of geriatric interdisciplinary programs is difficult to assess. Most clinical trials, for example, have been short-term—over 1 or 2 years. Given the trajectory of chronic illness, it is difficult to predict the impact of these interventions over time. It is also difficult to determine the type of program and intervention that produces favorable outcomes. In the Stuck and

Siu[19] meta-analysis, for example, only one-half of the included studies reported physical function outcomes for at least one follow-up period. Although the inpatient geriatric evaluation and management units had an overall beneficial effect on physical function at 6 and 12 months, a similarly favorable effect was not demonstrated for the other interdisciplinary programs. It is also difficult to predict the long-term impact of inpatient interdisciplinary programs. Benefits achieved during hospitalization, for example, may not be sustainable on return to the community or to a long-term care facility.[20] Cohen and colleagues,[25] in a study of frail geriatric patients in the VA system, used a two-by-two factorial design to determine the effects of care provided in both inpatient and outpatient units where a team approach was employed. Although patients in both inpatient and outpatient geriatric units demonstrated improved scores on some of the SF-36 subscales, there was no synergistic effect between the two interventions.

It is even more difficult to determine appropriate outcome variables. What variables should be measured? Is there a difference in effect on specific ADLs, rather than on ADLs as a whole? Are some markers of physical and cognitive function more amenable to intervention than others? Palmer et al.,[20] for example, noted that patients assigned to acute care for the elderly "prehabilitation" units showed improvement in some, but not all, ADLs. Patients at one site showed improvements in bathing, dressing, and walking; patients at a second site demonstrated a "trend toward better functional status" (p. 513) and improved mobility at hospital discharge. Other studies have shown mixed effects on ADLs. Participants in a VA interdisciplinary team inpatient unit[25] demonstrated improvement in four of the eight SF-36 subscales. Outpatients in the same clinical trial demonstrated improvement only in the mental health subscale of the SF-36.

Resources and Costs

The assumption is often made that interdisciplinary teamwork is resource-intensive and not cost-effective. As above, discussion of cost-effectiveness requires taking the "long view" when discussing cost benefits.[20,22] When factors such as fewer acute-care hospitalizations, fewer office visits, and fewer overall nursing home placements are considered, interdisciplinary team practice can reduce health-care costs. Resource dependency theory[29,45] proposes that organizations are more likely to collaborate if resources are reduced. Given the current health-care environment, where the fee-for-service system is being replaced by managed care, the team approach is especially relevant to consolidation of resources.[26] As Capitman notes in Chapter 7, coordinated systems of health care, like those proposed for expansion of Medicare services, address issues of equity as well as cost-effectiveness.

The time required for development and implementation of the interdisciplinary team is another oft-cited barrier. Team training and ongoing participation require meetings and time spent in case discussion. Cole and colleagues,[41] in evaluating the GITT project, noted that with the current emphasis in the health-care system on productivity and time-limited patient visits, the time-intensive nature of GITT was a potential barrier to its implementation. These authors recommended increasing the use of technology and the creation of "virtual teams" as one way of conserving resources.

The time commitment required for teamwork must be supported by both individual team members and the institutions within which they work. There must be "buy-in" by the organizations within which interdisciplinary teams function.[16,20,29,30] Palmer and colleagues[20] suggested that an inpatient interdisciplinary geriatric unit be started on only one selected nursing unit. From this unit, successful interdisciplinary interventions could be carried over to other nursing units.

Conclusion

The interdisciplinary team has been integral to the practice of geriatric health care. In its best form, the interdisciplinary team has the potential to provide cost-effective, comprehensive care over time to elders with complex health needs, as well as opportunities for optimal professional practice. In contrast to the multidisciplinary team, the interdisciplinary model offers opportunities for egalitarian collaboration among health professionals, with the goal of providing expert need-directed care for patients. Much work remains, however, in determining the situations in which interdisciplinary practice works best and the outcomes toward which efforts should be directed. Continuing efforts should also be directed toward improving interdisciplinary team training, with the goals of improving team function within the constraints of available resources.

Case Study

Although there are many scenarios of how a patient case may be integrated within the OACTRPP health-care/research/teaching and community initiative, we offer one hypothetical example of a clinical case applied to these initiatives. We first present the case and then demonstrate the application of the case to the OACTRPP. As you read through this section, you will see an example of how each of the four missions of the OACTRPP is addressed using this sample case study.

Sample Case Study

History

Sylvia Whelan is a 78-year-old female who sustained a right greater trochanteric fracture from a fall at home 3 weeks ago. She reports that she initially fell from tripping over a rug. She was able to crawl to the phone to call 911 and was taken to the local emergency room (ER). She reports that she was discharged home from the ER with a diagnosis of hip contusion. Her pain continued over the next week, so she followed up with her primary-care physician (PCP), who then referred her to an orthopedic doctor. She had repeat X-rays done, which revealed a fracture. She was taken to the operating room the following day for surgery, where she had a plate and screws put in her hip. After surgery, she was transferred to the transitional care unit in the hospital for 2 weeks and then sent home. She is now seen at home.

Past medical history includes hypertension, osteoporosis, alcohol abuse, and type 2 diabetes mellitus controlled by diet and medication.

Social

The patient lives alone in a two-story home with her bedroom on the second floor (she reports that she slept on the couch last night due to a fear of falling on the stairs). She is a retired librarian, who was never married and has no children. Her widowed sister is flying in from Florida tomorrow to help her for 2 weeks.

Insurance

Her insurance is Medicare.

Medications

Medications included hydrochlorothiazide 50 mg po q.d., enalapril 10 mg po b.i.d., calcium carbonate with vitamin D 600 mg po t.i.d., alendronate sodium (Fosamax) 10 mg po q.d. (patient has not filled yet due to high cost), glyburide 5 mg po q.a.m., metformin 500 mg po b.i.d., Tylenol 3 one tablet po q.i.d., ibuprofen one or two tablets po q.i.d. p.r.n., Tylenol PM one or two tablets po q.h.s.

Functional status

The patient ambulates with weight bearing as tolerated on the right lower extremity with a standard walker on level ground for 40 feet safely. She refused to negotiate stairs today secondary to fatigue. She was transported home from the hospital via ambulance yesterday and did not need to negotiate stairs; however, she practiced three steps in the hospital with the therapist. Prior to admission, she reports she was independent and safe with driving, ambulation outdoors with a cane, and safe with all ADL/IADLs. Currently, she needs assistance with bathing, laundry, shopping, meal preparation, housework, and transportation.

Application to the Case Study: The Older Adult Care, Training, Research, and Planning Program

Although there are many scenarios of how a patient case may be integrated within the OACTRPP health-care/research/teaching and community initiative, we offer this one example of how a clinical case may be applied to these initiatives. Chapter 16 offers a dialogue of an interdisciplinary team working toward carrying out the global missions of the OACTRPP, while this chapter offers a clinical example of the interaction between a patient in the community and the medical center, home health care agency, student teaching, and research initiatives.

Health care in a community setting

Ms. Whelan resides within the community that is served by the OACTRPP. She receives local home care clinical services upon discharge from the hospital to her home as well as community homemaker services for ADL and IADL needs. When she is discharged from home services, she will be referred back to the main medical teaching hospital associated with the OACTRPP for follow-up care by the orthopedic department and her PCP. She will likely need to ask for continued homemaker services and financial support for these services from the home-care division of the OACTRPP due to her limited resources and ongoing needs.

Provide community-based, multispecialty clinical care and referrals to academic medical center

Ms. Whelan initially received her ER care in a local hospital and was referred home. When she had ongoing symptoms, she went to her PCP, who referred her to the orthopedics department at the OACTRPP. At the medical center she received repeat X-rays, which revealed a hip fracture. She was taken to the operating room the following day for surgery, where she had a plate and screws put in her hip. After surgery, she was transferred to the tertiary-care unit in the hospital for 2 weeks and then sent home with follow-up services from the OACTRPP. Currently, she is being seen by an interdisciplinary team consisting of a nurse-practitioner, physical therapist, occupational therapist, social worker, home health aide, and homemaker. When she is discharged from home services, she will continue with follow-up care by the orthopedic department and her PCP through the OACTRPP. It is likely that Medicare and Medicaid are the primary funding sources for her clinical home care and outpatient follow-up appointments. Her homemaker services are likely funded in part from state aid and grant money from the OACTRPP.

Student training

Ms. Whelan is currently treated at home by an interdisciplinary team of health-care professionals and their respective students. During this time, she will interact with students in the following disciplines: nurse-practitioner, physical therapist, occupational therapist, and social worker. She will likely interact with medical students, residents, and fellows while in the medical center.

Research on Health, Functional Status, and Health-Care Service Utilization

Ms. Whelan has signed a consent form to participate in a recent OACTRPP research study which examines average length of services per diagnosis and functional outcomes based on independent and safety status upon discharge from home-care services. The study also explores funding sources which include grants and insurance, ethnic and cultural diversity, socioeconomic status, medications, and usage of ADL/IADL equipment.

References

1. Tsukuda, R.A. A perspective on health care teams and team training. In: Siegler, E.L., Hyer, K., Fulmer, T., Mezey, M. (eds.) Geriatric Interdisciplinary Team Training New York: Springer, 1998, pp. 21–35.
2. American Geriatrics Society Geriatrics Interdisciplinary Advisory Group. Interdisciplinary care for older adults with complex needs: American Geriatrics Society position statement. Journal of the American Geriatrics Society 2006;54:849–852.
3. Benson, J.D., Williams, D.L., Stern, P. The Good Beginnings Clinic: an interdisciplinary collaboration. Occupational Therapy in Health Care 2002;16:21–37.
4. Fulmer, T., Flaherty, E., Hyer, K. The Geriatric Interdisciplinary Team Training (GITT) program. Gerontology and Geriatrics Education 2003;24(2):3–12.
5. Gong, J., Greenwood, R. The business side of PACE, part 2. Nursing homes and long term care management. Nursing Home Long Term Care Management 2003;52(5):60–64.
6. Pfeiffer, E. Why teams? In: Siegler, E., Hyer, K., Fulmer, T., Mezey, M. (eds.) Geriatric Interdisciplinary Team Training. New York: Springer, 1998, pp. 13–19.
7. Satin, D. (ed.) Clinical Care of the Aged Person: An Interdisciplinary Approach. New York: Oxford University Press, 1994.
8. Williams, B.C., Remington, T., Foulk, M. Teaching interdisciplinary geriatrics team care. Academic Medicine 2002:77(9):935.
9. Holmes, D., Fairchild, S., Hyer, K., Fulmer, T. A definition of geriatric interdisciplinary teams through the application of concept mapping. Gerontology and Geriatrics Education 2002;23:1–11.
10. Hamel, P.C. Interdisciplinary perspectives, service learning, and advocacy: a nontraditional approach to geriatric rehabilitation. Topics in Geriatric Rehabilitation 2001;17:53–70.

11. Norrefalk, J. How do we define multidisciplinary rehabilitation? Journal of Rehabilitation Medicine 2003;35:100–101.
12. Zeiss, A.M., Thompson, D.G. Providing interdisciplinary geriatric team care: what does it really take? Clinical Psychology: Science and Practice 2003; 10(1):115–119.
13. Counsell, S.R., Kennedy, R.D., Szwabo, P., Wadsworth, N.S., Wohlgemuth, C. Curriculum recommendations for resident training in geriatric interdisciplinary team care. Journal of the American Geriatrics Society 1999;47(9):1145–1148.
14. Joint Commission on Accreditation of Healthcare Organizations. Comprehensive accreditation manual for hospitals: the official handbook. Chicago: Joint Commission on Accreditation of Healthcare Organizations, 2000.
15. Institute of Medicine, Committee on Quality of Health Care in America. Crossing the Quality Chasm: A New Health Care for the 21st Century. Washington, DC: National Academy Press, 2001.
16. Iutcovich, J.M., Pratt, D.J. Establishing geriatric health centers: can the aging network successfully navigate the changing health care system? Journal of Aging Studies 2003;17(2):231–250.
17. Scherger, J. E. Challenges and opportunities for primary care in 2002. Medscape Family Medicine 2002;2(1). Available at: www.medscape.com/viewarticle/420680.
18. Sommers, L.S., Marton, K.L., Barbaccia, J.C., Randolph, J. Physician, nurse, and social worker collaboration in primary care for chronically ill seniors. Archives of Internal Medicine 2000;160(12):1825–1833.
19. Stuck, A.E., Siu, A.L. Comprehensive geriatric assessment: a meta-analysis of controlled trials. Lancet 1993;342(8878):1032–1036.
20. Palmer, R.M., Counsell, S.R., Landefeld, S.C. Acute care for elders units: practical considerations for optimizing health outcomes. Disease Management and Health Outcomes 2003;11(8):507–517.
21. Rabow, M.W., Dibble, S.L., Pantilat, S.Z., McPhee, S.J. The comprehensive care team. Archives of Internal Medicine 2004;164(1):83–91.
22. Burns, R., Nichols, L.O., Martindale-Adams, J., Graney, M.J. Interdisciplinary geriatric primary care evaluation and management: two-year outcomes. Journal of the American Geriatrics Society 2000;48(8):8–13.
23. Kellogg, F.K., Brickner, P.W. Long-term home health care for the impoverished frail homebound aged: a twenty-seven year experience. Journal of the American Geriatrics Society 2000;48(8):1002–1011.
24. Wieland, D., Lamb, V.L., Sutton, S.R., Boland, R., Clark, M., Friedman, S., Brummel-Smith, K., Eleazer, G.P. Hospitalization in the Program of All-Inclusive Care for the Elderly (PACE): rates, concomitants, and predictors. Journal of the American Geriatrics Society 2000;48(11):1373–1380.
25. Cohen, H.J., et al. A controlled trial of inpatient and outpatient geriatric evaluation and management. New England Journal of Medicine 2002;346(12):905–912.
26. Castle, J. Planning GITT: the providers. In: Siegler, E., Hyer, K., Fulmer, T., Mezey, M. (eds.) Geriatric Interdisciplinary Team Training. New York: Springer, 1998, pp. 63–75.
27. Cleary, K.K., Howell, D.M. The educational interaction between physical therapy and occupational therapy students. Journal of Allied Health 2003;32(2):71–77.
28. Halm, M.A., Gagner, S., Goering, M., Sabo, J., Smith, M., Zaccagnini, M. Interdisciplinary rounds: impact on patients, families, and staff. Clinical Nurse Specialist 2003;17:133–144.

29. Harley, D.A., Donnell, C., Rainey, J.A. Interagency collaboration: reinforcing professional bridges to serve aging populations with multiple service needs. Journal of Rehabilitation 2003;69(2):32–37.
30. Sierchio, G.P. A multidisciplinary approach for improving outcomes. Journal of Infusion Nursing 2003;26:34–43.
31. Temkin-Greener, H., Gross, D., Kunitz, S.J., Mukamel, D. Measuring interdisciplinary team performance in a long-term care setting. Medical Care 2004;42(5):472–481.
32. Wieland, D. The effectiveness and costs of comprehensive geriatric evaluation and management. Critical Reviews in Oncology/Hematology 2003;48(2):227–237.
33. Gross, D.L., Temkin-Greener, H., Kunitz, S., Mukamel, D.B. The growing pains of integrated health care for the elderly: lessons from the expansion of PACE. Millbank Quarterly 2004;82(2):257–282.
34. Lee, W., Eng, C., Fox, N., Etienne, M. PACE: a model for integrated care of frail older patients. Geriatrics 1998;53(6):62, 65–66, 69, 73.
35. Farrell, M.P., Schmitt, M.H., Heinemann, G.D. Informal roles and the stages of interdisciplinary team development. Journal of Interprofessional Care 2001;15(3):281–295.
36. Leipzig, R.M., Hyer, K., Ek, K., Wallenstein, S., Vezina, M.L., Fairchild, S., Cassel, C.K., Howe, J.L. Attitudes toward working on interdisciplinary healthcare teams: a comparison by discipline. Journal of the American Geriatrics Society 2002;50:1141–1148.
37. Albinsson, L., Strang, P. Staff opinions about the leadership and organization of municipal dementia care. Health and Social Care in the Community 2002;10:313–322.
38. Clark, P.G. Service-learning education in community–academic partnerships: implications for interdisciplinary geriatric training in the health professions. Educational Gerontology 1999;25(7):641–660.
39. Clark, P.G., Leinhaus, M.M., Filinson, R. Developing and evaluating an interdisciplinary clinical team training program: lessons taught and lessons learned. Educational Gerontology 2002;28(6):491–510.
40. Rose, M.A., Lyons, K.J., Miller, S.K., Comman-Levy, D. The effect of an interdisciplinary community health project on student attitudes toward community health, people who are indigent and homeless, and team leadership skill development. Journal of Allied Health 2003;32(2):122–125.
41. Cole, K.D., Waite, M.S., Nichols, L.O. Organizational structure, team process, and future directions of interprofessional health care teams. Gerontology and Geriatrics Education 2003;24(2):35–49.
42. Mellor, M.J., Hyer, K., Howe, J.L. Geriatric interdisciplinary team approach: challenges and opportunities in educating trainees together from a variety of disciplines. Educational Gerontology 2002;28(10):867–880.
43. Reuben, D.B., Levy-Storms, L., Yee, M.N., Cole, K., Waite, M., Nichols, L., Frank, J.C. Disciplinary split: a threat to geriatrics interdisciplinary team training. Journal of the American Geriatrics Society 2004;52(6):1000–1006.
44. Fulmer, T. Curriculum recommendations for resident training in geriatrics interdisciplinary team care. Journal of the American Geriatrics Society 1999;47(9):1149–1150.
45. Jenkins, C.L., Laditka, S.B. Mental health care for older persons: networking as a response to organizational challenges. Policy Studies Review 2000;17:77–97.

13

Knowing the Individual Disciplines and Introduction to Team Development, Function, and Maintenance

JENNIFER L. KIRWIN AND TERESA T. FUNG

WITH MYRNA D. BOCAGE, SOCIAL WORKER; NANCY A. LOWENSTEIN, OCCUPATIONAL THERAPIST; SUSAN NEARY, NURSE/NURSE-PRACTITIONER; CLARE E. SAFRAN-NORTON, PHYSICAL THERAPIST; DAVID G. SATIN, PHYSICIAN; ANN STAHLHEBER, NUTRITIONIST

As described elsewhere in this text, care of the geriatric patient usually involves more than one, and often many, health-care providers and other professional consultants. Geriatrics practices in both ambulatory and inpatient settings have adopted a team approach to patient care. The interdisciplinary team model has been recommended by professional and accrediting bodies alike as the preferred setting for provision of this care. Chapters 1 and 12 of this text define and explore the differences between unidisciplinary, multidisciplinary, and interdisciplinary teams in depth. In short, the interdisciplinary team differs from the multi- and unidisciplinary team in two key ways: Members have overlapping and flexible roles, rather than performing only the established tasks of their discipline, and they learn and work together often on similar problems, rather than only on problems within their own "turf."

Successful interdisciplinary practices are the result of careful planning, substantial training, and ongoing adjustment. Professionals of different disciplines need to meet, learn, and work together.[1] Interdisciplinary practice is built on a foundation that is comprised of many different professional disciplines and the idea that the successful integration of these disciplines into a true interdisciplinary team will produce synergistic results. The keystone of this foundation is an understanding and appreciation for all the other disciplines that may be involved in the process. As described in the previous chapters, the current state of professional education does not necessarily engender this type of understanding. We feel that there is no better way to begin to understand the various professions than by discussing introductory information about each from educational programs and professional training to workplace roles and other relevant issues. In the first part of this chapter, core and module faculty from this course briefly describe their own disciplines, with the goal of providing a level starting place for students of interdisciplinary education to begin to develop this mutual professional understanding and appreciation.

When clinicians adopt the interdisciplinary model of practice, substantial organizational and administrative support is necessary to ensure effective clinical operation. In the second part of this chapter, we address interdisciplinary team development, membership, and issues around leadership and team member roles.

Knowing the Health-Care Disciplines

We now describe the scope of practice for major disciplines in geriatrics care. Team members are certainly not limited to what is listed below, though the professionals listed below are most commonly involved in clinical care of the patient. Understanding the expertise of different disciplines will help to illustrate the assets each professional brings and to highlight areas of cross-training needed for different team members, enhancing joint decision making and collaborative patient care. We review the training, clinical role, and team role of professional disciplines commonly involved in interdisciplinary geriatric practice.

Nurse/Nurse-Practitioner
SUSAN NEARY

Registered nurses are educated in diploma programs (30%), associate degree programs (40%), and baccalaureate programs (29%). Ten percent of them hold either a master's or a doctoral degree.[2] Nurses employed in geriatrics are concerned with physical, psychological, and spiritual care of the older patient, with an overall goal of preservation and maximization of function. Nursing's scope of practice in geriatrics may overlap with social work, physical therapy, and nutrition, as well as medicine. Reimbursement of nursing services is chiefly by bundling nursing care into overall hospital/nursing home fees.

A nurse-practitioner is "a registered nurse with advanced academic and clinical experience."[3] A master's degree is required for entry into practice. Although state regulations vary, certification by a national certifying body, such as the American Nurses Credentialing Center, is an additional requirement for practice in many states.

Nurse-practitioners practice both autonomously and in collaboration with other health-care professionals. Their scope of practice includes diagnosis and management of acute and chronic health problems, health promotion and prevention, ordering and interpretation of diagnostic tests, and pharmacological and nonpharmacological therapeutics.[4] They practice in nursing homes, ambulatory care centers, home health, and hospice. Nurse-practitioners are recognized health-care providers and are reimbursed by Medicare, Medicaid, and commercial insurers.[5]

Nutritionist
ANN STAHLHEBER AND TERESA FUNG

Registered dietitians (RDs) are a vital part of the medical team in hospitals, nursing homes, health maintenance organizations, and other health-care facilities. The RD provides medical nutrition therapy and specific nutrition services to treat injuries, illnesses, or chronic conditions. Medical nutrition therapy is nutrition-based treatment that follows evaluation of a patient's nutrition status. Evaluation may include services such as diet history, review of lab data, diet counseling of the patient and caregivers, detailed meal planning, observation during meal times, and conducting intake counts. This treatment can range from changes in diet to making suggestions for improvement of specialized treatments to providing therapies such as intravenous or tube feeding. It is a medically necessary and cost-effective way of treating and controlling diseases such as heart disease, diabetes, AIDS, cancer, and kidney disease.

The difference between an RD and the commonly used term "nutritionist" is lack of licensure or any form of regulation for nutritionists. At minimum, all RDs have completed a bachelor's degree in nutrition science, with extensive coursework in physiology and biochemistry; passed a national registration examination; and served an internship, often in a hospital or medical center. More than half of all RDs exceed these minimal requirements and hold a master's or doctoral degree.

Any member of the interdisciplinary team is able to refer a patient/resident to the RD. Since RDs do not receive reimbursement for inpatient services provided to patients/residents, they do not need a formal order to see a patient/resident. The RD might get a referral from a speech pathologist regarding a functional problem that a patient/resident might have with chewing or swallowing. Nurses often refer patients to RDs since they observe patients/residents while they eat and may identify a problem that needs to be addressed. The pharmacist may recognize that a possible drug–food interaction may require a referral to the RD. The RD may work with the social worker to plan for nutrition support resources upon the patient/resident's discharge.

Occupational Therapist
NANCY LOWENSTEIN

Occupational therapy is skilled treatment that helps individuals achieve independence in all facets of their lives. It gives people the "skills for the job of living," necessary for independent and satisfying lives. Services typically include creating programs to improve one's ability to perform daily activities, performing skills assessments and treatment, home and job-site evaluations, recommending adaptations, equipment usage, and providing training for equipment. The occupational therapist (OT) also provides guidance for family members and caregivers of clients.

The OT is a skilled professional whose education includes the study of human growth and development with specific emphasis on the social, emotional, and physiological effects of illness and injury. The OT enters the field with a master's or doctoral degree, after completing supervised clinical internships in a variety of health-care settings and passing a national examination. Most states also regulate OT practice. Reimbursement for OT services falls under most health insurance. It is a covered service under Medicare, for both parts A and B. There are usually monetary or number of visit caps on OT services, depending on the third-party payor.

Occupational therapy overlaps with many disciplines. Physical and occupational therapies are most closely aligned in people's minds, and this is probably due to the medical model of rehabilitation. Both the OT and the physical therapist (PT) will work on the body structure and function level, but the OT looks at the person in the context of his or her environment, supports, and barriers to function. Speech and occupational therapies often overlap in the areas of cognition and dysphagia. Occupational therapy and social work overlap in the area of psychosocial function. Occupational therapy has a long history of work with individuals with mental health issues, and this is still a strong aspect of the education of an OT.

Pharmacist
JENNIFER KIRWIN

Pharmacists work with other members of the health-care team to create, implement, and monitor drug treatment plans. In addition to dispensing medications for patients in the community and in health-care facilities, the pharmacist is available to provide information about diseases and treatments to patients and caregivers. In the clinical setting, pharmacists also advise members of the health-care team on the prevention and treatment of drug-related problems in order to optimize the use of medications and avoid medication errors.

The entry-level degree for practice in pharmacy is the doctor of pharmacy (PharmD) degree. This program includes coursework in the basic and applied sciences, with an emphasis on disease pathophysiology and applied uses of medications to safely and effectively diagnose and treat disease. Pharmacy students also complete one academic year of clinical rotations in a variety of settings. After graduation, pharmacists who successfully pass a state-specific licensure examination may use the designation "registered pharmacist" (RPh). Pharmacists may elect to complete postgraduate training programs in the form of pharmacy residencies and fellowships.

While patients or third-party insurers may pay the pharmacist for the cost of medications, currently the majority of pharmacists do not bill for the "cognitive" (i.e., clinical) services they provide, such as patient education and reviewing the drug regimen for problems. Pharmacists are not yet recognized as providers by Medicare, though this status is being actively pursued by the profession. Patients regularly "self-refer" to the pharmacist by approaching the counter to ask questions about medications and general health matters. Patients may also be referred to the community pharmacist by their health-care providers. In a health-care facility, pharmacy services are provided to the patient by pharmacists who are routinely members of the treatment team and are therefore involved in the care of all of the patients in the facility. In most settings, the pharmacist's services are not billed separately and, as such, do not require formal referral.

The pharmacist's practice overlaps with that of other health-care providers virtually every time a drug, whether prescription or over-the-counter, is recommended for patient care. For example, a pharmacist may help the patient select vitamins or nutrient supplements recommended by a registered dietitian, work with a rehab therapist to reduce the risk of falls or injury as a result of medication side effects, or explain information about medications or diagnoses to a patient or family in collaboration with the physician and registered nurse.

Physical Therapist
CLARE E. SAFRAN-NORTON

Physical therapists play active roles as independent practitioners as well as members of interdisciplinary teams. The common practice settings for working with an aged population include acute-care hospitals, nursing homes, home health care, inpatient rehabilitation clinics, and outpatient clinics. In acute-care and nursing home settings, therapists work closely with other team members on a daily basis, whereas in an outpatient setting the therapist may be the sole practitioner. In home care, the therapist is typically part of a team that meets weekly at the agency office. Home care is also unique for therapists as they are allowed to independently admit patients into an agency on behalf of other disciplines. Regardless of the practice setting or style of the facility, PTs still work as team members in optimizing patient care.

Typical treatments designed for elderly patients address functional problems such as difficulty with ambulation, safety, and patient education. Common impairments addressed in physical therapy include deficits in balance, range of motion, joint mobilization, muscle strength, proprioception, kinesthesia, and pain. Therapists involve the patient, their family, and caretakers by educating them about the treatment plan to optimize recovery and safe functional outcomes.

All PTs are licensed and have an entry-level doctoral or master's degree. Hands-on clinical training is also a part of the requirements for all degrees. In most of the United States PTs have direct access and do not need a physician's referral. However, most insurance companies and Medicare mandate this referral to be eligible for insurance coverage. In the elderly population, most therapy is covered under Medicare. When there is potential for overlap, it is typically with occupational therapy. When this occurs, team members decide who will cover which part of the intervention.

Physician

DAVID SATIN

Physicians are trained in basic sciences—physical, biological, and a variable amount of social. They are then trained in applied sciences—internal medicine, biochemistry, physiology, pharmacology, various surgical specialties, and psychiatry (from the biological, psychological, and/or social perspective). To varying extents, they are trained in health-related social systems perspectives and practices. Psychiatrists are physicians who focus on the basic sciences, clinical applications, or social system issues related to behavior, emotions, interpersonal relations, or societal processes.

Physicians (and psychiatrists in their specialty) deal with health, traditionally seen as abnormality or pathology. This may be broadly applied to normal human or social function; the causes or nature of dysfunction; diagnosis; prevention, cure, or rehabilitation; dealing with the health and illness of populations; or policy and administration of health maintenance, illness treatment, and health-related resources (including personnel). It follows that appropriate roles for them on the health team depend on the individual's capacities and the task's needs.

Physicians and psychiatrists are widely and highly reimbursed. At present, fee-for-service pays for a minority of health care, managed-care schemes pay for an increasing proportion (in some places a majority), and government programs pay for a large proportion. Psychiatry is often treated specially, with separate control bodies ("carved out" of general medical care) and given less financial support (through coverage of a smaller percentage of the fee—e.g., 50% rather than 80% in Medicare—fewer treatments or more limited total expenditure, larger payments required of patients, more resistance to approval of insurance coverage, requirement of more levels of approval before treatment will be paid for, etc.).

In clinical practice, referrals to other disciplines often originate from physicians or psychiatrists. Their special contribution may lie in the breadth of their understanding of basic science, clinical application, and planning/policy, as well as the interrelation of these fields. They may contribute this breadth of perspective to the health-care team and its members, and they may learn from other disciplines, which have primary competence in any topic.

Social Worker
MYRNA BOCAGE

Social workers fill a variety of roles and provide services to every age group from birth through the later stages of the life span. The entry-level degree for the profession is the bachelor's in social work. However, a master's degree in social work is the expected degree for clinical social work practice and usually for positions in policy, planning, and administration. Social work practice is regulated, most states offering certification or licensing; however, the type of credential varies from state to state. Licensed independent clinical social workers are eligible for third-party reimbursement.

Geriatric social work includes roles such as case manager, individual and group counselor, discharge planner, program administrator, liaison, advocate, and community resource expert. Although a unique attribute of the social work profession is working with the individual in her or his environment, many of the activities of social workers overlap with those of other professions.

According to the code of ethics of the National Association of Social Workers, the professional association for social workers in the United States,

> A historic and defining feature of social work is the profession's focus on individual well-being in a social context and the well-being of society. Fundamental to social work is attention to the environmental forces that create, contribute to, and address problems in living. ... Gerontological social work has a focus on prevention and wellness and is particularly concerned with ameliorating those physical, psychosocial, familial, cultural, ethnic, racial, organizational, and

societal factors which serve as barriers to physical and emotional well-being in later life." (Accessible at http://www.socialworkers.org/pubs/code/code.asp)

Some areas of expertise include crisis intervention and other forms of brief or short-term treatment, working with family systems to strengthen older adults' coping abilities and informal support systems, resolving barriers to service utilization.[6]

Introduction to Team Development, Function, and Maintenance

Organizational Support

At the outset of an effort to form an interdisciplinary team, consideration must be given to the team's role in the context of the larger organizational structure of the institution. Teams require time and energy to develop into productive groups. The organization should support the use of resources and time for team activities, rather than other patient care activities, and a method should be established to evaluate the performance of the team. Ideally, resources should exist for problem solving and other activities to support improved team function.[7] While time used for team development will almost certainly result in increased trust between two members of different disciplines as each learns and appreciates the skills of the other, both the team and the institution must acknowledge that this time will not be spent on other valuable (and profitable) activities.[8] In addition to considering the implications of time spent on team-building activities, the team and supporting institution must carefully consider space and facilities issues, including the need for places to house team meetings and family conferences as well as a workspace for each provider. Teams or team leaders should consider involving institutional administration as soon as possible into the process, to establish systems to address the team's space and facilities requirements.[9]

Administrative Structure

Traditionally, clinicians report to their discipline-based supervisors, who usually have infrequent contact with other supervisors. When additional opinion is needed, clinicians generally seek colleagues of the same discipline. Such diffusion of supervision and clinical decision making does not foster collaboration. Instead, the matrix organization may facilitate clinical effectiveness. In this model, an interdisciplinary team can be seen as an administrative unit and all members report to the same supervisor. Each supervisor can manage several teams and in turn report to the director of health services.[1] As a unit, members share the same budget, accountability for outcome, and office space.[10]

Team Membership

In order to be successful, an interdisciplinary team must be more than a simple group of professionals working in the same setting. Team members must both work together to provide care to patients and provide crucial support to each other. Those clinicians who do not appreciate the value of different perspectives or who have little interest in alternative viewpoints will not make the best team members. Team members need to be willing to work within the context of the group and move away from a discipline-centered practice in order to appreciate the contributions of other team members. Just as important, clinicians must also be motivated to participate in the team and be willing and able to make the time to participate in ongoing team activities. In addition to the clinical evaluation of the patient, each interdisciplinary team member should be able to take time to attend team meetings and conferences, teach and learn from fellow team members, and work with the group to achieve its goals. Lastly, while different perspectives and cultural diversity are assets to the team, it is important to consider team members who share a similar vision or mission.[10–12] Successful team members often share common philosophies, experiences, and a feeling of investment in the well-being of the team as a whole. This concept of "total stakeholder satisfaction" implies that the team strives for both patient satisfaction as well as the satisfaction of every member of the team.[13] When problems arise, the team members must assist one another to overcome the obstacle and ensure that the needs of the whole team (from the patient to each team member) are met.[13,14]

Team Goals

An effective team requires a common language and understanding of team goals, which include patient care philosophy and quality standards.[10] Once formed, the team should consider drafting goal statements that describe both general goals for the type of care the team can provide overall and, upon initial contact with new patients, specific goals for particular individuals or families, which consider the current situation and available resources. Philosophically, jointly developing a team mission and vision results in a unified approach to patient care. Practically, the process can clarify differences in terminology, and understanding the role and patient care approach of other disciplines can enhance collaboration and reduce redundancy and costs. Developing a common goal is an important step in starting an interdisciplinary team. New members of an existing team should be oriented to the team goal.

Goal development must go beyond simply coordinating each individual discipline's list of desired outcomes to offer truly integrated, interdisciplinary care.[13] The ideal team goal-setting situation would involve some form of open "brainstorming" session in which team members freely offer suggestions with a related discussion of the inevitable issues of overlap and conflict. Once all suggestions have been voiced, the team can refine this list and express specific performance goals. The team members must be able to focus on outcomes that are achievable in order to maximize use of the resources available.[7] Once common goals are established, individual team members can offer their unique services to contribute to the achievement of the overall goal.

Failure of the team members to integrate their plans into the larger common goals can result in turf battles and conflicts over prioritization and power.[13] As conflict over goals is inevitable, it is important for team members to consider how to deal with differences of opinion. One or more strategies may be utilized to manage the conflict, depending on the situation: negotiation and compromise, changing the structure of the system, or as a last resort, the loss of team members because of the conflict.[7]

Training Teams

Training needs include knowledge of tasks of other discipline as well as functioning collaboratively. As roles and responsibilities are overlapping in an interdisciplinary team, cross-training of similar tasks should begin before switching the mode of operation. Cross-training does not mean that each team member becomes an expert at the other disciplines. It means understanding the perspectives and basic content and being able to perform tasks of other disciplines that are similar to one's own. Take medical history interview as an example: Instead of each discipline collecting information that is relevant to that discipline only (which most certainly will overlap to some extent with other disciplines), a comprehensive interview would yield information useful to many. After the initial phase of cross-training, team members continue to educate each other as responsibility sharing continues. Initially, members may insist on their own interpretation and seek support from colleagues of the same discipline but outside the team. The goal is to foster acceptance of the team assessment.[10] A successful team is characterized by members' ability to incorporate each other's perspectives and to plan together.[1]

Leadership and Power Structure

The leadership and power structure of the team will have significant effects on team productivity and innovation. While there are usually several disciplines represented on the health-care team, in one survey physicians tended to influence the majority of treatment decisions, followed by PTs, speech and hearing therapists, and OTs.[15] In Chapter 12 of this text the authors discuss this as one of the main barriers to interdisciplinary health care, and it is specifically addressed later in this chapter. Although traditionally physicians have been solely responsible for medical decision making and legal liability, in the practice of modern health care other team members share the personal and legal responsibility for patient outcomes. Ultimately, all team members participate in the discussion of the clinical case and decision making at some point, though possibly not for every patient.[7,9]

The leadership role of the team may be undertaken by any of the members. While the leader or leaders may provide organization and structure to team meetings, he or she must also be able to execute goal-oriented tasks (encouraging discussion and expression of ideas about a particular problem) and team-supportive tasks (elaboration of various points of view, mediating differences, managing conflict).[7] Other tasks of the team leader include process analyzer, ambassador, facilitator, creator, follower, and reviewer.[16] Teams may choose either one person as a leader or to rotate leadership responsibilities. In some cases, leadership for a particular patient may change due to the needs of the patient. Regardless of the choice of the leader, research has supported the hypothesis that leadership must be clearly established and that failure to do so can be associated with lower levels of team innovation or reduced productivity.[7,17] The team leader is chosen based on rapport with the patient and the complexity of needs. Although the primary-care clinician will probably see the patient in the initial visit, it is not necessary, or even preferable, that he or she be the team leader as the leader needs to assume more than the clinical role.

Interpersonal Communication and Conflict

Even after the careful selection of team members and diligent efforts in team building and training, many factors can conspire to sabotage a successful team. Successful team members must have effective communication skills including a willingness to listen empathetically and demonstrate that they have indeed heard and understand the situation being discussed.[13] While they need not socialize outside of work, members must maintain mutual respect of each other's disciplines and opinions.[9] Interpersonal discord resulting in issues that cannot be resolved can affect both individual team members and the group as a functioning entity. The loss of a team member can affect the balance of an entire team. Likewise, once a team is developed, the addition of new members may result in the need to reestablish individual roles and interpersonal connections.[7]

In order for team members to carry out their assigned parts of the treatment plan, they must have access to information from other team members. Role conflict may arise as various team members struggle to determine who is best suited to offer a particular service, especially if more than one member feels qualified (or entitled) to do so. Likewise, it may also be difficult for individual practitioners who have an established relationship with a given patient to become accustomed to "sharing" the care of that patient.[9] An effective approach to dealing with these issues is to plan for conflict to occur and establish a well-defined system to address it when it does. The team should develop a formula or process which offers the freedom to bring up issues of role conflict, interpersonal differences, and other problems in a nonjudgmental manner in order to resolve these differences.[7] Some strategies for conflict management include setting standards for practice and norms for team behavior, encouraging each member of the team to contribute, listening to different opinions, and brainstorming solutions as a team.[18]

Interpersonal issues that harm team dynamics may result from personality incompatibilities or from differences in philosophies of practice and cultures. Each profession approaches the patient with an ultimate goal in mind, and this goal is sometimes in implicit or explicit conflict. The physician's goal may be to diagnose and cure disease, while the nurse may focus on patient comfort and the pharmacist may focus on safe and effective use of drug therapy. While none of these goals seems to be in direct conflict with the others, a lack of identification and appreciation of each different philosophy may result in the perception that other caregivers are not appropriately "focused" in their care of the patient.[8]

The fact that team members may come to the team with various levels of health-care experience and geriatric knowledge can pose a threat to the successful team. Members with more experience in health care will be more familiar with medical diagnoses and interventions and may inadvertently downplay the importance of contributions of less experienced members of the team. Likewise, some disciplines may incorporate more specific geriatric knowledge into curriculums than others, possibly resulting in feelings of inadequacy in those members with less specialized training. For example, medical and nursing team members may be well versed in physical changes associated with aging and social work or counseling team members, while less attuned to the physical aspects of aging, are well versed in the psychosocial changes associated with aging. Team development must anticipate that team members bring various levels of training and knowledge to the team, and care must be taken to ensure that all members of the team value the different experiences, education, and perspectives of the each team member.[8]

Lastly, failures of communication across disciplines can cause conflict within the interdisciplinary health-care team. Each discipline has a specific professional language and shorthand; a failure to clarify discipline- or pro-fession-specific terms can result in misinterpretation by other clinicians and possibly increase distrust among the team members. This sort of miscommu-nication can be avoided both by establishing a comfortable culture in which team members feel able to ask for clarification and by working to identify pos-sible language overlaps and inconsistencies as they arise.[8]

Decision Making

Decision-making styles vary from team to team; there are a number of deci-sion-making styles that can be effective in the interdisciplinary team setting, depending on team composition and goals of the team. A team may choose to use a democratic style, where decisions are based on the majority opinion of team members, or an autocratic or "executive" style, where decisions are ulti-mately made by one or two team members. Compromise or consensual deci-sion making is less common but involves treatment decisions that are ultimately accepted by all team members, if not preferred by everyone.[15] Teams may also use more than one style based on the needs of the particular patient case. The degree to which the members agree on a particular decision may affect their motivation to carry out a particular plan, and if a team cannot reach a compro-mise, it may delay the ultimate progression of objectives for the patient.[7]

Several reports describe the use of personality profiling questionnaires to help team members recognize individual character attributes that may affect team functioning. In one study, using the Myers-Briggs Type Indicator helped teams to realize the potential for conflict and assisted the team in developing ways to avoid conflict. These activities can also serve as an "icebreaker" for the team members to get to know one another better.[19] Another study found that the DISC Personality Profile helped team trainees both to understand their own personality type and work styles as well as to provide insight into the characteristics of other members of the team.[8]

Other Roles Within the Interdisciplinary Health-Care Team

Once team leadership is clarified, the roles of each of the other members must be defined. Ideally, the role of each member of the interdisciplinary team should be defined at the outset but remain flexible enough to allow for unan-ticipated situations. Many of these roles are interdependent, with members of the team relying on the information and expertise of other members to com-plete their own review. There is no set requirement for the type of disciplines involved in the interdisciplinary team.[20] Almost always, the team will include a physician or nurse-practitioner. These core members, although they may be responsible for assembling the team of professionals who will be involved in the care of a particular patient, may not necessarily act as team leader. The inpatient setting will also include a nurse. In geriatrics, extended team members would very often include a PT, OT, social worker, nutritionist, pharmacist, and psychologist; other clinicians are included as needed. Depending on the needs of the patient, nonclinical professionals, such as clergy and legal counsel, may also be involved. Individualization is the key to team composition. Even in the same work setting, different patients will be cared for by teams comprised of different disciplines. The size of the team should depend on patient need and characteristics, as well as logistical issues such as meeting space and administrative support. As assessment and care plans are done collaboratively, team members need to be available for meetings.[12] In addition, having a high motivation for the interdisciplinary approach is also essential.

Conclusion

As highlighted in several chapters of this text, geriatric care lends itself to working with a group of health professionals. The team-based approach to geriatric care was recommended by the National Institutes of Health in its 1998 Consensus Statement, which encouraged the involvement of clinicians from many health disciplines in the assessment of the geriatric patient, and likewise the Institute of Medicine's report *Health Professions Education: A Bridge to Quality* highlighted the need for health-care professionals to work in interdisciplinary teams to ensure that health care is continuous and reliable.[21,22] In order for these teams to be successful, health professionals need to be trained both in team development and in how to function within an interdisciplinary team.[8,9] Ideally, this training is initiated in an interdisciplinary educational setting and continues when professionals move from the academic setting into practice.[22]

This type of environment can be demanding but personally and professionally rewarding. The interdisciplinary model is an effective patient care model. It offers clinicians a refreshingly different practice mode and collaboration among different disciplines. It is also extremely valuable for clinician trainees to be exposed to this practice model as they can be the agents of change in their professions.

Application to the Case Study: The Older Adult Care, Training, Research, and Planning Program

There are three steps to forming an interdisciplinary team in the Older Adult Care, Training, Research, and Planning Program (OACTRPP). The first is planning and organization. This includes allocation of office and clinic space for the different disciplines; setting up billing procedures, especially if the patient is cared for by clinical specialists who are non-OACTRPP staff; and determining organizational structure and line of reporting. The second is to set aside time for the training of the team, and this mostly involves establishing interdisciplinary goals, developing team work, and training team members as preceptors. The OACTRPP may choose to hire professional team trainers or to invite members of established interdisciplinary teams from other institutions or to do a self-study with available curriculum.

Before forming an interdisciplinary team for each patient, the OACTRPP needs to identify a primary-care clinician who will see the patient in the initial visit. A case conference can be called to discuss and specify the initial role and responsibility of each discipline for the patient. Team members will also identify a team leader, establish an overarching goal, identify the patient's problems and their impact on health and quality of life, identify resources that the patient has for each of the problems, decide what additional information is needed, and form a care plan with expected outcomes. Additional disciplines may join the team depending on the team's assessment.

As the team evolves and matures, it would be desirable to conduct periodic evaluations on the functioning of the team as well as clinical effectiveness. In addition, regular further training would be beneficial for existing and new members as well as clinician trainees.

Classroom Exercise

1. Appreciating health-care disciplines begins with knowing the basics about each one. With an interdisciplinary group, have a representative from each discipline prepare a short summary addressing the following about their profession: didactic training, experiential training (if applicable), credentialing, professional scope of practice, possible overlap with other professionals. Have each person present a summary, and then open the floor for questions from other participants.

2. Review the case about Ms. Whelan in Chapter 12. Consider each of the issues or problems that need to be addressed in her care. Which profession(s) might be traditionally responsible for each issue or problem? Then, brainstorm and think of other disciplines that might be able to address the problem in an interdisciplinary team. Is there much overlap? Which professionals make up the core of your team? Which ones might you call in on a consultant basis? How would your team function?

Bibliography

Jablonski, R., Cifu, D.X., Boling, P.A., Slattum, P.W., Peyton, A.L., Netting, F.E., Parham, I.A., Wood, J.B. Case study: Geriatric Interdisciplinary Team Training. Age in Action 1999;14(Winter). Available at: http://www.vcu.edu/vcoa/ageaction/agew99.htm#Case%20Study.

Rush University Medical Center. Geriatric Interdisciplinary Team Training Program. Available at: http://www.rush.edu/professionals/training/geriatrics/index.html.

Siegler, E.L., Hyer, K., Fulmer, T., Mezey, M. (eds.) Geriatric Interdisciplinary Team Training. New York: Springer, 1998.

References

1. Satin, D.G. Theoretical issues of interdisciplinary education and practice. In: Satin, D.G. (ed.) The Clinical Care of the Aged Person: An Interdisciplinary Perspective. New York: Oxford University Press, 1994, pp. 404–425.

2. Spratley, E., Johnson, A., Sochalski, J., Fritz, M., Spencer, W. The registered nurse population: findings from the National Sample Survey of Registered Nurses, March, 2000. U.S. Department of Health and Human Services Health Resources and Service Administration, Bureau of Health Professions, Division of Nursing. Available at: http://bhpr.hrsa.gov/healthworkforce/reports/rnsurvey/default.htm. 2000. Accessed March 3, 2004.

3. American College of Nurse Practitioners. What is a nurse practitioner? Available at: http://www.acnpweb.org/i4a/pages/index.cfm?pageid=3479. 2004. Accessed March 3, 2004.

4. American Academy of Nurse Practitioners. Scope of practice for nurse practitioners. Available at: http://www.aanp.org/NR/rdonlyres/edhltucoxqd2xnrfwbve26d3cowleh5-rqqcfmhlcoi3sp7ihpzxry7rdqtkezw5zvpggxsuc7z4iao/scope+of+practice+v2.pdf. 2002. Accessed March 3, 2004.

5. Buppert, C. Billing for nurse practitioner services: guidelines for NP's, physicians, employers, and insurers. Medscape Nurses 2002;4(1). Available at: http://www.medscape.com. Accessed March 4, 2004.

6. John A. Hartford Foundation. Gerontological social work. Available at: http://www.gswi.org/. 1998. Accessed November 29, 2004.

7. Siegel, B.S. Developing the interdisciplinary team. In: Satin, D.G. (ed.) The Clinical Care of the Aged Person: An Interdisciplinary Perspective. New York: Oxford University Press, 1994, pp. 404–425.

8. Mellor, M.J., Hyer, K., Howe, J.L. The geriatric interdisciplinary team approach: challenges and opportunities in educating trainees together from a variety of disciplines. Educational Gerontology 2002;28:867–880.

9. Castle, J. Planning GITT: the providers. In: Siegler, E.L., Hyer, K., Fulmer, T., Mezey, M. (eds.) Geriatric Interdisciplinary Team Training. New York: Springer, 1998, pp. 63–75.

10. Bowers, B., Esmond, S., Holloway, E. Creating an Integrated, Consumer Centered Care Team. Madison: University of Wisconsin, 1996.

11. Cowell, J. Flawless teams. Executive Excellence 2000;17:3.

12. Hill, K. Build a dream team. Nursing Management 2001;32:37–38.
13. Gage, M.M. From independence to interdependence: creating synergistic health-care teams. Journal of Nursing Administration 1998;28(4):17–26.
14. Pfeiffer, E. Why teams? In: Siegler, E.L., Hyer, K., Fulmer, T., Mezey, M. (eds.) Geriatric Interdisciplinary Team Training. New York: Springer, 1998, pp. 13–19.
15. Fiorelli, J.S. Power in work groups: team member's perspectives. Human Relations 1988;41:1–12.
16. Drinker, T., Clark, P. Healthcare Teamwork: Interdisciplinary Practice and Teaching. Westport, CT: Greenwood, 2000.
17. West, M.A., Borill, C.S., Dawson, J.F., Brodbeck, F., Shapiro, D.A., Haward, B. Leadership clarity and team innovation in health care. Leadership Quarterly 2003;14:393–410.
18. Grant, R.W., Finocchio, L.J., California Primary Care Consortium Subcommittee on Interdisciplinary Collaboration. Interdisciplinary collaborative teams in primary care: a model curriculum and resource guide. San Francisco: Pew Health Professions Commission, 1995.
19. Clinebell, S., Stecher, M. Teaching teams to be teams: an exercise using the Myers-Briggs® Type Indicator and the five factor personality traits. Journal of Management Education 2003;27:362–383.
20. Wieland, D., Kramer, B.J., Waite, M.S., Laurence, Z. The interdisciplinary team in geriatric care (perspectives on chronic illness: treating patients and delivering care). American Behavioral Scientist 1996;39(6):655–665.
21. National Institutes of Health. Geriatric assessment methods for clinical decision making. National Institutes of Health Consensus Development Conference Statement October 19–21, 1987. Available at: http://consensus.nih.gov/1987/1987G eriatricAssessment065html.htm. Accessed February 2, 2004.
22. Greiner, A.C., Knebel, E. (eds.) Health Professions Education: A Bridge to Quality. Washington, DC: National Academies Press, 2003.

14

Functioning Interdisciplinary Teams

A. The Mt. Auburn Hospital Multiple Sclerosis Comprehensive Care Center

LINDA Y. BUCHWALD AND NANCY A. LOWENSTEIN

WITH KATHLEEN LEAHY, SOCIAL WORKER; DONALD MEYER, PSYCHIATRIST; STEVEN MOSKOWITZ, PHYSIATRIST; SUSAN NUTILE, NURSE/TEAM COORDINATOR; AND ANN PISANI, PHYSICAL THERAPIST

Rationale

Multiple sclerosis (MS) is a complex disorder which engenders a multitude of problems and needs, all of which present many challenges in the areas of medical management, psychosocial intervention, and neurorehabilitation. There are challenges relating to integration and use of community resources and advocacy and problems navigating the current health-care system with a complex, chronic disorder such as MS. Complexity is added by currently evolving criteria and guidelines set by insurance companies or health-care plans, as to different types and frequencies of covered services. The prescribing physician's care must be integrated with insurance plan eligibility. Information regarding eligibility must be kept updated and accurate.

There is need for cost efficacy and for comprehensive streamlined care. The interdisciplinary team approach to MS care has been proven to be cost-effective, with decreased complications, nursing home admissions, and acute hospitalizations. Also documented have been decreased disability and handicap with increased independence and decreased caregiver burden.

The health care of an individual with MS requires professionals from numerous different disciplines. It is important that each discipline knows what the others are doing. There are multiple multifaceted health-care needs that are interdependent and interresponsive. No one provider can encompass the depth of expertise required to deal with the range of MS needs effectively. One must eliminate problems from multiple perspectives and call for all professional expertise to be brought to the fore in order to be integrated into the evaluation, education, and intervention comprising effective health care. The nature of MS, its complexity and unpredictability, and the fact that there is no specific cure or prevention in the face of a disease which is compatible with normal life span calls for numerous professionals with new, ever-expanding, progressively more sophisticated roles in neurology, rehabilitation, and the psychosocial sciences.

The providers caring for persons with MS share common concerns and needs:

- Safety of patient, caregivers, and clinical professionals and paraprofessionals
- Fragmentation of care and lack of a cohesive care plan
- Conflicting priorities and goals
- Differing and perhaps unrealistic expectations on the part of individuals with MS and their families/caregivers
- Feelings of frustration and of being overwhelmed on the part of persons with MS, their families/caregivers, and professional care providers
- Lack of compliance
- Needs for education and communication
- Cost efficacy

Caring for patients with a disease with no cure or prevention yet compatible with a normal life span is challenging. A "wellness" approach—one that espouses the maintenance of optimal health within the physical and emotional confines of the disorder—manages the primary symptoms of the disease, those directly related to the disease process of inflammatory demyelination of the brain, spinal cord, and optic nerves resulting in symptoms such as weakness, numbness, tingling, difficulty walking, tremor, etc. Secondary symptoms must be addressed as well, including complications such as urinary tract and respiratory infections, skin breakdown, etc. There is need, as well, to address tertiary symptoms related to the MS such as loss of employment.

The best and most efficient way for multiple health-care professionals involved in the management of MS to deliver comprehensive care is with an interdisciplinary team working closely together with the inclusion of a principal care provider.

Problems and Obstructions

It is possible for one principal care provider, a neurologist with an interest in MS, to work alone and to create a miniteam of referrals; but it is difficult, often overwhelming, and unsatisfying for a variety of reasons. Communications are multitudinous and laborious. The various providers see different perspectives of the same individual with MS at different times. There is considerable duplication. Therefore, with some experience in medical training in the Albert Einstein Neurology training programs and Montefiore Hospital and Medical Center, where some of the earliest efforts in interdisciplinary care took place, the chief of Neurology at Mt. Auburn Hospital in Cambridge, Massachusetts (a Harvard Medical School–affiliated teaching hospital), embarked upon an initiative to institute an interdisciplinary team to care for individuals with MS. The care center initiative was discussed with key individuals within the hospital organization and, with the assistance of Labe C. Scheinberg, MD, dean and chair of Neurology at the Albert Einstein School of Medicine and cofounder of the Consortium of MS Centers, the leadership at Mt. Auburn Hospital was convinced to proceed with the MS Interdisciplinary Comprehensive Care Center. A proposal was written and presented to the Medical Executive Board and forwarded to the hospital Board of Trustees, both of which approved.

Getting started, even once there was approval, was not straightforward. An effort was made to assess the extent of the problem: How many persons with MS resided in the commonwealth? How many in the hospital catchment area? How many were unserved? How many underserved? The Central New England Chapter of the National Multiple Sclerosis Society was very helpful in providing figures from their needs assessment data and have remained an integral support ever since. In 1991 the Mt. Auburn Hospital Multiple Sclerosis Comprehensive Care Center (MAHMSCCC) became a reality, and in 2000 it became the first clinical center in the state of Massachusetts to affiliate with the National MS Society.

Space and resources needed to be allocated. Neurology at Mt. Auburn Hospital is a division in the Department of Medicine, and as a division, it had little political clout and access to resources. It had little representation on committees that allocate budget and space items. The space allocated was shared with the Division of Hematology/Oncology, with the only time availability for the MS Center being at night. The space was "perfect," with a comfortable, central waiting area surrounded by an adequate number of consultation and examination rooms. However, with the growth of hematology/oncology, the space was remodeled and the MS interdisciplinary team found itself with a new home in the general outpatient clinic area. Initially, the MS center was given the use of consultation and examination rooms, a place to store equipment, a filing cabinet, and a place for the high–low examination and treatment table purchased for physical therapy. The general waiting area was not amenable to the peer counseling and educational components of the team program, nor was it compliant with the Health Insurance Portability and Accountability Act (or HIPAA). Consultation rooms have been shifted and reduced in number, storage space has been taken away, equipment has been stolen since there is no space in which to lock it away, and even the high–low treatment table has been taken over and broken by the ambulatory clinic laboratory personnel. Our evening hours, we have discovered, have been helpful in enabling family and caregiver involvement in the client treatment. Multiple sclerosis impacts the whole family; it moves in with them. It is important to educate not only the patient but also the family and any other caregivers. It is important to identify those individuals who might support or sabotage team efforts and deal with them in a timely fashion. Having family members available in the evening to drive a person with MS to and from the clinic facilitates transportation.

The financial support provided to the clinic by the hospital, in addition to the space allocated, has included a half-time and later full-time nursing position, a portion of a social worker's time, and a small portion of secretarial/receptionist/clerical time from the Division of Neurology staff or from the ambulatory care staff. The medical director has had to become involved in fund-raising and grant requests in order to adequately complement hospital resources needed to support the center.

Recruitment

Once space and time were allocated, the team needed to be constituted. Ingredients for a successful team have included interest and availability to work with the team—at the Mt. Auburn Hospital team, this means working in the evening and staying for team meetings as well as being available for family/team conferences and for informal discussion with persons with MS, their families, and other team members. Experience has not been as critical for success as has interest and commitment. The physicians have worked on a fee-for-service basis, which has brought problems. The psychiatrists have not been enrolled in many health plans, and they have not generally billed for their services, nor do they have billing services. A psychologist is not covered by some insurers for outpatient services. For psychiatry and physiatry, hospital funding in addition to the grant money has been necessary to provide for contracted services. The physical and occupational therapists were initially on contract with the hospital; more recently, they have been hospital employees. Hospital billing has been a complex issue as well, with much time and energy devoted to developing proper billing for the MS clinic.

A seven-member team has met once a week, currently in the hospital ambulatory care area. The nurse coordinator has an office in the neurology division, and the neurologist and nurse see individuals with MS throughout the workweek in their offices.

The Team

The team size has varied, but it usually consists of seven members, generating 21 relationships. The primary team members include a neurologist who is the medical director, a nurse coordinator, a physiatrist (a specialist in rehabilitation medicine), a psychiatrist, a social worker, a physical therapist, and an occupational therapist. The team has had access to a speech therapist, a durable medical equipment vendor, an orthotist, and a chaplain to address the spiritual side of well-being. All team members define their roles, interests, and primary and secondary areas of competency. These areas may overlap; this helps team members to reinforce each other's efforts. All members share their impressions upon evaluation as well as their opinions and contribute to the overall evaluation and care planning for each individual with MS coming to the clinic.

How the Center Works

Evaluation and screening

Evaluation and screening of individuals with MS for referral to the MAHMSCCC is carried out by the medical director and principal care provider, a neurologist. This evaluation includes a detailed neurological assessment including review of past medical records. There is a focus on prior medical and pharmaceutical therapeutic management, the participation of the individual in past rehabilitation efforts, and their responses to interventions. The prescribing physicians are responsible for the ordering of medications, therapies, and durable medical equipment and for referrals, with input and decisions by the entire team.

Periodic neurological reassessment is carried out every 3–6 months by the neurologist, either in the center setting or in the private office, and, when necessary, referral back to the center is made if the individual is not concurrently followed there. If the patient has remained active in the center, then follow-up by neurology as well as other disciplines is scheduled there.

The nurse coordinator receives the initial referral to the clinic and performs an in-person or telephone assessment interview with the individual. She then schedules the appointments with the necessary team members.

Each individual with MS is referred into the center with a medical record, which includes the initial neurological/neurorehabilitation assessment and the coordinating nurse interview materials. The individual is then seen by the remainder of the team of health-care professionals in order to address his or her needs with as much breadth and depth as possible. As much as is feasible, "one-stop shopping" is achieved. In between appointments individuals with MS and their family members can participate in educational and peer counseling programs.

Team leadership

As with all teams, the interdisciplinary team needs leadership. At the MAHMSCCC, the principal care provider, the neurologist, is the medical director of the center. This person is the prescribing physician of record and is held accountable for the care, services, and therapies ordered and the education of individuals with MS with regard to clinical issues and any educational initiatives of the center.

Leadership is also provided by the nurse coordinator, who arranges the clinic schedule and coordinates and case manages the care. She also attends to a variety of nursing needs, such as teaching immune modulation therapy, injection technique, other self-care skills, and primary health-care needs such as exercise, bowel and bladder habit, and skin care. The leaders must be the keeper of the vision, which is the safe, optimal function and independence of individuals with MS, with reduction of disability and handicap and the maintenance of optimal health given the physical and emotional confines of the disorder. This overall goal must be considered in terms of quality of life—the fulfillment of potential, life goals, and roles of the individual with MS—at home, within the community, and in society in general. The vision includes the reestablishment of psychological equilibrium of the individuals with their disorder, the maintenance of their relationships, and, finally, the encouragement of a creative and productive life.

The medical director must facilitate relationships among team members, set the agenda, address team conflicts with consensus, and keep the team on track. The leader must make sure that all team members have expressed their opinions, have been heard, and are valued.

The leadership should function to keep members communicating: to make sure that planning is cohesive, logical, and progressive; that the team is oriented to the individual with MS and their families/caregivers; and that the team remains on task. When dealing with complex problems, team members must communicate in order to make sure there is integration of care and that they don't go in multiple directions and produce "comprehensive fragmentation." It is important, too, that there is a liaison with any institution, agency, or group dealing with the individual with MS, such as a home-care team, a rehabilitation hospital staff, or a hospital discharge case manager. This liaison person is most often the nurse coordinator.

Team conflict must be handled at team meetings under the leadership of the medical director and generally by consensus building.

The process

All team members complete an assessment, and each MS center session concludes with a team meeting. All team members present the results of their assessments, problems are identified, and solutions are offered. All aspects of the care of each person with MS are discussed. The individual with MS, the family, and other caregivers are considered essential consultants to the team; and the values, interest, goals, and priorities of the individual with MS are all taken into consideration. Assessments and recommendations of consultants to the primary team are integrated into the assessment and planning. From the in-depth comprehensive assessment comes a consistent, logically therapeutic approach and, with it, a comprehensive care plan. Solutions of problems are assigned to members of the team on the basis of interest, competence, and specific circumstances. The disciplines might work individually or jointly. The roles and assignments might shift with new resources and as new needs arise. The team encourages the interest and expertise of its professional members, and together the team enjoys cross-stimulation with enriched creative problem solving.

Assumptions

The individual with MS is expected to be a responsible team participant. Care plans encourage independence and self-reliance and foster the individual's independence, which allows the individual with MS to cope successfully and to learn from and feel supported and encouraged by the team.

The individuals with MS must be considered within the context of their environments and their society, particularly within their community of care. At times there is need for outreach to be made to other services (legal, advocacy, family, educational, architectural services, commissions of protection of persons with disability, etc.).

The team must make an effort to improve health maintenance because staying healthy impacts positively on the course of the disease. The team encourages active participation and responsibility on the part of individuals with MS in areas such as stress reduction, regular exercise, energy conservation, healthy diet, reduction of unhealthy habits such as smoking and overeating, and, finally, adhering to medical and other therapeutic regimens.

Team mainstays

Comprehensive teamwork. Comprehensive evaluation, problem identification, cohesive planning, and case management collaboratively promote the overall health care of individuals with MS to keep them safe, independent, and in control, fulfilling their roles as individuals and leading productive and creative lives. Follow-through is a requisite for success. Periodic evaluation is necessary; in addition, follow-up is done when there is a change in condition or an increase in impairment. There is need to monitor the effects of the disease upon the nervous system (impairments), on physiological and psychological functioning (disability), and on function in terms of family, community, and society (handicap).

Communication. Channels of communication must be kept open, including informing the prescribing physician, primary-care physician, and consultants of the team's work. There must be communication between home health aides and personal care attendants and their supervisory professionals. Communication among team members is a prerequisite for success and includes the following:

a. Team meetings: There is a need to "team up" once a week after individual assessments are completed.
b. Other interteam communications, such as e-mail, conference call, or fax.
c. There is a need to keep informed and communicate with primary-care physicians, particularly if they are the prescribing physicians and are held accountable for ordering the care and services managed by the team.
d. Family/team conferences: In addition to regular team meetings and informal communications, there is sometimes need for family/team conferences. At the MAHMSCCC this is generally orchestrated by the social worker. It is important that everyone is getting the same information at the same time, particularly in regard to goals and priorities, and it is important that patients and families have had input into the setting of goals and priorities as this is essential for adherence and success.
e. Team meeting conference notes: Details of decision-making, task and role assignment, responsibility for solutions, and other interventions are recorded in the team meeting conference notes. These, along with reports from each discipline, are sent to primary-care providers, referring neurologists, and pertinent consultants.
f. The team or its representative, the medical director or nurse coordinator, at times need to communicate or even meet with insurance company personnel, case managers, or other administrators to facilitate support, especially for financial coverage of services.

Outcomes anticipated

The health-care professionals working as a team provide hope, counsel, guidance, and treatment, which can have an invaluable impact on the lives of people with MS in their quest for independence. It offers control over the negative aspects of the disease. The team aspires to meet complex challenges efficiently and comprehensively. It helps people with MS to develop skills and strengths, to compensate for lost function, and to establish a healthy, positive attitude. We attempt to give these people the feeling that the team is with them to go the distance to wherever that may lead. It offers a hopeful, supportive environment and a comprehensive consistent therapeutic approach while encouraging independence and self-reliance.

In regard to the team itself, members experience the fostering and enrichment of professional practice and growth as multiple needs, systems, and disciplines interact. The team itself has had an ongoing development of competence, style, and identity. It has progressively functioned more as a whole, with the whole being greater than the sum of its parts. The several instances in which a team member has been lost have been traumatic. It can take 6–12 months to rebuild equilibrium and establish new identity. With time, teamwork has become more streamlined and understanding of the clinical problems more comprehensive as identified from multiple disciplinary perspectives. There has been enrichment of the care given upon exposure of one discipline to another, one talent to another, with deepening of insight and appreciation into the professional needs and practice of individual team members. There is cross-stimulation, with progressively greater creativity in problem solving.

The commitment and motivation of team members have been infectious, particularly in the face of improved outcomes in regard to individuals with MS. Growth and morale have been maintained by expanding the program with new challenges and new associations, such as a durable medical equipment vendor and orthotist willing to come to team sessions. It has also come with new programs, such as a caregivers' support series done in conjunction with the Boston University occupational therapy program and an all-day symposium offered by the team to those with MS and their families under the sponsorship of the National MS Society. Growth has occurred through team members attending continuing professional education programs. And most of all it has come through positive outcomes, that is, through the improvement and function of individuals with MS, reduction of their impairment, increased activity and participation, and the resolution of the problems they encounter on a regular basis.

Advocacy

Most programs and services for the neurologically impaired and disabled cannot function without financial resources. It has been important for professionals and other advocates for individuals with MS to become aware of funding mechanisms. In a country in which basic services and delivery programs are heavily subsidized by federal and state funds, it is important to understand the basics of public funding systems as well as private funding resources. The federal and state budget systems define and reflect our priorities as a nation, and provision for the chronically ill and disabled has depended on a complex interaction of private citizens and organizations, state and local governments, executive branch policy makers, and members of Congress and state legislators. (This is discussed in detail in Chapter 6.) As advocates for individuals with MS, team members have needed to understand the budget process and how to influence it so that appropriate services and benefits are included in federal and state budgets. Not only has the MS team reached out to community services for equipment, housekeeping, medical, and other funding, as well as for the protection of disabled individuals, but team members have also become involved in assisting individuals with MS in navigating the health-care system and in enjoying their due rights. The team has found itself also engaging, along with persons with MS and their families and with the National MS Society, in lobby efforts.

In these times that are so tumultuous in health care, the MAHMSCCC is appreciative of the support of its hospital system, particularly of its chief executive officer, in allowing the team to persevere in what it believes to be a model of care for those with chronic illness and disability in this country in the twenty-first century. This is the interdisciplinary care model which offers a coordinated problem-solving and therapeutic effort so that those with MS may achieve more functional, safe, healthy, productive, creative, and satisfying lives.

Specific Roles of the MAHMSCCC Team Members

Role of the neurologist/medical director
LINDA Y. BUCHWALD

The specific role of the physician/neurologist/medical director is to provide the overall medical care and symptomatic medical treatment for the person with MS and to alert team members as to the implications of other health problems, current treatment, and past response to medical, psychosocial, and rehabilitation interventions.

The role of the physician/neurologist begins with an initial comprehensive evaluation of the individual with MS. This must include the collection and review of past medical records, a comprehensive history, and a general physical and neurological examination. A summary and formulation with impression and plan of management is prepared. The management includes initial medical treatments of the disease (immune modulation, immunosuppression, etc.) and the initial symptomatic (pharmaceutical and therapeutic) management, with specific referrals to the MAHMSCCC (providing the patient is deemed suitable for interdisciplinary care), prioritizing appointment scheduling.

In the neurological assessment, the history of the present illness is elicited, including the history of onset and evolution of the disorder, prior workups, and all prior interventions and responses. The history should include place of birth, family history of MS, all symptoms of the disorder, the evolution of any disability, and how it has impacted activities of daily living. The history should target the impact of the disorder upon roles in the family, at work, and in the community. It should include any primary, secondary, or tertiary complications of the disorder. The history should elicit information regarding the acquisition of assistive devices to substitute for failing or lost function.

Past medical history addresses any other prior diagnoses, injuries, surgical procedures, etc. Family history includes not only MS but also other neurological and systemic disorders such as hypertension, diabetes, and Lyme disease.

Social history targets aberrant behavior such as tobacco, alcohol, and drug abuse; exercise or lack of same; exposure to HIV, Lyme disease, or other infectious disorders; medication allergies; living conditions, especially factors of accessibility; work history; and support systems.

Review of systems includes screening of all neurological symptoms, assesses sensorium and affect, and screens for symptoms of systemic diseases.

A general physical examination is performed. A neurological examination is carried out in depth, including mental status, examination of cranial nerves, motor examination, sensory assessment, cerebellar function and coordination, reflex examination, and ambulation or gait.

Summary and formulation should address all impairment, disability, and handicap as well as primary, secondary, and tertiary complications of MS. Formulation should include areas of involvement (visual system, spinal cord, cerebellum, cortical, etc.) and disease characterization as to progression (relapsing remitting, benign sensory, primary or secondary progressive disease). Any other etiological factors regarding the patient's impairment should be noted. Finally, in regard to impression, other concurrent medical diagnoses and significant past medical encounters should be enumerated.

A plan is made with regard to initial management including any further workup indicated, the initiation of medical treatment of the disease with immune modulators/immunosuppressant medications, and symptomatic medical management. Referrals for psychosocial and rehabilitation assessments are made to the MAHMSCCC with prioritization of appointments.

The neurologist provides the nurse coordinator with the neurological assessment and collection of past medical records. The nurse then goes forward with an initial nursing intake.

The patient is referred to the center for an initial evaluation by other team members, after which an initial detailed care plan is drawn up by the entire team, including follow-up appointments.

The patient is referred back to the MAHMSCCC by the neurologist at any time as needs arise. Follow-up is also carried out in the office of the neurologist, performed with or without nursing participation. Teaching and review of immune modulator injection with the person with MS is done by the nurse coordinator in her office.

The neurologist/medical director, with the assistance of the nurse coordinator, completes paperwork, which includes insurance preapproval forms, appeals of denials, letters of medical necessity, letters in support of disability, status and support.

Additional Roles of the Neurologist

1. As team leader/medical director, facilitates open discussion and communication in goal setting
2. Supports patient values and goals of the team
3. Alerts to treatments that may counteract one another
4. Assumes responsibility for overall health care and writing of orders
5. Evaluates ongoing team progress
6. Supports educational programs
7. Relates the team to the hospital Department of Medicine and, with the nurse coordinator, relates the team to the hospital administration
8. Raises funds for the MAHMSCCC
9. With other team members, advocates for the patient (letters and testimony) and advocacy programs (education, national and state MS lobby days, etc.).

Role of the Nurse Coordinator
SUSAN NUTILE

Quality nursing care of individuals with MS requires expertise in the disease process, disease-modifying agents, symptom management, and an appreciation of the impact of MS on individuals and their families. Nursing care for MS utilizes the full spectrum of nursing skills, including assessment, direct care, education, patient and family support, and collaboration with other healthcare professionals.

At the MAHMSCCC, nursing care begins with the neurologist fully assessing the person with MS, creating a medical file, and making referrals to the center for initial evaluations by one or more of the following disciplines: nursing, occupational therapy, physical therapy, social services, psychopharmacology, and rehabilitative medicine. The nurse coordinates the scheduling of these recommended evaluations and obtains health insurance authorization.

In preparation for the MS center visit, all patients undergo a nursing assessment. The nursing assessment interview can take place in the neurology office or via telephone. The goal of the nursing assessment is to gain further understanding of the patient's current status in regard to MS; other health-related problems; impact of the disease on personal, social, and employment lives; and the patient's expectations in regard to the visit. Neurological evaluation and nursing assessment reports are available to the interdisciplinary team members at the time of the patients' first visit.

In addition to the traditional areas of nursing assessment, there is emphasis on the patients' eating patterns and habits; bladder, bowel, and sexual function; skin care; sleep patterns; alternative or holistic remedies; adherence to prescribed medications; and problems in access to diagnostics and therapeutic services. The nursing assessment also includes information on the patient's living situation and support system, use of adaptive equipment, safety concerns, and emergency preparedness. Current and past MS medications are reviewed, as are the responses to those medications. A review is made of the patient's current MS symptoms and how these symptoms are being managed. Psychosocial issues are explored, as are the patient's perceptions and understanding of symptoms and their management. Clarification and education target the patient's knowledge and understanding of MS and the goal of fostering healthy behaviors.

Based on the MAHMSCCC team comprehensive care plan generated at team meetings, the nurse coordinator documents recommendations and facilitates implementation, communicating the plans to the patients and any caregivers and facilitating follow-up appointments and referrals made to providers outside of the center, such as referral for more intensive rehabilitation or for neurourology and neuro-ophthalmology assessments. Nursing is also responsible for liaisons with other institutions in which the patients are involved, such as the various visiting nursing associations, insurance companies, or hospital case managers. Nursing plays a significant supportive role in immune modulator therapy in the treatment of MS. Once an immune modulator is agreed upon by the individuals with MS and their neurologists, nursing facilitates insurance approval for this costly therapy. Then, with the initiation of immune modulation, nursing provides education in regard to the self-injection procedure, management of side effects, and reinforcement of the rationale and expectations of therapy. Periodic follow-up by neurology and nursing helps to promote proper injection technique and management of adverse side effects, including skin site reactions.

There are occasions where a patient issue may be addressed by any one of several team members, such as the home situation: Is the patient living alone in the home on multiple levels, and how are the household chores managed? These are all areas where any or all team members can intervene as the more input, the better the problem solving. Nursing may overlap with neurology, psychiatry, and rehabilitation medicine in regard to reconciling medications; this may appear reduplicative, yet often clients report different information to different providers. Team members freely confer, and there may be a need to redirect client issues to a more specific discipline. Important messages are reinforced when reiterated by different providers. Historical information is enriched, is more comprehensive, and has broader perspective when elicited by each of the different disciplines.

The neurologist and nurse follow patients admitted to the hospital for acute care to assure their needs are met, to serve as advocates, and as a resource to the nursing and medical staff.

The focus of the nurse should be on assisting patients in the development and maintenance of an independent, satisfying, and healthy lifestyle. The nurse gives support to patients throughout the disease course and deals with unnecessary misconceptions and with patients' concerns and frustrations. The patients' sense of control is enhanced through participation in their own care and as members of the interdisciplinary team. Patient independence is encouraged.

Interdisciplinary Team from an Occupational Therapy Perspective
NANCY LOWENSTEIN

Health professionals often see occupational therapy as the profession that addresses activities of daily living (ADLs) and adaptive equipment. This misunderstanding of the unique skills that occupational therapists bring to the interdisciplinary team could significantly limit the contributions that these professionals can make to the care of patients.

Occupational therapists look at the "occupations" that individuals must do, want to do, and are expected to do and how the individuals view their abilities and priorities. An occupational therapist asks individuals to look at their daily and weekly routines and indicate in what ways their deficits and strengths inhibit or facilitate their abilities to perform these occupations. For instance, people may feel that being able to make meals for themselves is more important than what they wear. The occupational therapist would, therefore, tailor treatment toward meal preparation and not dressing. Occupational therapy looks at the occupational areas of ADLs, instrumental ADLs (IADLs), education, work/volunteer activity, leisure/play activity, and social participation. As a member of the MAHMSCCC, the occupational therapist contributes in many ways to the interdisciplinary team in all those areas.

Primary responsibilities of the occupational therapy professional on this interdisciplinary team are to address the areas of ADLs and IADLs. These include bathing, dressing, hygiene, functional mobility, meal preparation, driving or community mobility, adaptive equipment and assistive technology needs, cognition, perception, and energy conservation and ergonomic issues around use of the body in everyday activities. For individuals who have MS, two important areas that are regularly addressed are fatigue management and cognition. Individuals with MS often have fatigue that significantly impacts their daily functioning. It might influence their ability to work, care for others, and enjoy social time with family and friends. Occupational therapists play a major role in teaching individuals techniques that help them manage fatigue and continue to participate in family life and work. These techniques are called "energy conservation." This often involves teaching new ways to do ADLs and IADLs, supporting patients in implementing exercise programs that the physical therapist gives them, or perhaps working with the social worker in developing new interests and hobbies to pursue in leisure time to help combat depression.

Occupational therapists look at people's psychological well-being and see this as a key component for their ability to engage in their daily occupations. Occupational therapy sessions often build on psychopharmacological or psychiatric findings of the social worker about depression, lack of motivation and hope, family supports, the individual's emotional status, past and current interests, and financial supports. For instance, individuals who are depressed because they are too tired to make meals for their family and are feeling that their role as a caretaker is diminished would benefit from occupational therapy in order to look at how to continue to engage in this important life role. Occupational therapists look at the environmental barriers in the home, work, and community that hinder people from fulfilling these roles. Also, vocational issues, seating, positioning, and mobility needs are addressed. Knowledge of community resources is important in order to be able to connect an individual to appropriate vendors for proper equipment such as wheelchairs and assistive technology, to connect the client to support groups, and to access other community-based activities.

Occupational therapy overlaps with many of the other disciplines that are members of the MAHMSCCC interdisciplinary team. Each discipline is able to support the recommendations of the others. For example, occupational therapy overlaps with physical therapy in the areas of seating and positioning, transfer training, and safety training. Additionally, when a patient wears an ankle–foot orthosis (a brace for the foot) on the right foot, it is important for the physical therapist to know if she or he still drives as she or he may need adaptations in order to use the gas pedal and brake. Occupational therapy often overlaps with social work in the area of support networks, vocational needs, and volunteer activities and may collaborate in dealing with psychosocial issues. Overlap with neurology and nursing occurs around medication management. It is important for the occupational therapist to know what medications patients are taking and in what way they take these medications (injection, pill, liquid, eyedrops, etc.) as the occupational therapist, physician, and nurse may work together to make sure that the people are able to manage their medications from both cognitive and fine motor perspectives. Speech therapy and occupational therapy both work on cognition and swallowing, and collaboration among these team members leads toward more integrative intervention.

The ability to go to another team member and learn is an ongoing process that a good interdisciplinary team engages in. The greatest strength of a good interdisciplinary team is the lack of individual ego and exclusive professional roles, recognizing how disciplines can augment each other's treatment effectiveness and put the patients in the center of the team.

The Role of Physical Therapy in the Interdisciplinary Team for Individuals with MS

ANN PISANI

Quality physical therapy in the care of the individual with MS requires expertise in assessment and treatment in neurological disorders and especially in MS, which might represent one of the most challenging professional experiences due to the variability of the disease process. Almost all individuals with MS may benefit from physical therapy treatment from the time of diagnosis. An exercise program recommended early in the course of MS will help patients have a sense of control over their physical well-being. In addition to a home exercise program which targets flexibility, balance, strength, and gait training, MS issues and cardiovascular well-being are important to address. A home exercise program should be initiated as early in the disease process as possible. Also, the appropriateness of recreational activity should be reviewed by the therapist. The unpredictability of MS makes the development of a treatment plan challenging. Safety and independence should be emphasized. Training should include the use of devices such as scooters, wheelchairs, and orthotics; and education should include the proper care of such devices. The therapist will need to help patients adjust to the equipment as resistance on the part of the patient might be a barrier to successful implementation. The emphasis needs to be on the replacement of failing or lost function, which will allow patients to go on with their lives. Again, the role of the team in reinforcing this message is key.

Initial evaluation by physical therapy should included assessments of strength, flexibility, balance, gait, etc. Manual muscle testing is included, as is examination for contracture (limited motion at major joints), which jeopardizes skin integrity and functional mobility. The Berg Balance Scale is a useful tool to assess balance. Factors such as posture, pain, and fatigue are assessed, especially as they impact mobility.

A comprehensive physical therapy treatment plan is designed to address all identified problems and is discussed during the team meeting. Written instructions are provided for a home exercise program. The adverse effects of deconditioning are stressed, while regular exercise up to an individual patient's specific capacity is encouraged. Especially for the more severely physically impaired, stretching and physical exercise are emphasized in order to avoid contracture. It is important for caregivers or family members to understand the home exercise program in order to achieve maximal benefit. Attention is also given to exercise options in the community: the use of exercise equipment at gyms, yoga and tai chi classes, and aqua therapy programs.

The physical therapist works closely with the physiatrist, a physician whose area of expertise is rehabilitation medicine. Decisions regarding braces, assistive devices, wheelchair modifications, as well as specific exercise suggestions are discussed and finalized when the team meets as a group. In regard to wheelchair planning, factors such as posture, skin integrity, pain, and respiratory status are considered. Education by the physical therapist about correct techniques for exercising, correct use of orthotics, as well as proper use of ambulatory devices is essential for the achievement of optimal results in terms of safety and maximal functional mobility.

The physical and occupational therapists confer in such areas as wheelchair seating, transfers, home modifications, and fatigue management, particularly in regard to their impact on ADLs. Functional mobility skills are also addressed because of the impact on daily living skills. Organizational skills and cognitive issues are discussed as they relate to daily functioning and with regard to exercise.

Physical therapy and social service provide emotional support, especially in regard to changes in mobility. This is compounded by changes in body image with the use of a mobility device. Social service helps patients and families deal with these feelings as well as helping to convey the importance of the role of physical therapy. Patients often can feel overwhelmed or experience depression, which the social worker and psychiatrist address. As a team member, social work also alerts physical therapy to changes in living situation which may have impact on functional mobility.

Compliance issues with regard to exercise programs are often elicited during conversations between the neurologist, nurse, and patients. Nursing also provides information regarding health insurance coverage and limitations that could impact necessary follow-up care.

All team members work together to reach the goals set for patients. Communication is a vital component of our good team, as well as confidence in the judgment of the various team members. Team members need to feel confident in their skills and to be willing to share their knowledge. They also need to be able to accept differing opinions and not allow differences to affect the overall function of the team. Peer support and respect are vital for success. Each clinician must be able to appreciate the opinions of the other team members. Disagreements can be handled in a constructive way. Working as a team requires patience, independence, and self-confidence. Team members who can work together provide exceptional patient care as well as personal satisfaction.

The Role of the Physiatrist in the Interdisciplinary Team for Individuals with MS

STEVEN MOSKOWITZ

A physiatrist is a physician specializing in physical medicine and rehabilitation. Physiatrists treat a wide range of medical problems, with a focus on restoring function. There is significant clinical overlap with other medical specialties, though the physiatric approach is often centered on rehabilitation. The physiatrist looks at the overall framework for intervention by the rehabilitation team. In addition, this discipline offers expertise in regard to the rehabilitation of medical issues such as musculoskeletal and neurogenic pain management, specific orthotic concerns in people with diabetes or peripheral vascular disease, and orthopedic issues which may complicate the course of MS.

Since the education and training of the physiatrist involves the rehabilitative care of a wide variety of medical, orthopedic, and neurological conditions, it allows for an overview of how various impairments combine to create disability. Clinically, the physiatrist might make recommendations regarding a sore shoulder, low back pain, the specific prescription for customized orthoses, etc. In regard to a sore shoulder in individuals with MS, paralysis, the use of crutches, impaired sensation, etc. contribute additional stresses to the shoulder and affect treatment options. An individualized approach to combined impairments is necessary. The physiatrist will help define a rehabilitation strategy for complex MS patients with multiple needs. Administratively, the clinic team identifies and coordinates with external rehabilitative resources off-site and facilitates the acquisition of durable medical equipment such as wheelchairs and rollators. Often, the prescription of a specific wheelchair requires the combined efforts of all team members, patients, and their caregivers. The physiatrist in the Mt. Auburn clinic assisted the team in the acquisition of an appropriate and compassionate durable medical equipment vendor, who attends clinic and participates with the team in the acquisition of equipment. Likewise, the physiatrist has introduced an orthotist who is willing to attend clinic and participate in the team effort. The addition of both of these vendors has enabled the team to ensure the acquisition of proper bracing and durable medical equipment.

The Role of Social Work in the Interdisciplinary Team for Individuals with MS
KATHLEEN LEAHY

The social worker brings expertise, training, and experience in assessing individuals, couples, and families who are living with MS, a chronic illness. The initial evaluation involves a psychosocial assessment within the context of a medical history (impairments, disabilities, and handicaps). The social worker makes recommendations and educates patients and their families/caregivers regarding resources such as agencies, commissions, federal and private insurance, financial consultants, consumer organizations, etc. The social worker facilitates family team meetings and, at the MAHMSCCC, such support groups as Mothers with MS. There is need to investigate underlying vulnerabilities as well as to determine coping mechanisms and strengths. One determines what coping mechanisms are working or have worked for individuals and or families, currently and in the past. For example, where activity has been an important coping mechanism, the consequences of fatigue may be particularly distressing to patients. If self-sufficiency is a value, then the acceptance of a brace or cane may be perceived as a threat to independence and sense of self, including body image, thus posing a barrier to the utilization of any such device despite frequent falls. This kind of knowledge is important in devising treatment plans acceptable to the patients. Families can learn what feels supportive to patients. Helping couples to identify underlying feelings about MS can sometimes facilitate better relationships and family function.

What is stress for some people may be perceived as a blessing for others. Dealing with the diagnosis and changes may become a positive experience for some. Identifying the strengths in individuals and/or families is often the beginning of that process.

The diagnosis of MS is a crisis for patients and families, a narcissistic injury that attacks people's self-perception. It changes expectations and life goals. Relationships are altered on a personal basis at home, at work, and in the community. Priorities are changed and goals revisited. The social worker helps in this process.

B. Sawtelle Hospice House
EDITOR DAVID G. SATIN
WITH JANE DUGGAN, CHAPLAIN; TERRY FALLON,
NURSE/COORDINATOR; JOAN KEY, VOLUNTEER; PAT KUMPH,
ADMINISTRATOR/MANAGER; DEBORAH MOORE, HOME HEALTH AIDE
AND SUE BERGER, VOLUNTEER AND DISCUSSION COORDINATOR

TERRY FALLON/NURSE: *When I started working at Sawtelle I was working in the homes. We would go to people who might be appropriate for hospice program but might not be quite ready for it and get our whole team involved and maybe prevent them from going back to the hospital so much and do hospice care. Hospice, if you don't know, is for people who have less than 6 months to live. Doctors are trying to spread that out a little bit because one of the biggest problems is that we get referrals very late. In fact, we had a referral very late today: A patient came to our house and died 3 hours later. That's a little late as far as we are concerned. We'd rather have referrals earlier in the disease so that we can get them comfortable and they can enjoy whatever time they have left. That's our philosophy and of hospice in general. The Sawtelle Hospice House came about because we were finding that we had a real problem: We had people at home alone—not just elderly but younger people, especially women. A lot of these women had been taking care of their husbands, and then the husbands died, and then they're all by themselves. And they were fiercely independent for so long before they get some kind of illness and then find that they just can't take care of themselves. So, as visiting nurses we would go in to try to help them out in any way we could: We interfaced between the patient and the doctor's office, we ordered medication sometimes if they need that, we decided if they needed physical therapy, occupational therapy, if they needed a home health aide, for hospice patients if they needed volunteers or if they needed our chaplain. The nurse—the case manager—goes in, assesses all of that, and then follows patients throughout the course of their lives. What we were finding, especially for a lot of these elderly women, is that all of a sudden they were at a point where they couldn't take care of themselves and they needed another option besides the nursing home. We cringed when we had to send our patients to nursing homes. To those who work in nursing homes I apologize, but the nursing homes are just not set up to take care of dying people. They're just way too understaffed. People aren't going to get the kind of TLC [tender, loving care] that we really want them to get. So we started a hospice house. Nine beds at present, and it's been working out really great. We're just trying to get the word out there so that more and more people know about it. Hospice care is covered by Medicare and most insurance plans. A lot of insurance plans for people under 65 actually cover a little more of it. And we have donors who will help pay if someone can't afford to pay. The process of entering the hospice house usually starts when we get a telephone call. The call would go to Pat Kumph [administrator] and she'll find out if they're appropriate for hospice. For instance, if we found out one of our patients was scheduled for radiation therapy next week, that's not really the hospice philosophy. We're hoping to make people feel comfortable here, and radiation therapy means that person is not at the point of hospice care. So Pat'll find out what doctor you're going to, make sure that the people get "do not resuscitate" orders, and kind of get a feel for what's going on with that patient, what the diagnosis is.*

PAT KUMPH/ADMINISTRATOR: *At the very beginning, right from the very start, we're actually discussing the patients before they even come in the house.*

FALLON/NURSE: *Right, absolutely. Pat and I talk about it. We'll also get the hospice manager at the main agency involved. We'll get our social worker involved right away: She'll do a financial evaluation to see if they can afford to pay. If not, we would look to other sources to try to pay for care. So before they even come into the house we've already talked to each other and conferenced to see if they're appropriate for the house. Once they arrive Pat does the financial piece. I want nothing to do with money. I'll meet with the family and have them sign consent forms and figure out what's been going on. The stuff we get from hospitals we know most of the time is no longer valid. The patients have had a big change. Now they're our patients—here, today. Then I'll decide if the patients need certain services, like the therapists. We tend not to do a lot of physical* therapy, occupational therapy, things like that at hospice house, but sometimes we do. Our home health aides are always there and they will always take care of all the physical needs the patients have and a lot of the extra TLC that we like to give these people. Deborah [home health aide] will talk a little about her piece. Our volunteers are always there: The volunteers are constantly checking on people, making sure they're OK, seeing if they need anything. And many times, as Joan [volunteer] will tell you, she'll hear things that she thinks are important to me and she'll come back down and tell me, "I was up talking with Helen today and she mentioned this, that, and the other thing." And I'll respond, "OK, that's great." Volunteers are like another set of eyes for us as a team, and they find out a lot of information sometimes that we don't hear about because we're not in there just sitting down and relaxing: We're usually managing medications, managing services, and such. If our social worker needs to be involved, she will be. Helen, that patient we were talking about, did need the social worker: She had one daughter who was very much on board with what was going on and another daughter who pretty much wanted nothing to do with her. She also was a very spiritual person. We had Jane, our chaplain, involved. She went up to talk to her. We arrange for a Greek Orthodox priest to be there for people, and whatever religion people are a part of, if they want to continue that, we try to contact people from the community to help them out.

So my role is the case coordinator: I figure out what everybody needs, what the patient needs. All people in the house get volunteers. All people in the house get the home health aide care that they need. Everybody needs Pat for any other kind of business-type stuff. They'll all meet me. A lot of what I do is not just for the patients but more for the families, so there'll be a lot of teaching of the families. This is what's going on right now. I'll give an idea of how much time the people have, especially if I think it's going to be really soon. I'll give them an idea of what we're doing to help manage their symptoms. I see where the families are at and just try to get in the door with them to make sure they understand what's going on and that we're all on the same page. And probably the most challenging part of the job is breaking news to families that their loved ones are a lot sicker than they think and try to make sure they understand this is what's happening right now. You just need to be prepared and get them to a place where they're as OK with that as they can possibly be. I'll let Deborah tell you about the kinds of things she does as a home health aide. I would have to say that the home health aides and the volunteers really make up so much of the care at the house, the kind of care they're not going to get in the hospital or a nursing home or in their own homes. They really make such a difference.

DEBORAH MOORE/HOME HEALTH AIDE: Like Terry said, I give personal care. I think I have the best job because I really get to connect with each individual on a personal basis. When they come in sometimes they're anxious and they're scared and they're nervous, not knowing what's going to happen to them. Half an hour I just sit and talk to them, giving them a back rub or giving them a shower, combing their hair, or maybe cleaning their fingernails. You know you get to hear their whole life story most of the time, and it's really nice because when the families come in the one part Terry didn't get to tell you was it gives them an opportunity to be their families and not their caregivers, and it takes a big burden off their shoulders. Once they get past that door we can't change their diagnosis but we certainly change their level of comfort, and that gives you so much gratification. And those are the types of things I provide: their personal care, I become their friend, and make their last days comfortable.

FALLON/NURSE: You know, you really are the first caregiver. People come through the door sometimes and they haven't been shaven and they cannot bathe and shower, their *nails are black and filthy, and they haven't been out of bed, and they come in the door uncared for. Then I see a gleam in Debbie's eye.*

MOORE/HOME HEALTH AIDE: *I first introduce myself as Deborah, but then I tell them I'm better known as Fluff and Buff. They just call me Fluff and Buff and that's what I do. Whatever they need is what they get.*

FALLON/NURSE: *It's great because I know Deborah's taking care of that patient. I'm just going to give her an hour to take care of that patient unless they're in pain or have some kind of symptom management problem, in which case I'll jump on it right away. But I'll know Deborah's in there getting them cleaned up or sometimes getting them in the shower. And just taking a shower for these people sometimes is the best thing. They'll say, "Oh, this just feels so good!" Or get them a wheelchair, get them outside. We've had families come in and say, "Oh my gosh, they're outside! Look at this—they haven't been outside in months!" Families are so happy. You see relief in them. You see them relax for a little bit. They're just so happy when they come in and see how clean their loved one looks. She's washing their hair. One of our patients she's blow drying every day and curling and everything else. Families come in and they just feel like their loved one is being so well taken care of by the personal care that they're getting—that Deborah gives. And she's got all kinds of special things for people: If people like their nails done, if Deborah's there, she's cleaning them and manicuring them and there's this kind of nail polish and matching this with that and just all those little extra things that make their life just so much better at that time. A lot of patients just want to look good—even if they don't feel good, they still want to smell good.*

We do a lot of personal care. Our other aides are just fantastic; we have an unbelievable group of people. And Deborah tells me things all the time. She'll come down and she'll say, "You know what? When I was moving him, he was in a little bit of pain." OK, that's good to know. Next time we put him in the shower we give him medication, we'll prevent that pain. That way we understand his needs and help a little bit more. So Deborah and I are talking back and forth all the time. I call her my right hand—some days my left hand, too.

KUMPH/ADMINISTRATOR: *While she's in the room she's not just taking care of their personal needs; she's finding out information. They're talking to her, emotional stuff, telling her things that there are times they don't tell anybody else. But then she's able to tell us so we're able to help the families. It's a huge element.*

FALLON: *And while she's doing all that I'm helping the people to function better, so we're sort of tag team. The patients have been in the hospital, been sick, and they just couldn't do all this stuff. The families are just so appreciative, and the patients too. And then Deborah's always watching out for any kind of skin problems—the skin breaking down or anything like that—and we work together: "What do you think is going to work best? An alternating air pressure mattress? Maybe an egg crate?" We work back and forth a lot. Deborah's always repositioning people who are bed-bound. And when Deborah comes down for instance in the case of Helen: "You know, she was talking a lot about God or forgiveness, or whatever." The first phone call is to Jane, our chaplain. Jane, I'll let you talk a little bit about Helen and about spiritual care.*

JANE DUGGAN/CHAPLAIN: *What I try to do is help people to access whatever it is that gives spiritual meaning to their lives, which is very interesting right now because so many people are not connected to a church. Where 25 years ago there'd be a minister from each church visiting, a lot of people are spiritual but not attached to a community, so I try to help people identify what it is that gives them courage and strength.*

Sometimes it's very traditional. We are next door to a Catholic church. If someone comes in who is Catholic, it's easy, it's prescribed. We offer and sometimes the answer is "Yes," and sometimes the answer is "No, thank you." So you feel your way in. Terry has a very nice way of often saying to people, not so much "Do you want to see the chaplain?"—it's "Have you met Jane?" and that sometimes is a lot. It's disarming for people who are close to death, who sometimes don't want to see a person who's a chaplain—it's getting a little too near to the end, it feels spooky for them. So I try very hard to meet people just where they are and help them to use the strength that they already have. Sometimes that means praying with people or talking with people. I'm learning a lot about different faith systems and rituals and traditions and things that people hold dear. Just this year we had new families: a Muslim family, a Buddhist family. And here we are out in the suburbs of Massachusetts, so it's very interesting. I'll come in one day and introduce myself to the new patients. I spend time with families. Often, I'll come in and Terry or Debbie will tip me off that so-and-so had a real tough night or I think I heard her crying. That's so helpful to me. And I'll go in and try to find out what's going on.

I'm developing a thicker skin. Some people want to see me and some people....My first day—my very first day in the house—I came and met this wonderful guy who was, sadly, leaving us because his family wanted to move him down south to be near them. He gave me a tour of the house, and he introduced me to a couple of the other patients and brought me down to the kitchen. They have a beautiful kitchen: great big, open, in a great room, and all who are up to it come down for their meals. And there's this nice guy sitting there reading the Boston Globe and eating his bacon and egg (which I learned was his staple meal) at 3:00 in the afternoon. And I was introduced to him, so I said, "Hi, how are you?" And he put his newspaper down for a few minutes and talked to me. And I said, "So I'm the chaplain. Maybe we could pray or we could read scripture." And he picks up his paper and ignored me. And I said, "Oh, OK. I'll take that as a no." We ended up being good friends. Each time I came in I'd visit him and we'd talk about whatever was happening and no God stuff. Toward the end of his life I went by and his door was closed, so I knocked and he says, "Yeah?" and I said, "Oh, hi, it's Jane. Could I come in?" And he said, "Yeah," in a very grumpy voice (he was kind of grumpy, gruff guy). So I came in and he was listening to this beautiful piece of classical music, and he said to me, "Do you know what this is?" And I said, "No. I can appreciate it. It's beautiful, but I don't know too much about classical music." He said, "Well, sit down." And we just sat in silence and listened to the music. And when it was over, he said to me, "That's where I get my peace." And I took that as such a wonderful, wonderful gift, that if I'd come on too strong with him I would never have been privileged to find out what gave meaning to him. And again I was able to be there as he was dying, just to be there. So it's wonderful work we do. We function very much as a team. Pat has taught me some of her administrative things. If I'm there and the house is hopping there are other things that I can pitch in and do. I think that we don't so much sit down and have formal meetings; it's very much on the fly, but I like that. I like the spontaneity and the informality of that. The house is very homelike, and I think we function in a family kind of a way too. Say, you go do this, or whatever needs to be done.

FALLON/NURSE: *And she provides a lot of support for the staff.*

DUGGAN/CHAPLAIN: *I try to do that. I try to be there to support the house.*

KUMPH/ADMINISTRATOR: *If the team functioning were more formal, the difference in the house would be that every other Thursday we would get together as a team to case conference about the patients who are in the homes. The same workers would be sitting around the table, going around the table, maybe giving 3, 4, 5 minutes—whatever is needed—to each patient. In our house we're able to do that constantly. To my way of thinking it's better because it's hard to wait for every 2 weeks to bring something to the table without having dealt with it. You have to deal with it when it happens. So the interdisciplinary collaboration gets done.*

FALLON/NURSE: *This way is effective.*

KUMPH/ADMINISTRATOR: *This continuous interaction to us is the way we conference. I feel it accomplishes more than sitting at the table formally going over patients in order.*

Joan is our volunteer. Volunteers are wonderful in this house. We have 35 to 40 volunteers. They are at the house from 8:00 to 8:00 every day—sometimes one, sometimes two, sometimes three. I sometimes pick up the phone and go, "Help," and they are incredible. We could not run the house the way we do without you all. Joan will just give you a little feel for what she does.

JOAN KEY/VOLUNTEER: *My background is with hospice. This is my 26th year. I used to do the home route. I babysat animals. I've taken care of babies so the patient can go visit somebody; I've been all through the whole gamut of volunteer work. And then when I found out that you were going to have a hospice home so close to mine, I jumped to it. I've been with them now for over a year and I love it. All patients, as far as I'm concerned, are the greatest people there are because they know why they're there. A big percentage of them come to the realization that their time is short. I don't know why but I stumble into relationships with them. I just—boom! I'm there for them. I love each one of them, and I go twice a week. I spend about 8 hours a week. But there's been times when my favorites are fading out and I'll be up there Sunday morning or I'll sneak in Friday night and check on them. But we do everything that the girls don't have time for. I do some shopping, grocery shopping. I change bedpans I clean up the vomit. I do it because it needs to be done. I don't chase them down and tell them there's something that has to be done; I do it myself just as long as I don't endanger the patients.*

FALLON/NURSE: *I always think of the volunteers not doing the stuff that Deborah and I can't get to but doing all the extra stuff. So we'll see volunteers setting up a CD player, picking out music that this patient really likes from the assortment that we have that our friend Bob left for his aunt; he left a lot of CDs for us. And I see the volunteers doing things like reading to them. Just finding out what special things that they really like. Getting them that ice cream sundae: That's all they can think about is that ice cream sundae, that's the only thing they want to eat.*

KEY/VOLUNTEER: *Or giving them a back rub.*

FALLON/NURSE: *Find the right channel: They can't deal with these remotes. All those little things that people would just like around.*

KUMPH/ADMINISTRATOR: *And again, finding out concerns that they're not afraid to tell Joan or Deborah because they're in there just to be with them.*

KEY/VOLUNTEER: *I've had them open up to me and tell me things about their private lives that I stand there amazed; I'm startled at times. And I just appreciate the fact they can trust me at the end stage of their lives, that they can tell me things. Now this was a particular experience. A hospice patient of mine left town when she was diagnosed. She didn't want anyone to know that she was ill. She finally found herself in a nursing home and that's where I used to hospice. And when her end was coming, she wanted me to sit down and write her fiancé and her mother and father what she did, why she did it. And she didn't want me to mail the letter in Newport; she wanted me to mail it in Boston, where they couldn't find her. I'll never forget her because she put her trust in me. Those are the little things that I take away. That's my reward for being a hospice volunteer.*

KUMPH/ADMINISTRATOR: *The difference in the hospice kind of visiting nurse care is there has to be a skilled need in the home. In the hospice, as long as people are diagnosed as having 6 months or less to live they can get someone to visit them as often as the nurse feels is needed.*

FALLON/NURSE: *The nursing visits covered under Medicare and under most insurance plans are very limited, so there's not going to be someone there 8 hours a day. The nurse goes in there, she sees what kind of services are needed, and then goes back to the office and puts all this paperwork through. If we check on the insurance and if it's not covered, the doctor has to refer for those services: If we had a doctor, for example, that said, "This patient should be on home health services for this, this, this, this, and this," the insurance company has to cover that. Now if the nursing services go in and then they say, "What she needs is continual care and the only way she can have that is in a skilled nursing facility."*

KUMPH/ADMINISTRATOR: *But we couldn't go in there until the doctor orders that. We can't just go in the door and hope the insurance company will pay.*

FALLON/NURSE: *We never denied people care because they can't pay. Never. So we usually know up front that they don't have insurance, they can't pay, and then we go to alternative sources. We have one woman who is willing to pay for not the insurance part of it, but room and board for up to 2 weeks at the hospice house. We have a couple of other funds we know of: People happen to be a patient at Lahey Clinic and they happen to have a cancer diagnosis. They'll pay for 2 weeks for someone to be at the hospice house. We can eat the cost of the insurance.*

KUMPH/ADMINISTRATOR: *The medical order has to come from the doctor for hospice, and once that happens, there's no way we can refuse it.*

FALLON/NURSE: *The policy is for Medicare to pay for hospice for a maximum of 6 months, but I had a person in hospice for 3 years. The doctor said, "This woman needs to be in hospice. She's 95 years old, she has aortic stenosis, she's going to drop any day. I want her on hospice." And we have another patient in our house right now that's been on hospice for over a year. Her body has learned to coexist with her disease. You look at her blood counts and everything else and you say, "She should be one sick woman." But she's up, she's walking around, we have her doing jobs, she helps, she does the laundry. As long as her doctor says in most cases this person would have less than 6 months to live, as long as her doctor still appeals that, that person can stay in hospice program.*

KUMPH/ADMINISTRATOR: *Hospice nursing and medications is paid for by the Medicaid benefit at our house. We will not refuse anybody and never have. We have to have it down on paper that they need financial support. We take their word for it. We don't have to have evidence. But I don't know; I think some of them should.*

FALLON: *Last month alone we gave 18 days of free care to those who didn't have financial coverage.*

KUMPH/ADMINISTRATOR: *Most people have some sort of resource for their nursing care. The room and board is very inexpensive: $150 a day, about half-price compared* *to nursing homes. But we just don't refuse people. That's part of our director's philosophy. That's what we're there for: people who really need it. Doesn't matter where they live.*

KUMPH/ADMINISTRATOR: *We're just going to bring up a patient who we all really got involved in, as we do. She really needed a lot of support in the house because she didn't have a lot of outside supports. One daughter was available if she could be. Another daughter was at quite a distance and really didn't want to get involved at all. So we tried as a team to figure out how we could help her not only with the clinical piece but the emotional piece. And I don't know who wants to discuss this—just go around the table and speak up.*

FALLON/NURSE: *I took care of Helen's medical needs, most of her nursing/medical needs. She was a diabetic who was used to doing all the testing and everything herself. So one of the things I had to do was convince her that it was time for her to hand that over to us because she wasn't doing a very good job of it; she was getting a little bit more confused. So I talked with Deborah. Deborah made her meals, and I said, "Since I have to take her blood sugar, make sure you let me know before you feed her, and let me know if you see her getting more confused, if she's starting to drop things," on and on. She didn't want a whole lot of home health aide stuff at first: She wanted to do some care for herself, take her own shower and everything else. So we were always very much on guard for her safety, that she might start feeling weak, she might fall, whatever. So Deborah was always on hand. She said she could go outside herself. When she started to decline, I made a lot of medication changes, kept in contact with her doctor.*

When people come to our house, some people know they're dying. Some people want to think they're in rehabilitation, and if they're really set on getting a little bit stronger, they want that physical therapy. I call the physical therapist and I say, "Can you help this person?" You know, let them have physical therapy, let's see if it helps them. If it helps them mentally, it's worth it.

But quite often, the family doesn't want the patient to know because they're afraid of hurting their feelings or they're afraid they're going to be sad. The person in the bed knows what's going on, they just don't want the family to know because the family is going to be upset. So it's that elephant in the room thing where nobody wants to talk about it. I'll wait for the patient to open the door and then start talking about it little by little. With families, too. They don't believe that their husbands are going to die. They think he needs to do his physical therapy exercises every day, he needs his cholesterol medicine. I have to say, "He really can't swallow right now. You try to give him a pill, he'll aspirate on the floor. He'd be so much worse. So we're not going to do that." You have to meet them where they are and not say, "What, are you stupid? He can't swallow! Who cares about his cholesterol? He's got cancer from head to toe!" You just have to let that stay inside—I call it in a little bubble. But that's what you say.

The social worker will talk with the family first of all about finances and see if they can afford to pay for the room and board there. She'll help them out with any other kinds of situations that are going on. We had a patient who had a lot of family issues wrapped around drug abuse, alcohol abuse, things like that. She'll help with funeral arrangements. Jane will also help with funeral arrangements. I'll help with funeral arrangements. Pat does that sometimes.

KUMPH/ADMINISTRATOR: *Everybody does a little bit of everything. That's why it works in this setting.*

FALLON/NURSE: *The social work will help with a lot of family issues. As far as the patient goes, if they have any things on their mind that they want to get settled. We've had her help people hook up with a lawyer, get stuff down on paper because they're not going to be able to relax until they have their heads clear of all that stuff. She's done legal maneuvering for us. We've had patients where those last few days family members were fighting over what to do with them; she'll intervene and have family meetings and go over things to make sure that it all works out the way they really need it to for that patient.*

KUMPH/ADMINISTRATOR: *At one point Terry might say, "I think they could use volunteer services. They could definitely use a chaplain. They are naturally going to need Deborah." So she might give everybody a little bit of information of how they would be helpful. I run the volunteer program also, so I will talk with Terry about the patient. Then I might go out if it's in the patient's home, or see them if it's in the hospice house. I'd find out a little about the patient before I asked a volunteer to get involved. Jane will come into the office and ask, "Does anyone need to see me?" If I've had a chance, I tell her; if I haven't had a chance, she'll go in very gently and see for herself. But we usually get most of our information from the nurse case manager. And at a round table when we talk about the community patients, our social worker is there and every nurse that works at the agency is there. So if Terry had a concern or problem or questions, something she needed to bounce off us, there's a whole table full of case managers at the table. Just today when I was there one nurse there was struggling because the medication she was using didn't seem to be helping the patient. So she'll mention that at the table, and they went around in a circle trying to figure out what might help depending on how long that nurse has been there or maybe her experiences using other medications. That's the case conference, and it's helpful. In our house if Terry has a concern she might call one of her coworkers and just bounce something off somebody. We have a wound specialist at the agency. If there's something going on with wounds that Terry feels she might need more help, she might call that person. Terry will start it because this is her patient. She's going to take care of all their needs. She'll also call people out. She might say, "No volunteers here. No chaplain here. Leave the social worker out because they will close the door." That's basically how we case conference.*

FALLON/NURSE: *As for Helen, she wanted to stay alone. But she really liked having company. So when the volunteers came in, we'd always have a patient information sheet which says what the patient's interests are, what kind of foods they like, what kinds of foods they don't like, what kind of concerns we have: safety, things like that. And the volunteers will look at all those sheets for all the patients before they go in and see a patient. If I think Helen needs a little bit of extra time, I'll say, "Joan, could you go up and see Helen? She's just not quite herself today. I'm not sure what's going on, what's on her mind. I don't know if she's worried about things, if she's not feeling good. If you could just go up and spend some time with her." And Joan will go up and then spend more time with her. And then Jane, of course, does so.*

DUGGAN/CHAPLAIN: *Helen was a very spiritual person, so when you said, "Who should we talk about?" Helen's a piece of cake to talk about. She was just so funny! She had a great sense of humor. She'd lived three generations in the same house. She had a whole sense of history. She was kind of a gentle matriarch. She was a very interesting person and with enormous peace and kind of ready—fearless, ready to die. Not in the least bit worried about that.*

MOORE/HOME HEALTH AIDE: *She was very happy in her room. It was like she was in a country club. She loved her room.*

KUMPH/ADMINISTRATOR: *What we're doing here by telling you about this person is what we would do amongst ourselves to get to know the person better. Right now, it just sounds like we're telling you about our family, but by Jane saying that she was spiritual we became aware of that. We may have not known that had Jane not gone in and talked with her. The fact that she was very private she made very clear to Terry right from the very beginning. We were able from that information to make sure we didn't bombard her with people coming in. Some people can be very chatty, think that you need a lot of conversation. Well, that's not true of everyone. So by explaining all that to each other, in not a round table way but the way we do it now, we do get to know the patient, and we feel that way we can give the best care.*

MOORE/HOME HEALTH AIDE: *Helen was very set in her ways. Even though there's no rules, she was used to having her breakfast at 8:00, having her insulin at 8:00, she wanted to be woken up. So I'd say, "Terry, Helen wants her insulin at 8:00 'cause she has her breakfast right after." I would send Terry up to give her insulin. And she'd say, "Deborah's making your omelet." And I'd make her that omelet every single day. But she'd have her insulin at 8:00. If Terry said, "Deborah, I have a meeting, so-and-so's coming over from the office." "Well, you'd better give Helen her insulin at 8:00 for us before you go in that room." And so we communicate constantly.*

FALLON/NURSE: *If the nurse goes in the home and she finds that it's an unsafe situation, such as this woman who can't walk by herself, her sister is out working, she's here by herself, she's in pain, she's trying to get up to go to the bathroom, she's falling. We get our social worker involved right then. And the social worker will work with them and say, "You've got to look at other alternatives. You've got to quit work for a while, take a family leave, or we've got to find a different situation for her because she's not safe."*

We do one another's job all the time. I mean, I'll do all the medicating and all the nursing care and the more medical stuff as the nurse case manager, and I'll work with the doctor. That will always be my job. But quite often if I go in and see that a patient needs some personal care, I can do that or I can call Deborah to do it or I can call a volunteer to do it. So some of those types of things absolutely are shared. Psychosocial support, we all do it. If I know someone needs psychosocial support, I don't take that on myself; I get the chaplain involved right away or our social worker. So we do each other's jobs a lot, but there are certain boundaries. I'm not going to have Deborah decide to give this patient 20 milligrams of morphine. That's not her decision to make; that's mine. So there's where you can see the boundary. But Deborah might say to me, "You know what? They need some kind of pain medication." And I'll pick up on that and take over from there. When it comes to personal care, I've got eight other patients that need medication; chances are I call Deborah to do it. Or if Joan is available, I'll say, "Joan, this person just needs some mouth care. Could you please go do that?" So our roles cross over a lot, with the ultimate goal of making sure this patient is as comfortable as possible and their families.

KEY/VOLUNTEER: *I know my boundaries. I know that when it comes to nursing care, that's Terry. I'll help with turning patients, I'll help make the beds, I'll help clean up the messes. I'll do those things to help ease her load when the time comes, but I think we all know our boundaries.*

MOORE/HOME HEALTH AIDE: *We're all good at multitasking. We run our hospice house like we run our home, not a facility. Think of your household containing nine bedrooms.*

I'm the cook, I'm the bed maker, I'm the butt-washer, whatever it takes. We do it all. Today Pat and I was putting extenders on a bed because one of our residents was too long for the bed. So we had to take the bed apart, get an extender, put it on. I mean, we do whatever it takes to make that individual comfortable. I could walk into somebody's room and see that they're very congested. Now, Terry was in there 20 minutes ago; maybe she didn't hear it or it wasn't there at that time. I'll say, "Terry, Mrs. Johnson is very congested." She'll say, "OK, thank you for telling me." She'll go in and she'll take care of it. They might need medication, whatever it takes. We multitask.

KUMPH/ADMINISTRATOR: *We're in our element. When it comes to saying the rosaries or something, Jane…*

MOORE/HOME HEALTH AIDE: *I say "Amen" a lot.*

DUGGAN/CHAPLAIN: *If I'm there and the house is really busy I'll answer the door, I'll sit with the family, I'll do a tour if someone's coming to look at the house, answer the phone, empty the dishwasher. We do interchange.*

FALLON/NURSE: *One thing we learned when I started hospice that I learned very quickly is as a nurse going in you tend to think you can do everything. You can't. And one can either very quickly want to say, "Get that social worker in there fast, otherwise I'm going to be sucked dry. Get the chaplain in there fast. These people need this." You can't do everything by yourself. You've got to call on your resources and use them.*

DUGGAN/CHAPLAIN: *What we were trying to do was have conversations with people that help them move from where they are. We don't do anything in terms of formal groups, although we've had informal groups around that kitchen table many times.*

FALLON/NURSE: *And our social worker oftentimes will have a family meeting to make sure that everybody kind of is working in the same direction.*

KUMPH/ADNINISTRATOR: *Last week Terry and I went in and talked with one of our patients because we were told by the family that he wanted to go home and they couldn't tell him he couldn't go home. We really felt he knew that he wasn't doing well, but they couldn't say it together. So we went up to the room and Terry opened the conversation up and said, "Do you know why you're here?" And he said, "I'm not doing well." "And you're probably not going to get any better." And he said, "OK." And we said, "Your kids want you to go home but we don't feel you can." "OK." I mean, we really felt all along he just needed to hear that.*

FALLON/NURSE: *And then he said, "I guess I better figure out what to do with the house, then, huh?" And he was fine.*

DUGGAN/CHAPLAIN: *Sometimes just saying, "What do you think is going on?" and they'll tell you. Or "What do you think is going to happen next?" Just that little opening all of a sudden…*

FALLON/NURSE: *Opens the door.*

DUGGAN/CHAPLAIN: *Or "What are you worried about?" They'll ask for the social worker, call in a lawyer. It's a great grace when people do have that time to get stuff together.*

FALLON/NURSE: *Sorting out team problems and disagreements has taken a while.*

KUMPH/ADMINISTRATOR: *I think because we each have our own roles and our own jobs. We sometimes bump heads, for sure. My job as the manager of the house is to fill the house and keep it filled, and we often have a waiting list. Terry's job as nurse and case manager is to take care of her patients. Everybody else has that function of taking care of all the people. And I'm sometimes the bad guy because I have to fill the house, because I'm under pressure from the agency. So once in a while if I say, "We're getting some new patients today," I get a bad look. But she also understands that that's my job. Terry and I, depending on how we're both doing that day, we may walk away from each other, or we may just say we understand that this is our job, this is what we have to do. Doesn't always work that easy, but we work it out because she knows it's my job; I know it's tough on her when she's got admissions and deaths and everything going around in circles. Today, for instance, we had three admissions and two deaths. That's terrible for a case manager to be put through in one day.*

FALLON/NURSE: *We've got two admissions tomorrow to fill those two beds because we had those two deaths. There are different expectations and pressures that can be in conflict with one another. Absolutely.*

KUMPH/ADMINISTRATOR: *But we know in our hearts what our job is. We'll call in extra help if Terry's really stressed out from all the admissions and deaths she's had. We have the ability to just pick up the phone and try to get extra help and we'll do that. If we see that Deborah's really overwhelmed with what she's doing—we did it today— we call in extra help to help her.*

FALLON/NURSE: *It's been a process, though. It got rough because all the stress is on me to do the patient care, the family care. I've got two people actively dying, a new admission, and Pat's talking about filling up the rooms before the person is even out of it. I said, "Pat, they're not even dead yet. Will you give me a break?" So we lock horns quite a few times. And part of it was the pressure on me to hurry up and take care of these patients, take care of these families, get them out. That was very hard for me. And we had quite a few meetings with our supervisor, too, the three of us trying to work things out. Now we're much better at predicting when we're going to need extra help so that I don't bite Pat's head off and so she doesn't end up biting my head off.*

KUMPH/ADMINISTRATOR: *Or we walk away and we discuss it when we know we can calm down.*

KEY/VOLUNTEER: *Or we learn to hide.*

FALLON/NURSE: *It really takes a lot of maturity in people to be able to go and talk to each other after you've had a major disagreement, and that's something that Pat and I have worked a lot on. It's been a whole process. And even with the hospice manager at the agency. And with home health aides—before Deborah sometimes I had priorities in my mind: This person needs this, this person needs that. And I might throw them out to the home health aide and she's busy doing something else. So sometimes we'd lock horns. But we just learned after a while: I learned to look at things from her perspective, and she learns to see things from my perspective. I explain to her why I want this done first: "The family's coming in an hour and this person's going to die. Get in there now, take care of this patient." So we talk to each other and we're honest with each other; that's the most effective kind of communication that we've learned we really have to do at the house. It's just really effective communication and being willing, being open to hearing somebody else, trying to see it from their eyes.*

KUMPH/ADMINISTRATOR: *I don't believe there's any job where you work closely like we do that there wouldn't be problems because we all have our different roles and responsibilities. We all answer to different goals.*

DUGGAN/CHAPLAIN: *There are certainly days when people growl and snarl at you and bang into each other, and then hopefully they'll draw on mutual respect and trust. At the end of the day someone might say, "I was really such a bitch today. I'm sorry."*

Or someone might say, "You really took my head off. I was just asking...." So it's an ongoing thing. It's not euphoria.

KUMPH/ADMINISTRATOR: *It's a home. It's kind of like in your home. And people have to deal with problems.*

DUGGAN/CHAPLAIN: *And you have to factor in, too, that often we're sad. People have formed different degrees of relationships with the patients, and sometimes they're difficult, and sometimes we're not all on the same page with them. There might be a person you resonated with and somebody else found very difficult. So there's all this emotional stuff too. So there has to be a willingness to work it out.*

FALLON/NURSE: *We learn each other's personalities. Volunteers learn that "I'm not mad at you if I'm barking. I've got a million things on my mind. I'm just trying to get this and then get that done." And the volunteers now understand that about me, which is so helpful. I hear through the grapevine, maybe they'll go and complain to Pat, "She was mad at me." I'll go to them and say, "I'm so sorry. I didn't mean for you to think I was mad at you. I'm not mad at you at all. I'm mad because that husband just blah blah." So it's really a lot of open communication.*

MOORE/HOME HEALTH AIDE: *We deal with sadness and remembering past patients on a daily basis. We know what the outcome is right from the set-on. We know what they're coming here for. We can't change their diagnosis. But we change their level of comfort. And at the end of each case we all get gratification because we see them through their process. And we do it in such a dignifying way that it helps us. Before we came here tonight we lost two patients 20 minutes apart from each other, and that was just the end of a very draining day for me. The second one who passed, I walked in there and I saw that she wasn't breathing and I was like, "Aw," and tears came to my eyes.*

DUGGAN/CHAPLAIN: *And she killed an ant.*

MOORE/HOME HEALTH AIDE: *I saw this ant and I thought, "I don't have time for this now," and I just smacked it. And I went out and I got a hug from Terry and I got a hug from the other Terry—we have two Terrys—and we do that all the time. You're happy that that person's suffering has come to an end, but you're sad because you're not going to see that person again. But we're able to separate that. And we do—we get hugs from each other. Terry can read my face; as soon as I walked out of that room, she read my face and she hugged me. She could tell at that point I needed that hug, she could tell I was drained, it was the end of the day, and that was like the frosting on the cake. And we had to put on happy faces and get in the car and do this presentation. But did we do a good job?*

FALLON/NURSE: *We are able to give one another emotional support. I think it's because we work in such a homelike environment. But there are some people in the house I'm not going to hug; they're not the huggy type. Some other people I work very closely with and I'll go up and give them a hug after a hard day or difficult event. That's part of my team member role. We used to have volunteer support meetings once a month. Since we opened this house up, the attendance at them is very low. I believe the reason is that people are getting enough support in the house themselves. They're there, they're overlapping shifts. If at any point in the day you need to speak with someone, there's always somebody there that can help you. When Jane walks in the door oftentimes we just sit in the office and I will just unload on her what's frustrating me that day or making me feel sad and she would do the same with me. And so I think we have those resources right here in the house.*

One time there was a particularly difficult patient. We went out to an area out back that's a garden and has a palm tree and everything. A bunch of us went out there with Jane and we just did a little support in a circle, just out there, and the wind was blowing, our hair was blowing all over the place. It wasn't quiet as we wanted, but still we had that little bit of time just to talk about this one patient, just to talk about what kind of day that was. Our agency has support meetings every other week. But I find that every other week is not enough. You know, I've got five deaths and I've got to wait for the following week? I have to move on, I don't have time to still talk about people who died before.

SUE BERGER/OCCUPATIONAL THERAPIST/DISCUSSION COORDINATOR: *I have volunteered at Sawtelle Hospice House and I know Pat well. I asked the staff to come because I am always amazed when I go there and I see everyone doing just anything. It seemed to me just a wonderful model of an interdisciplinary team: Knowing your roles but really being able to blend them. I think you've exemplified that here.*

15

Policy Making and Policy Changing

THEODORE CHELMOW

This chapter explains the context which governs social policy and our role as interdisciplinary workers to be agents of social change. Policies grow out of the experience of our daily lives, which includes individual perspectives and values, family experiences, cultural history, and economic forces.

This context impacts the social policies, services, and ultimately the clients we serve. Dr. Margaret Lawrence, the first African American to attend the Columbia Psychoanalytic Institute and dedicated therapist to the families of Harlem, urged fellow practitioners to work from the following standpoint: "Know the long sweep of your own history…know the values embedded in your cultural perspective; know the inner workings of your own psyche…" (p. 2).[1] The helper's role "is not designed simply to maintain the status quo, to make impoverished people feel comfortable with their deprived state. When therapy is successful there will be social and cultural ripples, if not waves. Individual health inspires a changed view of old, unproductive conditions. There is a strong, if complicated, relationship between psychotherapy (insight) and social change" (p. 3).[1]

Learning about social policy and government by examination of our social context and values may increase our effectiveness as client advocates and collaborative team members. This chapter will focus on the following topics: government and social policy, homeostasis, and strategies for change.

272

Governance and Social Policy

Government can be defined as the act or process of governing, especially the control and administration of public policy in a political unit. Readers should consider "the people" as integral components of both the organization and outcomes of government. A general outline of government structure is provided.

State Government

Executive branch
Governor
Secretary of state
Attorney general
State auditor
Government council
"Secretariats and agencies" (Public Health, Human Services, Transportation, etc.)
Judicial branch
Supreme court, superior court, appeals court, district court
Legislative committees that report to:
House of Representatives (160 members/160 districts)
Senate (40 members/40 districts)

Government as an ideal can express human rights, democracy, equality, civic participation, and a growth-promoting society.[2] Many factors create barriers to this ideal.

Government is inherently complex, much like explaining how a switch turns on a lightbulb. We cannot see the array of parts comprising the electrical system. There are a fuel source, a generator, distribution of power, wiring conduits, and a target appliance in the home. Government and legislation have multiple steps and utilize a language that is not clear to the average citizen. All manner of human interactions both precede and follow the process of governmental decisions.

Understanding the structural functions of government, though helpful, is not essential to making policy change. Knowledge of the process is gained in increments, much like peeling an onion. As an advocate, you may use the structure of government as a directory to focus advocacy and social action. It may be more pragmatic to consider national, state, and local governments as large, complex organizations made up of thousands of people. This oversimplification directs our attention to an essential variable in policy making and policy change, the human element. People, in large part, shape society, which in turn influences government. Government in turn largely shapes the thoughts and actions of the people (Fig. 15.1).

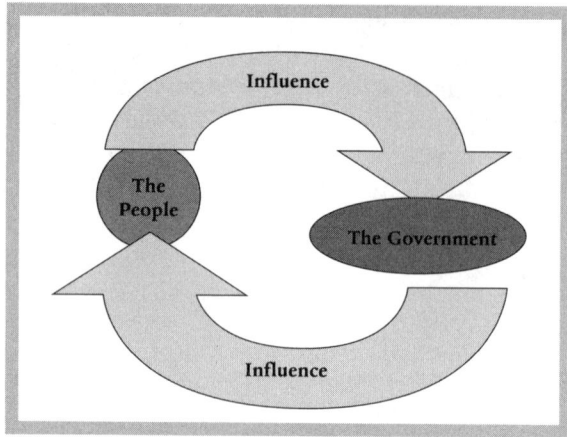

FIGURE 15.1 People and government influence one another.

Social Context

Social policy evolves from government. *Social policy* can be defined as policy management or procedure based primarily on material interest, a definite course or method of action selected from among alternatives and in light of given conditions to guide and determine present and future decisions, and a high-level overall plan embracing the general goals and acceptable procedures especially of a governmental body. Broad examples of social policy include our constitution, state constitutions, human service agency guidelines, and general law.

Those who administer policy (i.e. government officials, appointees, and employees) are essentially ordinary people. They drive, use public transportation, watch movies, shop at supermarkets, own pets, and use bathrooms. They are neighbors, parents, teachers, contractors, legal and medical professionals, and perhaps film actors.

Interdisciplinary workers are also people living in the same culture as our officials. Policy makers and human service workers operate from neighborhood values or the values of our families.[3]

History

Institutional or social knowledge is comprised of common, shared information including wisdom, myths, and practical information. This knowledge is passed on through time, which guides our thoughts and conduct (Fig. 15.2).[4]

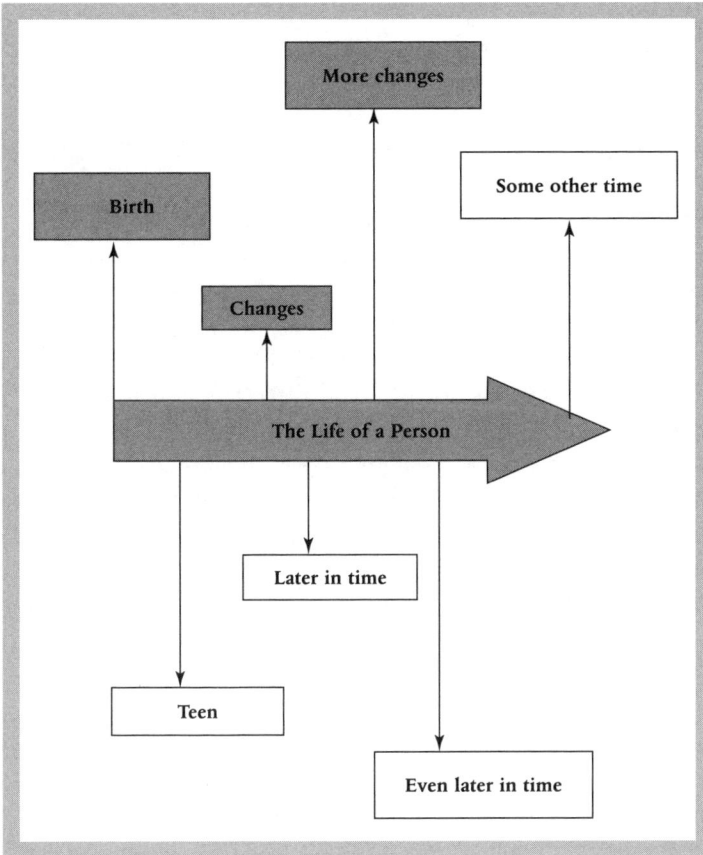

FIGURE 15.2 Evolution of knowledge.

History can serve as a powerful guide to the interdisciplinary worker for policy solutions. Many of the problems and solutions for today were identified and established long ago. Most of the scholarly work cited in this chapter is well over two decades old as the insights seem stronger with the passage of time. A variety of historic human service lessons are summarized to display a potential failing to learn from the past.

- Louis René Villermé (1782–1863), a founder of epidemiology, challenged 2000-year-old premises for disease causation. Social factors, as opposed to strict environmental factors, were found to correlate with neighborhood mortality in Paris. Wealthy neighborhoods had lower mortality than poor neighborhoods.[5]

- In 1939, differences in rates of mental disorders in Chicago were described as the result of socioeconomic conditions. Stress related to certain neighborhoods increased the likelihood of having a mental health problem.[6]
- In 1953, poverty was again reported to be a factor in mental illness.[6]
- In 1967, Burton Blatt, assistant commissioner for mental retardation at the Massachusetts Department of Mental Health, urged the governor and state legislature to "develop a network of small community centered residential facilities.... Without such approaches we will continue to fund new curtains, and paint jobs and once or twice in a century we will demolish old buildings" (pp. ix–x).[7] In December 1986 the governor of Massachusetts cited expenditures of $240 million over a 10-year period to improved buildings at five institutions for mental retardation. This came to $76,000 per resident, for building improvement, curtains, and paint jobs. Community residence development was kept to a minimum in that time frame.
- Titmuss[8] reported in 1968 that the war on poverty launched in 1964 was failing due to a lack of opportunity for participation by those in need of services in the government structures that promulgate their impoverishment.
- In 1990 Brody reported that caregiving for an elder or disabled adult or child can cause mental stress and other physical health problems. Approximately 50% of the caregivers reported concerns.[6]

The revelation of social problems and potential solutions does not prevent their reoccurrence. Our society stresses values of caring while continually showing resistance to social solutions. If we recognize mechanisms of resistance, homeostasis, we may increase the likelihood of developing a means to change these situations. "It's a mistake to assume it could never happen again" (p. 59).[9] Anyone who studies the language of the Navajo–Athabaskan confronts the reality of conceptual repetition. What was can be again.

Homeostasis

> For the human mind, generally speaking, does not just think: it thinks with ideas, most of which it simply adopts and takes over from its surrounding society (p. 44).[10]

This section deals with understanding mechanisms that sustain social practices and policies (Fig. 15.3). This can be positive if the condition we are sustaining is "good" for the people. Promoting the use of sidewalks is a good practice. Sustaining negative conditions is problematic. A worker's lack of an adequate wage not only compromises his or her day-to-day life but has a direct impact on his or her elder years. This section will review homeostasis and its

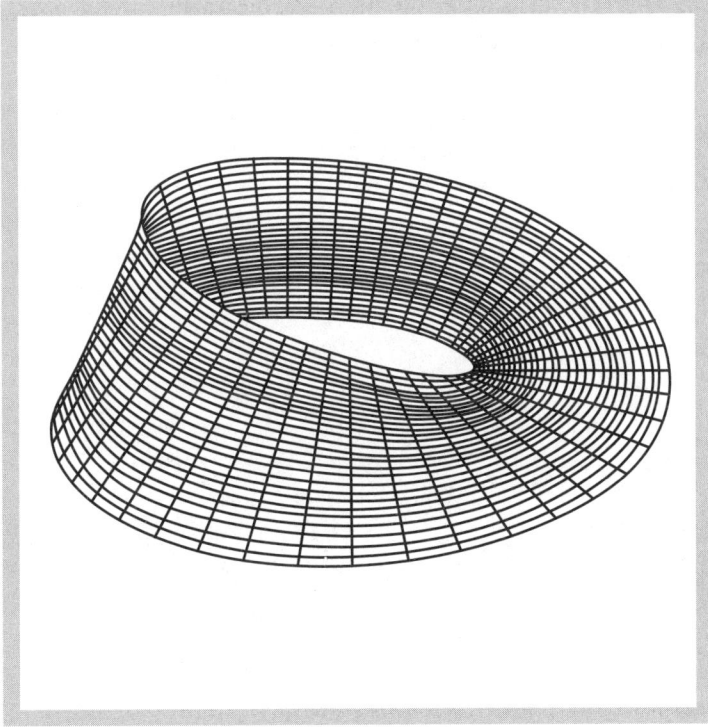

FIGURE 15.3 Continuity of social practices and policies.

relationship to social change through the following topics: power and privilege, homeostasis via policies and industry of care, homeostasis through the human service economics, and invisibility.

Homeostasis is a process of keeping things the same, which includes maladaptive or counterproductive policies and social practices. We participate and live in a world that supports the status quo.[11] If a person deviates from the ongoing pattern, society tends to push back and shape the individual back into habit.[12,13]

Power and Privilege

Homeostasis in society can be attributed to individuals' attempts to maintain their power and privilege. Rousseau states "Law is a very good thing for men with property and a very bad thing for men without property" (p. 44).[2] The tone of a culture is largely determined by the ruling factions. A ruling class usually comprises a minority of the population and holds certain advantages. Our government is purportedly democratic but relies on representation by a privileged minority, which does not allow full participation by all sections of society. Government action may not reflect the needs of the general populace.[14]

It is interesting to pause and reflect on what society is being conditioned to and who determines our social agenda.[15] He who pays the piper calls the tune. *Elites* get to define what is a problem.[16] Elites, or "haves," possess power, money, and security and want to maintain this status.[17] In order to broaden the base of social change, we need to understand some of the established mechanisms elites use to maintain power.

Homeostasis via Policies and Industry of Care

We maintain dependent populations and live off their social problems through the creation of human service industries. Max Weber stated "There are two ways of making politics into one's vocation: Either one lives 'for' politics or one lives 'off' politics" (p. 84).[18] This same premise holds true for the policies and services we develop. Government and its designated agencies keep control over services and the potential to create solutions, yet clients need solutions to their specific problems.[19]

Governments pay workers to appease segments of the population and support the status quo.[12] As human service workers, we serve corporate, agency, and government interests. Analogous to therapists working in prisons, much of the endeavor essentially assists the inmates in staying adjusted to the milieu. We also may be working to assist people to cope with life rather than to change the context where their problems may originate. People conform to institutional arrangements which disempower or enmesh them and "appear" to be the only way of life. Poor people are led to believe that their poverty is deserved and riches are deserved by others of differing classes.[20] Social Darwinism sorted and sifted people much like plants: Those who climbed had better natural talents.[11] Early eugenists identified the "fit" with the upper classes and the "unfit" with the lower classes. "Morons," pooled from lower classes, were generously categorized as such. Fit, college-educated "well-to-do" were at the upper end of the spectrum of wellness. Biology was seen as the root of poverty, rather than socioeconomic conditions. By focusing on the physical and mental aspects of people in need, we consequently distract public attention from the broad problems of social welfare.[21]

Adam Smith, the economist, is well known for his concept of the "invisible hand." People's interests are led in the direction that contributes to the well-being of the whole society.[11] Given that a portion of society are considered clients, and not by their own choice, what question does this raise? Human service workers deal with nonvoluntary clients.[19] When one's choice is no choice, our notions of equality and democracy are in question. Did the poor, unfed, and "stressed-out" choose this place in society? If this condition exists, is it in the interest of the whole society? We should perhaps put a glove on the invisible hand to see it more clearly.

Inherent in being poor is a lack of capital resources and guidance to direct change efforts. The poor misdirect action at agents who are part of the system. They may show a great deal of anger at a local welfare office as opposed to directing their protest at Washington, D.C. Without funds for transportation, hotels, or the freedom to take time off from work, they are limited in their initial efforts to voice change.[20] The sheer energy of living one day at a time is directed at basic survival. It is an "overwhelming present" (p. 98).[22] "Small marginal revisions in public assistance, job training or health insurance can not change environments fast enough to do much" (p. 7) for individuals affected by poverty.[23] Marginal interventions are just that, marginal. The other way to keep a group dependent is to offer charity. Charity acknowledges a social problem while sustaining both the social problem and individuals dependent on "hand-outs." The assistance, though well intentioned, is ameliorative at best. It reduces the acuity of problems such as hunger or short-term material needs but does not provide any longer-term solutions. Dependence is one of the structures our society relies on to keep the economy just the way it is.

Homeostasis Through the Human Service Economics

The presence of a dependent population serves the economy by creating a service industry. The workers, "experts," are a type of elite and hold solutions for dependent clients. Ryan[24] sees the mechanism evolving through identifying a social problem, defining individuals with the problem as different, and attributing the cause of the social problem as related to the individual's problem nature. The service formula is simple: Work to change the victim. This essentially means "serve people."

Bailey and Brake cite Bill Jordan (1973): "Be aware of artificially created financial problems as suitable material for social work intervention" (p. 126).[25] Poverty can be seen as an artificially created, though very real, social problem. If we look at our minimum wage and its associated hardships, we can simply change conditions by raising the wage to correlate with the actual costs required to live comfortably. Issues related to lack of health care could be solved by providing health care. Workers within the system talk about the need for services for their clients but do not voice the need to change the social context that is at the root of their clients' (and their own) problems.

Gunnar Dybwad talks of system maintenance in the form of institutions. These institutions represent past investment of hundreds of millions of dollars "but are still today considered by legislators and politicians as ideal receptacles for new construction funds...they employ large groups of people who have come to feel that their employment in the institutions is a vested right" (p. 175).[26]

Nursing homes are not simply private institutions when viewed through the flow of public dollars that support them. The government discharges its obligation to serve elders and disabled individuals to nursing homes. Gaylin et al.[27] report that the public, in the form of state government, holds the burden, through 1115 waivers, to prove to the funding agents, the federal government, that providing noninstitutional support costs less than or as much as the current modes of support authorized by the Centers for Medicaid and Medicare. Those forms of support are most commonly long-term care facilities.

Aging, a natural phenomenon, is now a service commodity. The workforce to serve elders includes physicians, lawyers, housing officials, and care managers. Despite their status as competent free citizens, nursing home patients share much with children and incarcerated individuals. Control is one of the most prevalent features of a nursing facility. Elders must frequently sign over their assets. Privacy is compromised and autonomy short-circuited through regimens of medication, care, and privileges. The elderly person is dependent upon the institution for food, clothing, recreation, and companionship. Can an institution really provide what humans are biologically wired to do?[27]

Part of the industry exists to provide jobs. The salaries of street-level bureaucrats make up a good portion of nondefense government expenditures.[19] Welfare recipient organizations state that their workers receive more money to help the poor than the poor receive in yearly welfare payments from the same welfare office. In many states the budget for Medicaid services to poor individuals is larger than the budget for direct cash to those recipients.[16]

The inequality embedded in public wealth distribution has been demonstrated through studies in New York City and Chicago. Both studies show that over 60% of all public funds in those cities for poor folks are allocated for services versus direct income to those in need.[16] This means that less than 40% of the overall funds to serve people actually go to these same people. There are other mechanisms that keep problems static. The inability to see problems needs examination.

Invisibility

This section defines "invisibility." We consider the concepts of complexity and consciousness as elements of making a problem invisible. The emperor believed he had clothes even though all evidence showed otherwise. An entire village rallied around him with full knowledge that he was nude. They complimented his nonexistent clothes, as finery no less, for fear of reprisal. Groups can coalesce both consciously and unconsciously around certain realities. Policies can lead us to feel secure or dressed, yet with examination they may prove to do just the opposite. "Like the natives of Lewis Carroll's remarkable Wonderland, they saw nothing strange or incongruous in their surroundings" (p. 2).[11]

Complexity

Problems can also be hidden in layers of carefully articulated complexity. Complexity can include numbers or language to veil social challenges.

Complexity in numbers

Problems can be made invisible by hiding them in vast numbers. Vast numbers can make us numb or desensitized. There is a saying about war: One death is a tragedy, a thousand deaths are a statistic. We tend to cleanse a problem with numbers (Fig. 15.4).

Homelessness serves as one example: 20–25% of individuals who are homeless meet criteria for serious mental illness; 66% of homeless report substance use and/or mental health problems.[28] Another study states that 40% of homeless individuals have a mental illness and 91% have serious emotional difficulty which shows the need for mental health services.[29] On top of this there are approximately 1 million individuals who are homeless in any year. Given this "fact," we have an unaddressed epidemic.

Another example relates to the fact that over 1 million elders in Massachusetts have Alzheimer's disease. This number may not strike some as significant. If we picture other cities—such as Hartford, Connecticut, Memphis, Tennessee, or Providence, Rhode Island—we get a much deeper sense of the magnitude. Add to this number the family members and friends of the person with the disease, and you may double or even triple the number of people who are impacted.

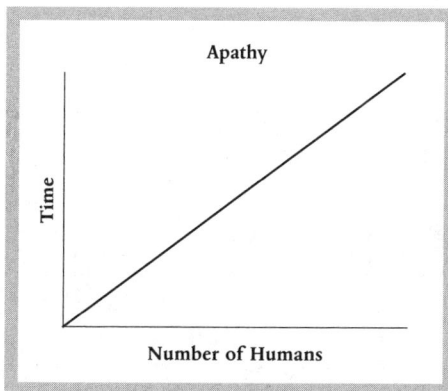

FIGURE 15.4 Overwhelmed by mass.

Complexity in language

Language can also create distortions in our perceptions. The meanings of words or processes have changed through social use. On a simple level, words have both a denotation and a connotation. Examples that come to mind include the following:

America versus the United States. America consists of two continents and 16 nations.

Sex is a word that can mean a pleasurable and loving activity or gender.

Cool is used to describe a less than warm temperature or a person's calm disposition.

"What we call normal is a product of repression, denial, splitting, projection, introjection and other forms of destructive action on experience" (pp. 27–28).[30] It is radically estranged from the experience or structure of being. Normal men have killed over 100 million of their fellow normal men in the last 50 years. This figure was cited by Laing[30] from 1917 until 1967. The world has had at least seven more major military conflicts since 1967. Think of many of the daily behaviors we call "normal." If we call something "normal," rather than a "problem," it fails to be problematic.

Language can clearly reduce the impact of a problem. We refer to "defense" as aggressive actions against others. We refer to a "poverty level," without looking at the true cost of living. We talk of "noninstitutional settings" for care while creating mini-institutions such as assisted living facilities and group homes. We work in "not-for-profit" institutions, but someone clearly profits. We must be permitted to allow certain problems to exist by using appropriate descriptors and plain English in order to prevent them.

Prevention has been reviewed in a previous chapter. We mislabel many of our services as "prevention." We actually mean secondary or tertiary prevention, when real prevention is primary prevention. A simple Google search using the words "prevention" and "organization" revealed over 70 million instances. The first 20 citations noted child abuse, crime, pollution, and health. Two examples of the mislabeling of prevention are provided: caring and prevention.

"Care is the consenting commitment of citizens to one another. Care cannot be produced, provided, managed, organized, administered or commoditized. Care is the only thing a system can not produce" (p. x).[16] Love is a facet of caring. It is normal for parents to love their children, but it is not "normal" for society to care for or love the mentally ill, troubled children, individuals experiencing homelessness, or the abjectly poor.[27]

The Society for the Prevention of Cruelty to House Plants deals with plants after they have been neglected, after the soil was left arid or overwatered, after the pot tipped over (due to being left on a precarious edge), after being left in the sun or shade too long. Real prevention would involve circumstances where the plant (and its owner) was given full knowledge of how to care for itself, adequate water, and adequate housing to provide sunlight. We generally treat elders or others after they fall in a cramped, ill-equipped bathroom or on a slick walkway. We have not gone out and waged a full-scale policy initiative to identify risky bathrooms or walkways.

Consciousness

Invisibility is also largely a matter of how we direct our conscious attention. We may fail to think of something as a problem simply because we fail to think about it, out of ignorance. Other problems are invisible through conscious action, disregard, or denial.

Ignorance

Note: The most dangerous assumption is the one we don't know we are making.

The impact on certain social problems could be reduced simply by changing how we use resources. We don't examine our personal and national buying habits. SUVs, luxury cars, fancy offices, and lavish homes are expensive. Government contributions to football stadiums, helicopters, and stealth bombers also eat up a good amount of cash. The cost of pollution and wasted electricity and water further decreases the available resource capital that could be used alternately for a social good. The redirection of these resources could provide a tremendous wealth to those in need. The playing field could be leveled.

We may not understand that the convenience and low price of a product, designed to increase profit, are related to the low wage we pay workers involved in the manufacture and supply of that item. Many of us don't understand what it means to work for minimum wage. When I purchase a can of beef soup for a dollar, I do not see the beef factory or the farms which exist to produce grain for the cattle. I don't think about the fact that 1 pound of beef is raised through at least 6 pounds of grain. That grain could feed hungry people. I don't see the people raising the cattle, the can factories, the paper mills, the chemical plants to make ink for the paper labels, the delivery trucks, and the stock people and cashiers at the supermarket. The low price of soup represents hundreds of workers.

R. D. Laing[30] cites the example of pâté de foie gras. A worker stuffs things down a live goose's neck with a funnel. We don't see this or try to think of this. We instead eat the pate spread on bread or crackers. Chicken farms and beef ranches are equally notorious.

Disregard

We can also make certain problems invisible by ignoring them. Our family once had a contractor whose work was dodgy. His common refrain, for leaky pipes and wobbly walls (delivered with a smirk), was "You can't see it from my house." How many problems can we disregard from our "house" or car, job, or vacation spot? Deforestation is another example. We consume wood and paper goods but "can't see it from our house." The logging roads of Washington, Maine, or the Amazon are far away. We drive large cars, consciously aware of the diminishing supply of fuel. Workers in urban settings become desensitized to walking past homeless elders.

Not only may we not see things from our house, but we may also disregard problems from the perspective of our lifetime. The polluted rivers of the United States are largely due to industrial and sewage practices set in motion well over a century ago. Individuals concerned with their immediate needs are not thinking enough about the future.[11]

An Eastern parable comes to mind. A little boy laughs as he watches his grandfather plant saplings. "Grandfather you are a very, very old man. Why are you planting trees that you will not see?" The grandfather rests his hand on his grandson's shoulder and replies, "So you will have trees."

Our society believes in its humanitarianism and altruism. It is very hard to accept that the same culture has effectively blocked much needed social change. The subsequent brief history captures many of the dynamics of invisibility and intractability.

Conquering the Invisible

Dr. Ignaz Philipp Semmelweis was a Viennese obstetrician who made an incredible medical breakthrough in 1847. During this time, having a baby at a hospital significantly increased the likelihood of death or the childbearing disease *kindbettfieber*. Doctors were primarily men, gentlemen, clean, well dressed, and well mannered. Semmelweis began to study the practices within his own profession after the death of a colleague echoed the symptoms of dead mothers. Were doctors in some way responsible for the deaths of women despite their good intentions?

He found that doctors were not washing their hands between examining the women. Their hands could not possibly be dirty as they were gentlemen. A cloth was used to wipe the doctor's hands between patients and, thus, hands appeared clean. Semmelweis found the mothers' deaths could be traced by following physicians through a ward. He suggested that unseen germs were the cause of the women's deaths—that, in fact, doctors were inadvertently killing the patients. The potential infection from one patient was passed to another via the open birth wounds. The unseen, unthinkable, and ultimately changeable factors were variables in the mortality of mothers. When he presented his findings with regard to doctors being agents in these deaths, he was met with incredible resistance and defiance.

The Semmelweis story underscores two issues. (1) It is possible to partake in governance, services, policy, and daily life in ways that hurt others as opposed to helping. Medical processes that cause harm are referred to as "iatrogenic practices." Infections that are related to hospital treatment are referred to as "nosocomial infections." Structural processes or policy processes, including our failures to respond, may be the policy equivalent of iatrogenic illness.[16] (2) We can fail to see that our practices, despite evidence, are harmful. What causes us to disregard "evidence"? Our failure to see may be rooted in personal gain or fear of some loss, such as income, status, or social position.

Strategies for Change

Once we are aware of the mechanisms that create or sustain social problems, we may be able to engage in more effective change. As an individual or part of a team, we should first discard the notion of a perfect approach to change. There will be times when there is a clear goal, times of trial and error, and times when the process is of greater relevance than the outcome. This section will address the following practices to engage in change: lens, questioning, role of dialogue, role of language, groups, research, action, and powerlessness.

The important question isn't so much the "rhetoric" of the policy but the social outcome. In order to understand social outcomes, we need to become aware of our perspectives, our lens, to subsequently examine and better understand social conditions.

Lens

Your way of seeing and framing a problem greatly impacts your approach to solving it. You are the sum total of your experiences and the experiences of others around you (Fig. 15.5).

Try on a different lens to bring a problem (or solution) into focus. There are many modes which can assist us in the identification of problems: sociologic, frames, social problems, social constructionism, meritocratic, social Darwinism, economic, philosophic, the work of Heidegger (intention and being) and Jacques Derrida (deconstructionism), psychological, family systems theory, cognitive behavioral therapy, humanistic psychology, and self-actualization.

More basic understandings of one's thinking may also be of value. Do you look at the world in an overly concrete fashion, as blacks and whites, or glasses

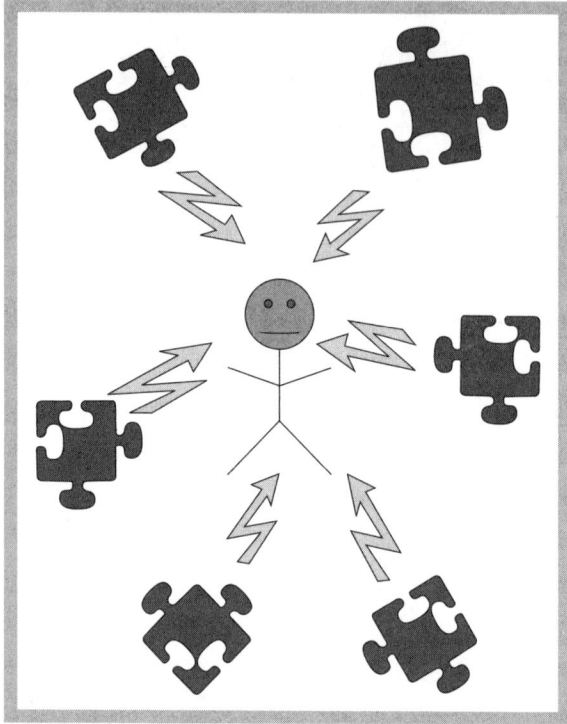

FIGURE 15.5 Experiences shape attitudes.

half empty or half full? "There is nothing more difficult than to become critically aware of the presuppositions of one's thought. Everything can be seen directly except the eye through which we see" (p. 44).[10] Learn about your perspective.

Some people talk of solution-focused work, as if "problem-based" work is pejorative. In order to identify a course of action, we must identify what isn't working. The next step is to hone one's lens, to focus it.

Questioning

The act of reasoning or questioning of social structures and life can be an additional tool in social change.

An example of effective reasoning is borrowed with gratitude from Louise Day Hicks. Hicks battled against school integration through the practice of bussing students outside of their own neighborhoods: She was profound in her austere statement, "The culturally deprived children need education not transportation" (p. 32).[24]

We must not be concerned with questioning the status quo, which includes social, political, religious, and moral values. We must also not shy away from our conclusions, drawn from our questions. These questions, proverbially "outside the box," may provide a course of action for social change. We must also give consideration to the reasons that problems are repeated or, more accurately, left unsolved for so long.

McKnight[16] poses five questions that help us penetrate social policy:

1. What are the negative effects of services designed to help?
2. Where might an intervention be paired with other services? What is the conjoint impact of combined services or services existing in relation to one another?
3. How would a focus that builds on human capacity be different from serving client needs or deficiency?
4. Will giving direct funding to those in need ultimately be more beneficial than funding an array of services?
5. Is community integration a better approach than institutional or fragmented services?

The way to reveal a problem or solution may involve engaging in paradox or contradiction. What would happen in the absence of a given intervention or situation?[19] Examples of paradoxical questions include the following:

If we live in a democracy, why are people choosing poverty, lack of education, and rough neighborhoods or institutional settings?
Why are we resourcing education when our children are learning less?
Why are we putting resources into criminal justice when society seems less safe?[16]

On a larger scale, our social energies and resources could be placed elsewhere. What can we do as an alternative to mainstream actions such as wars, building sports stadiums, or outer space development? Though we can engage in war, put men on the moon, rove mars, guard our southern borders, we can't seem to prevent the tragedy that recently affected New Orleans or the blight of many other communities in the United States.

Marx stated that if somebody who knows the laws of gravity finds himself in deep water and cannot swim, his knowledge will not prevent him from drowning. A Chinese proverb states, "Reading prescriptions does not make one well."[15] The power of questions or reasoning is enhanced when practiced with others, such as interdisciplinary teams. A team assisting elders possesses a wealth of diversity and wisdom.

Role of dialogue

Deep questions asked to one's self potentially breed insight. Questions asked in partnership with others can bring a much broader perspective. We need to understand our own actions in trying to influence policy. Alone we may not be aware of our own roles, incompetence, or ideologies. "Even facts become fiction without adequate ways of seeing the 'the facts'" (p. 17).[30] Experience, which involves history, helps build new theories for change, especially when experience is "felt" as a discourse or dialogue. As the reader may note, much of the material in this chapter is based on the experience of past decades. Teaching as a process of dialogue builds human experience through active learning, group and personal recognition of knowledge. We build the road as we travel, correcting the course as we may need.

In contrast to dialogical teaching, institutional learning relies heavily on "banking education." *Banking education* is essentially a process of filling a student up with knowledge and rote facts which can be memorized. The teacher is seen as the leader or boss. The student is seen as ignorant or subordinate.[22] Curriculums are developed outside the classroom by specialists.

Dialogical teaching, in contrast, creates a base of common knowledge among all participants—activists, social workers, or students. A facilitator engaged in dialogue and conjoint learning may greatly enhance the learning process. All participants work to insure that the teaching does not revert to banking education. The process of dialogical teaching, praxis, has two stages, reflection and action, which can lead to social change.[22]

Dialogue paired with insight frees those in their communication. They can see neighbors—people with lesser, greater, or equivalent means—as connected to them. Disregard for anyone is counter to being civilized or humane. Dialogue leads us to consider ourselves in a larger group context.

Role of groups

> No Man is an Iland, intire of it selfe.
> —John Donne (1572–1631), cited by Schumacher (p. 84)[10]

As we've noted earlier, social policy and governance are social or group activities. Social change is most effective when we work in a group toward a common goal.

We cannot create social transformation alone. Groups possess the strength to challenge institutions and the government. With regard to group processes, Hegel and Freire's thoughts are particularly poignant. Ideas generate ideas, counter ideas, and dialogue is an instrument of change.[11,22]

It should be noted that there is also an alarming tendency for groups to isolate from one another or fail to collaborate. Policy and social agencies have a tendency to form silos, to exist in separate fields. For example, many groups, such as elders and individuals with disabilities, share the need for decent housing. Resources are constrained through our overall Health and Human Service Administration budget. This agency serves multiple peoples within our country. Any groups, in order to meet their needs, must compete with each other for resource capital to create services. Education may garner more support than health insurance.

Our culture must learn that we have to share part of the wealth or lose all of it. We must endeavor to learn to respect and live with other political ideologies if we want our own culture to prevail.[2] Currently, the government is funding initiatives to facilitate communications among aging and disability resources. It is ironic, albeit positive, that the very silos we created are now being funded to talk to one another via grants representing millions of dollars.

We frequently fail to acknowledge the interrelatedness of most social problems. The problems of the young, if not treated, become the problems of the old. Some of those who are old may develop changes in their physical health, for example, mobility challenges, that can be supported through our existing disability network. The work of one group to better insure the needs of the developmentally disabled may have success that can be translated into helping elders with cognitive problems. We do human service a disservice when we set up a system where one well-intentioned interest group competes against another to meet its needs.

The interdisciplinary worker must consider him- or herself as an agent of change. The team itself, the support from others, is an indispensable resource to sustain transformative action within a rigid system. To join with others in a manner that has greater meaning and potential impact, interdisciplinary workers require a tool to discuss the basic needs of their clients.

Role of language

The use of a common language and lens to examine the practices of government and other organizations is essential. Policy viewed through a human-needs lens may significantly enhance our ability to become agents of change. Basic human needs can be characterized as biological, material, psychological, social, productive, creative, security-providing, and spiritual.[31]

Policies must provide an accessible, equitable means for people to eat, drink, sleep, and have shelter. Humans need a means to work and produce goods for the sustenance of life.[3] With this common language we can enhance our ability to work in partnership, frame our questions, and partner with or pilot research.

Group work insures that solutions are ameliorative and to what degree. It may also help with the acquisition of multiple perspectives to insure that the solution does not generate new problems.[17] With a solid sense of partnership and power, we can begin to launch on research more affiliated with primary prevention.

Research

The mission to probe deeply and to work and dialogue in community places us in a position to better engage in or consume research. Policy and service research should involve the evaluation of events that have affected the past and present and the process which impacts workers in the service of elders and others across all community settings.[8]

Research requires probing with the types of questions we discussed earlier. Numbers such as social statistics and census data identify populations but do not tell us why they are encountering certain challenges. Fragmentation of research poses another challenge. We may only look at one facet of a service. We may refer to a whole battery of support as community service with little examination of which parts of the service are included, excluded, of impact, or hindering effectiveness.

Ryan[24] identifies three potential research pitfalls:

Centralization. The research may be removed from the sources of data. This includes distance, whether physical or intellectual, between the researcher and the subject. Sharing of information among researchers and participants may also be limited.

Lack of comprehensive planning (reactive or ameliorative planning)

Accountability (all words but no music—absolve of responsibility to solve problems in meaningful way)

The research methods to gauge quality or effectiveness point to values but not to multipronged solutions. Solutions exist, but the current research paradigm does not reveal them. Measuring "the efficacy of various social and economic interventions will identify the piecemeal failures, but do not guide us to the situations in which simultaneous, multifaceted interventions would work" (p. 9).[23] "Various groups find it to their advantage to promote and call attention to some antecedents of any condition and to ignore or dismiss others as insignificant" (p. 69).[17] Examples include elder safety program measurements. Abuse reduction does not usually look at the idea of a particular episode or typology of abuse being of profound impact to an elder. Routine descriptive statistics which report cases responded to do not get at whether the problem is being eradicated. Another example is the evaluation of employment agencies. When placement of employees was examined, counselors shifted their work to the more placeable clients. In a similar fashion, when monitored, individuals who work with elders tended to disregard more difficult cases.[19]

Gunnar Dybwad, former director of the National Association of Retarded Citizens, has been cited as saying, "Every time we identify a need in this field we build a building" (p. 14).[23] Existing research can guide social policy and the solutions to social problems. Justice William Douglas, stated in 1954 with regard to urban renewal that it "was not enough...to remove existing buildings that were unsanitary or unsightly. It was important to redesign the whole area so as to eliminate conditions that cause slums....It was believed that the piecemeal approach, the removal of individual structures that were offensive, would only be palliative. The entire area needed redesigning" (p. 24).[32]

Research regarding the effectiveness of service delivery, though effective for secondary and tertiary prevention, distracts attention from the potential to deal with the roots of a given problem, which is why we need service in the first place. Research investigators tend to use complex theories. Clinicians and street-level workers, as well as the clients themselves, need simple solutions. Clinicians do have the ability to simplify problems or look at the social context. The challenge is to identify and engage the social factors most relevant to change a client's circumstances.

Action

Interdisciplinary workers are important agents of social change. Using some of the tools we've identified—praxis, group work, and research—we can next embark on organizing for social action. Social workers urgently need an education in how to place themselves in the world of politics.[25]

Alinsky cites Burke: "The only thing necessary for the triumph of evil is for good men to do nothing" (p. 20).[2] Another story helps, in the abstract, to move to social change. The first story involves a social worker at the scene of a terrible flood. A river is overflowing and displaying uncharacteristically strong rapids. The social worker sees two people struggling in the water, jumps in, and pulls them to safety. A crowd begins to form and cheers for the social worker. Three more people float downstream and the social worker again jumps in and pulls them out—one, two, three. Four more people are struggling in the water. The social worker pulls each of them out. An incredible, deafening cheer is heard. The social worker starts to run away. The crowd yells, "Where are you going?" The social worker yells back, "I'm going upstream to find out where all these people are coming from."

There are a range of specialists who write about social organizing and social action. For the purposes of this chapter, I use Saul Alinsky's[2] guide for social action (pp. 127–130).

Power is essential whether via numbers, group affiliation, or the illusion of a large group.

Let your group's experience guide your action.

Use facts. This can include research, testimony, and the government's own tenets, which include the constitution and law.

Promote community and support while engaged in change (and afterward).

Build a platform of change on multiple issues, builds group, encourages longevity, reinforces interdependence of social problems and solutions.

Keep pressure on. Alinsky[2] cites Franklin Roosevelt: "Okay you've convinced me. Now go on out and bring pressure on me!" (p. xxiii).

Pose alternatives to the problem (solutions).

Direct actions toward specific agents or agencies and hold to the target.

Powerlessness

As one organizes, one should also be aware of mechanisms which may hamper initial efforts to organize and mobilize change. There are two modes of rendering the organizer powerless, externally generated holdups and internally generated holdups, which relate more to the psychology of team members.

External removal of power

The government and other institutions use an array of tactics to maintain the status quo. Being attuned to these devices will afford groups that are in action opportunities to anticipate and continue moving forward.

Debora Stone[33] identifies the following stasis-producing modalities:

State goals ambiguously.

Shift goals and redefine goals as politics indicate.

Keep undesirable alternatives off an agenda by not mentioning them.

Make alternatives seem as if they are the only ones possible.

Focus on one part of the chain and ignore others that may cause political problems.

Use rhetorical devices to blend alternatives, don't appear to make a clear decision.

Select from a range of consequences whose costs and benefits will make your course of action look best.

Choose a course of action that hurts powerful constituents the least but creates a maximum good social impression.

Additionally, be aware of the following devices. Watch an organization for blame shifting or minimizing a problem.[2] Governments and institutions may use an array of terms and phrases to create stagnation. These include saying an issue is:

In discussion

Going or gone to committee

Moving or moved to a different agency

Offline
Under the radar
Off the record

Other ways of decreasing worker effectiveness include making an individual feel inexperienced. "You need to be here a while and learn *the way it really is*." Tell someone that he or she needs to "learn the ropes." Instruct new employees to not make waves or go through channels and reinforce that they read the whistleblower policy. The only ropes learned here are equivalent in effect to pushing a rope. An activist who heeds these messages to any extreme becomes like a dead atheist, all dressed up with no place to go.

Internal removal of power

Surplus powerlessness is a manner of thinking which relies on the understanding that people or a context will never change.[34] Being aware of the mechanisms which we individually engage in will also assist us in avoiding them.

> The most common way people give up their power is by thinking they don't have any.
>
> —Alice Walker

Michael Lerner[34] presents 10 tenets he defines as surplus powerlessness.

Victim blaming (William Ryan)

Overinflating achievements because small change doesn't feel like "success"
Setups for battles they will lose and using those losses to justify giving up.
   With regard to client advocacy (self-advocacy), this can be seen as previous experience dictating not trying.
Forcing ideas
Discrediting peers working toward similar goals (through "isms")
Excluding people who don't have the same goals (They won't understand)
Toning down one's objectives for fear of rejection or alienating people

Social workers are part of large organizations (including society) and are subject (as are doctors and nurses) to regulations requiring political neutrality (which in and of itself is a fallacy). Titmuss,[8] citing C. Everett Hughes, reports that codes or expectations required by professional and employing organizations call for objective attitudes which demand neutrality toward problems where neutrality renders the worker almost ineffective in changing root causes of problems.

To launch workers into action, I've provided some simple examples of argumentation which can garner the attention of groups, agencies, or government. Research is one tool to help shape and apply social welfare measures. We must also cite data and historic events and create convincing arguments to capture the attention of those in power. The following example illustrates a sound provocative policy argument.

Redistribution of about $15 billion a year (less than 2% of our gross national product, which is now pushing toward $1 trillion annually) would bring every poor person above the present poverty line. This is less than half of our annual expenditure on the Vietnam War.[24]

We now have two subsequent wars on which to compare costs. Instead of funding the wars, we might have allocated these funds for other endeavors. Other facts can be used to help illustrate inherent challenges in our democratic structures. Essentially those with the most assets are less of the overall population and hold most of the wealth.[11] Even during democratic control of the White House from 1932 to 1959, 15 people with an annual income of $1 million to $28 million had no federal income tax obligations, while those with less than $1000 per year were liable for a tax of $13.50.[11] Advocates can show how the interests of the few may play out in the larger society.

One can also help illuminate the growing disconnect between the design of welfare programs and the cost of living. We would include elders, workers, and anyone who has to exist on a limited income. We would also help illuminate the harsh realities of what constitutes a limited income in the year 2007.

Assume you are a couple of social workers in the city of Boston. You have a 1-year-old child. You have decided to let your husband stay home and be with the child. Your family income is $45,000 per year.

Expenses:	Annual
Rent: $1600 per month for a two bedroom apartment	19,200
Utilities: $120 per month (gas, electric)	1440
Auto insurance	1000
Auto maintenance, gas, oil	3000
Health insurance	3000
Food	3000
Phone (land line and cell)	1200
Appliances	1000

We're already at $32,840. This leaves us with $12,160. We haven't figured in taxes, clothing, diapers, one dinner out per month, two emergency plane flights out of state to elder relatives, books, newspapers, pharmacy copayments, and anything else you'd care to add to the list. The median household income for Boston is approximately $38,000. One can feel the strain of life if one is at the median, slightly above, or below. A family income can imply that both parents are working or someone is working one or two jobs. Where would college tuition or training for a trade come in for the child?

Conclusion

Social policy and government, in theory, exist for the common good. It is up to us to help define, mobilize, and monitor this good. We must approach the system from a variety of perspectives, which include client, consumer, patient, worker, entitled, disenfranchised, of means, and without means. We must continually work to engage the system. This can be in our jobs and in our communities. It can be as simple as gently talking about social issues with a stranger on a train.

Maintaining an understanding of complexity, of multiple factors influencing social problems, is also essential. We must understand that we partake in a daily reality where, as we work for change, we are also reinforcing certain oppressive values. It is better to work for change, while understanding one has to eat, than to not work for change at all.

There are a range of possibilities for partaking in a changing world. These include checking on our neighbors, learning about green energy, and questioning the expenditures of government. My partner taught me a Japanese expression: The nail that sticks up gets hammered down. This is fine when we are looking for a code of conduct conducive to safety. It is agreeable when crossing a busy street and following the flow of pedestrian traffic. We must also understand that social change depends on nails that stick up. The nail can serve as a hook. The nail can also serve to fasten one of the boards of a public meeting house.

> Acknowledging that patients are people with their own rights, autonomy and power of making choices could lead to a very different atmosphere in hospitals and clinics. It could also stimulate a more active role for the community in health care. A new partnership between health workers and the community will depend on fundamental and lasting shifts in attitude. In some countries such shifts have accompanied or followed radical political change.[35]

A student of mine, who was also a grade school teacher told me an interesting story. A woman is observed at a beach after a terrible storm. She keeps bending and picking up object after object and throwing it back into the ceaseless surf. A mother and daughter stroll the beach. The daughter sees that the woman is picking up starfish. The mother notes that for every starfish she picks up, five more replace it. She asks the woman, "Why do you bother doing this? It does not seem to matter." The woman breaks from her work only briefly. "It matters to the starfish."

> It is not only for what we do that we are held responsible, but also for what we do not do.
>
> —Molière

Application to the Case Study: The Older Adult Care, Training, Research, and Planning Program

The premise for the Older Adult Care, Training, Research, and Planning Program (OACTRPP) is to engage in community health care. The community includes the local community improvement association, the Gray Action Coalition (a state older adult advocacy group), the city Health Department, the state Department of Elder Services, the federal government via the Centers for Medicare and Medicaid Services (CMS), and the National Institute on Aging.

This diverse and enriching community brings a range of perspectives to the OACTRPP project. The group decided at the onset to document its process of development and required a model of participatory action research to accompany the development of the OACTRPP. The group required a mission statement that defined certain terms associated with the project.

Community was carefully defined as the residential area surrounding the OACTRPP. *Health* was defined as a condition governed by social and economic factors, not simply the presence or nonpresence of a disease or injury.

Diversity was also considered an essential feature of the OACTRPP. An advisory council was established "across the life span." Though the focus of the care was directed at elders, the nature of care in the new millennium had to be flexible, to address a range of issues including younger clinicians caring for elders, ageism, elders at work, elders caring for their grandchildren, involvement of youth in the center, and a mission to insure diversity that crossed racial, social, cultural, and economic domains.

The advisory council, in concert with the community and the service community, held several meetings to discuss issues of power and autonomy. The center was to be run by individuals from the neighborhood. This presented a direct challenge to the range of funding agents that included a pharmaceutical research company and the medical center itself (a nonprofit) with an incredible amount of revenue at stake. Engaged elders conducted dialogue with the planners and future care providers, to insure everyone understood their roles and the potential impact the new center would have on the community. Old memories were rekindled from a period two decades ago, when the neighborhood consisted of older apartments, homes, and businesses. The promise to engage in efforts to create affordable housing by the medical center and the federal government was empty. To add insult to injury, the cost of medical care was prohibitive for certain elders just above the income cut-offs for public health disbursements.

These "contradictions in terms" were to be addressed up front. Currently, there is a unique symbiosis: The medical center needs the elders, and the elders need the medical center.

HealthCo, an entirely profitable venture, had to learn partnership. The community input into the development of the health center was framed as mutually advantageous. HealthCo could display the center as one of its beneficent ventures; the neighborhood could have greater discretion over the array of services the OACTRPP provided. The CMS was interested in supporting medical community partnerships in the form of resource centers. The community helped identify existing service resources in the neighborhood and city at large that could provide additional services. This would free up grant money for developing an array of community resources. The resource center became a "health care for all" facility. It also was for community meetings, groups, elder–youth mentoring programs, tutoring, Alcoholics Anonymous meetings, community message boards, a small computer lab, and volunteer opportunities for local kids after school. Medical students gained practical experience at an earlier point in their careers and were proximal to their residential facilities.

House-bound elders and disabled individuals were identified, and through the residency training program, the medical students, and a partnership with local nursing institutions, home-based services were created. A network of gatekeepers were also mobilized, enhancing the neighborhood's intactness and rebuilding a sense of community missing for 20 years. The medical center became a true health center, and the OACTRPP was conceived of as a phase one unit. The OACTRPP satellites were formed in neighborhood buildings and a school, and a homeless outreach unit was developed.

Bibliography

Aaron, H. J. (The Brookings Institution, Director of Economic Studies). Strategy vs Tactics in Designing Social Policy. Waltham, MA: Brandeis University, The Florence Heller Graduate School for Advanced Studies in Social Welfare, Arnold Gurin Venture Fund. Speech, April 28, 1992.

Alinsky, S.D. Rules for Radicals: A Pragmatic Primer for Realistic Radicals. New York: Vintage Books, 1972.

Allard, M.A., Howard, A.M., Vorderer, L.E., Wells, A.I., Braddock, D.L. (eds.) Ahead of His Time: Selected Speeches of Gunnar Dybwad. Washington, DC: American Association on Mental Retardation, 1999.

Bailey, R., Brake, M. (eds.) Radical Social Work. New York: Pantheon, 1975.

Bassuk, E.L., Rubin, L., Lauriat, A. Is homelessness a mental health problem. American Journal of Psychiatry 1984;141(12):1546–1549.

Berger, P.L., Luckman, T. The Social Construction of Reality: A Treatise in the Sociology of Knowledge. New York: DoubleDay, 1966.

Durkheim, E. On Morality and Society. London: University of Chicago Press, 1973.

Freedman, L.P. Reflections on emerging frameworks of health and human rights. In: Mann, J.M., Grodin Gruskin, S. (eds.) Health and Human Rights: A Reader. New York: Routledge, 1999.

Freire, P. Pedagogy of the Oppressed. New York: Continuum, 2000.

Fromm, E. Escape from Freedom. New York: Avon Books, 1969.

Fromm, E. The Anatomy of Human Destructiveness. Greenwich, CT: Fawcett Crest Books, 1975.

Gaylin, W., Glasser, I., Marcus, S., Rothman, D.J. Doing Good: The Limits of Benevolence. New York: Pantheon, 1978.

Gerth, H.H., Mills, C.W. (eds.) From Max Weber: Essays in Sociology. New York: Oxford University Press, 1958.

Gil, D. Unravelling Social Policy. Rochester, VT: Schenkman Books, 1992.

Haley, J. Problem-Solving Therapy: New Strategies for Effective Family Therapy. San Francisco: Jossey-Bass, 1978.

Hofstadter, R. Social Darwinism in American Thought. Boston: Beacon, 1958.

Laing, R.D. The Politics of Experience. New York: Ballantine Books, 1967.

Lawrence, S.L. Balm in Gilead: Journey of a Healer. Reading, MA: Addison-Wesley, 1988.

Lenski, G.E. Power and Privilege: A Theory of Social Stratification. New York: McGraw-Hill, 1966.

Lerner, M. Surplus Powerlessness: The Psychodynamics of Everyday Life and the Psychology of Individual and Social Transformation. Amherst, NY: Humanities Press, 1999.

Lipsky, M. Street-Level Bureaucracy: Dilemmas of the Individual in Public Services. New York: Russel Sage Foundation, 1980.

Majone, G. Evidence, Argument and Persuasion in the Policy Process. New Haven, CT: Yale University Press, 1989.

McKnight, J. The Careless Society: Community and Its Counterfeits. New York: Basic Books, 1995.

Nasdijj. The Blood Runs Like a River Through My Dreams. New York: Houghton Mifflin, 2000.

National Resource Center on Homelessness and Mental Illness. Available at: http://mentalhealth.samhsa.gov/publications/allpubs/KEN95-0015/default.asp. 2001.

Piven, F.F., Cloward, R.A. Poor People's Movements: Why They Succeed, How They Fail. New York: Vintage Books, 1979.

Ryan, W. Blaming the Victim. New York: Vintage Books, 1976.

Schon, D., Rein, M. Frame Reflections: Toward the Resolution of Intractable Policy Controversies. New York: Basic Books, 1994.

Schumacher, F.F. A Guide for the Perplexed. New York: Harper and Row, 1977.

Spector, M., Kitsuse, J.I. Constructing Social Problems. New Brunswick, NJ: Transaction Publishers, 2001.

Stone, D. Policy Pardox: The Art of Political Decision Making. New York: W. W. Norton, 1997.

Tausig, M. A Sociology of Mental Illness. Saddle River, NJ: Prentice-Hall, 1999.

Taylor, S., Biklen, D., Knoll, J. (eds.) Community Integration for People with Severe Disabilities. New York: Teachers College Press, 1987.

Titmuss, R.M. Commitment to Welfare. New York: Pantheon Books, 1968.

Tucker, C. (ed.) The Marx Engels Reader. New York: W. W. Norton, 1978.

World Health Organization. Social Dimensions of Mental Health. Geneva: World Health Organization, 1981.

References

1. Lightfoot, S.L. Balm in Gilead: Journey of a Healer. Reading, MA: Addison-Wesley, 1988.
2. Alinsky, S.D. Rules for Radicals: A Pragmatic Primer for Realistic Radicals. New York: Vintage Books, 1972, p. xxiv.
3. Fromm, E. Escape from Freedom. New York: Avon Books, 1969, p. 305.
4. Berger, P.L., Luckman, T. The Social Construction of Reality: A Treatise in the Sociology of Knowledge. New York: DoubleDay, 1966, p. 65.
5. Freedman, L.P. Reflections on emerging frameworks of health and human rights. In: Mann, J.M., Grodin Gruskin, S. (eds.) Health and Human Rights: A Reader. New York: Routledge, 1999, pp. 228–229.
6. ausig, M. A Sociology of Mental Illness. Saddle River, NJ: Prentice-Hall, 1999.
7. Taylor, S., Biklen, D., Knoll, J. (eds.) Community Integration for People with Severe Disabilities. New York: Teachers College Press, 1987.
8. Titmuss, R.M. Commitment to Welfare. New York: Pantheon Books, 1968, p. 100.
9. Nasdijj. The Blood Runs Like a River Through My Dreams. New York: Houghton Mifflin, 2000.
10. Schumacher, E.F. A Guide for the Perplexed. New York: Harper and Row, 1977.
11. Lenski, G.E. Power and Privilege: A Theory of Social Stratification. New York: McGraw-Hill, 1966, p. 41.
12. Haley, J. Problem-Solving Therapy: New Strategies for Effective Family Therapy. San Francisco: Jossey-Bass, 1978), p. 124.
13. Durkheim, E. On Morality and Society. London: University of Chicago Press, 1973, p. 51.
14. Majone, G. Evidence, Argument and Persuasion in the Policy Process. New Haven, CT: Yale University Press, 1989, p. 2.
15. Fromm, E. The Anatomy of Human Destructiveness. Greenwich, CT: Fawcett Crest, 1975, p. 58.
16. McKnight, J. The Careless Society: Community and Its Counterfeits. New York: Basic Books, 1995, p. 48.
17. Spector, M., Kitsuse, J.I. Constructing Social Problems. New Brunswick, NJ: Transaction Publishers, 2001, p. 51.
18. Gerth, H.H., Mills, C.W. (eds.) From Max Weber: Essays in Sociology. New York: Oxford University Press, 1958.
19. Lipsky, M. Street-Level Bureaucracy: Dilemmas of the Individual in Public Services. New York: Russell Sage Foundation, 1980, p. 60.
20. Piven, F.F., Cloward, R.A. Poor People's Movements: Why They Succeed, How They Fail. New York: Vintage Books, 1979, p. 6.
21. Hofstadter, R. Social Darwinism in American Thought. Boston: Beacon Press, 1958, p. 163.
22. Freire, P. Pedagogy of the Oppressed. New York: Continuum International, 2000.
23. Aaron, H.J. Strategy vs Tactics in Designing Social Policy. Waltham, MA: Brandeis University, The Florence Heller Graduate School for Advanced Studies in Social Welfare. Speech, April 28, 1992.
24. Ryan, W. Blaming the Victim. New York: Vintage Books, 1976, p. 8.
25. Bailey, R., Brake, M. (eds.) Radical Social Work. New York: Pantheon, 1975.

26. Allard, M.A., Howard, A.M., Vorderer, L.E., Wells, A.I., Braddock, D.L. (eds.) Ahead of His Time: Selected Speeches of Gunnar Dybwad Washington, DC: American Association on Mental Retardation, 1999.
27. Gaylin, W., Glasser, I., Marcus, S., Rothman, D.J. Doing Good: The Limits of Benevolence. New York: Pantheon, 1978, p. 110.
28. National Resource Center on Homelessness and Mental Illness. Available at: http://mentalhealth.samhsa.gov/publications/allpubs/KEN95-0015/default.asp. 2001.
29. Bassuk, E.L., Rubin, L., Lauriat, A. Is Homelessness a Mental Health Problem? American Journal of Psychiatry 1984;141(12):1546–1549.
30. Laing, R.D. The Politics of Experience. New York: Ballantine Books, 1967.
31. Gil, D. Unravelling Social Policy. Rochester, VT: Schenkman Books, 1992, p. 26.
32. Schon, D., Rein, M. Frame Reflections: Toward the Resolution of Intractable Policy Controversies. New York: Basic Books, 1994, p. 24.
33. Stone, D. Policy Paradox: The Art of Political Decision Making. New York: W.W. Norton, 1997, p. 254.
34. Lerner, M. Surplus Powerlessness: The Psychodynamics of Everyday Life and the Psychology of Individual and Social Transformation. Amherst, NY: Humanity Books, 1999, p. 3.
35. World Health Organization. Social Dimensions of Mental Health. Geneva: World Health Organization, p. 22.

16

An Interdisciplinary Case Conference

EDITOR DAVID G. SATIN

PARTICIPANTS TERRY R. BARD, PSYCHOLOGY-PASTORAL CARE;
SARITA BHALOTRA, PUBLIC HEALTH; MYRNA D. BOCAGE, SOCIAL
WORK; LAURENCE G. BRANCH, PLANNING; ELLEN A. BRUCE,
LAW; JOHN A. CAPITMAN, POLICY; TERESA T. FUNG, NUTRITION;
JENNIFER L. KIRWIN, PHARMACY; NANCY A. LOWENSTEIN,
OCCUPATIONAL THERAPY; RALPH RANALD, LAW; CLARE E.
SAFRAN-NORTON, PHYSICAL THERAPY; DAVID G. SATIN,
PSYCHIATRY; AND MARK SCIEGAJ, MANAGEMENT

Introductions

RALPH RANALD/LAW: *I'm a lawyer in New York City and I've been a fellow at Harvard for 5 years. I'm interested in elder law and have been teaching at Fordham University Law School in New York, and also teach at the City University of New York, where I do elder law and some humanities. That's my source of interest in humanistic medicine, something quite different.*

MYRNA D. BOCAGE/SOCIAL WORK: *I'm Myrna Bocage. I'm a social worker, and my interest is in health care, older adults, and policy issues. I'm going to represent the social work perspective and also the interdisciplinary perspective.*

MARK SCIEGAJ/MANAGEMENT: *I'm Mark Sciegaj, and I have a focus on social policy and long-term care. Tonight I will represent issues related to elder autonomy and touch upon health-care management and political science.*

NANCY LOWENSTEIN/OCCUPATIONAL THERAPY: *I'm Nancy Lowenstein. I'm an occupational therapist, and I will be representing interdisciplinary issues of teaching and training students of interdisciplinary care.*

JENNIFER L. KIRWIN/PHARMACY: *I'm Jennifer Kirwin. I'm a pharmacist, and in this textbook I'm working with the chapter on individual health-care disciplines, team development and functioning, and issues around personnel.*

CLARE E. SAFRAN-NORTON/PHYSICAL THERAPY: *I'm Clare Safran-Norton. I'm a physical therapist. In this book, I'm contributing a chapter on the various models of disciplinary practice, with a specific focus on comparing and contrasting interdisciplinary and multidisciplinary team approaches to health care of the aged. My current interests in gerontological research are directed toward environmental and housing issues.*

SARITA BHALOTRA/PUBLIC HEALTH: *I'm Sarita Bhalotra. I'm at the Florence Heller School at Brandeis University, and I am going to be talking about prevention and health promotion in older adults. My interest in this arises from my knowledge of epidemiology, dementia, and the history of aging as a physician. I also understand from my health administration and health policy research background that the current configuration of both our service-delivery system and the way it is financed does not meet the needs of an aging population that is completing both a demographic transition as well as an epidemiological transition.*

DAVID G. SATIN/PSYCHIATRY: *I'm David Satin. I'm a psychiatrist. I'm representing the interest in models of disciplinary working relationships and differences among them.*

TERRY R. BARD/PSYCHOLOGY-PASTORAL CARE: *I'm Terry Bard. I'm a rabbi and clinical psychologist. I'm interested in how aging manifests itself in the community and how interdisciplinary care presents proper alternatives for this population.*

ELLEN BRUCE/LAW: *I'm Ellen Bruce. I'm an attorney and I'm interested in the legal perspective on this project as well as community advocacy.*

JOHN A. CAPITMAN/POLICY: *I'm John Capitman. I'm a social psychologist. Most of my research has been about community-based systems of care for older adults and issues of disparities by race and gender. I'm going to represent these perspectives in terms of addressing disparities and creating fair systems of care.*

LAURENCE G. BRANCH/PLANNING: *I am Larry Branch. I am trained as a social psychologist and have done gerontological health services research for more than 30 years. Several times I have provided invited testimony to Congress on issues related to Medicare and the health-care needs of older people. I am representing the interests of integrated health care for Medicare beneficiaries.*

TERESA T. FUNG/NUTRITION: *I'm Teresa Fung. I am a registered dietitian. I am the coauthor with Jen Kirwin of the chapter on building an interdisciplinary team.*

Case Conference

SATIN/PSYCHIATRY: *My concern in terms of interdisciplinary approach is disciplinary contributions to the OACTRPP project. Who are going to be the program planners and administrators? Remember, the overall management is chosen by the medical center, but the program planners and administrators for research, training, and clinical work are yet to be chosen. How do you pick those people? Are they going to be by discipline? Are they going to be by past experience? Are they going to be by nomination from the stakeholders, the advocacy groups—"I want my man in charge of something or other and representing my interests and my emphases!"? One thing that we ought to be aware of is that the medical center has the grant and the medical center has the overall administration, so is the medical center going to be exerting some influence or some expectations about who's going to be in charge of decisions? Will these decision makers be medically or biologically oriented, or can they be other professionals? How does that get done?*

BARD/PSYCHOLOGY-PASTORAL CARE: *It seems like one of the things that must be discussed first is, is this center going to be located within a community, and is it supposed to interrelate with the community? If so, the community's needs probably need to be represented, so individuals from the community ought to be invited to participate. And I'm thinking that not just people from the health community but certainly, from my perspective, people from the religious community ought to be consulted because they see many individuals on a week-to-week—sometimes day-to-day—basis. They certainly have a sense of what's going on and what are problems for members of the community that might be of use.*

SCIEGAJ/MANAGEMENT: *It seems to me that as we develop the governance structure, we need some sort of advisory group that would include people from the community, not just the institutions. It should include the people that the center either serves or conducts its research on. People of different races, ethnicities, age groups, etc. would be important, particularly if we're going to try to create a linkage with the community instead of just maintain ourselves as an academic institution that's providing these things for them.*

BHALOTRA/PUBLIC HEALTH: *I very much agree with the concern about community representation on the governing board. I suggest that in order that we do this most efficiently we look at best-practice models showing how governance is done effectively when there are community and academic health center collaborations like this. As part of the planning process, I suggest we engage in that search so that we're not inventing from the ground up.*

SAFRAN-NORTON/PHYSICAL THERAPY: *In looking at the goals and the missions of the medical center and in support of issues others have raised, it seems to me that there are four qualifications to consider when choosing advisory board members. They include (1) represent the community's needs, (2) represent the needs of the academic medical center, (3) an administrative background, and (4) research experience.*

CAPITMAN/POLICY: *Building on some of those comments, it seems to me that we really have to think about how to engage not just representatives of the community but also a substantial mix of people from the community. If we are not quite active in thinking about what this program is really about and not just say we know what's needed here, we're in trouble. This is important both in terms of setting up some needs assessment research that is based on real active community engagement and also, right from the outset, setting up a governing structure that shares power between this institution and the community. I understand that that's very complex since the hospital is the recipient of the funding and that we're working in the context of federal funding with specific requirements. Still, there seem to me to be many examples in other settings where organizations like this make a real, explicit effort to share the power with the community. One possibility is to think very actively about what kind of leadership we're going to appoint. Do we want leadership that is known only to the hospital? I think not. I think we want in a role as a leader for the program somebody who maybe would come as a representative of the elders in this community.*

BRUCE/LAW: *I would really like to know what this grant says and also get some input from the university medical center because it seems to me we're working within some restrictions and we need to know what they are. Clearly, there are going to be financial restrictions here. We know that there are problems with Medicaid, we may or may not have problems with Medicare, and we need to know what the money in the grant is telling us. I don't know for sure, but I assume the medical center—or whoever is responsible under this grant—is not going to easily share power or the direction of the program, and they're the ones responsible for whatever they said was going to come out of it. So, at a minimum, we have to be cognizant of what their obligations are and then try and figure out how to work within them to accomplish some of the goals the community puts in.*

BRANCH/PLANNING: *I agree that we will be working within a set of constraints that at present exert very real limitations on what providers can do. We indicated in our chapter that over 10% of Medicare reimbursements are judged to be fraudulent by the General Accounting Office, but part of this "fraud" represents well-intentioned providers who are simply trying to get the services that they judge their patient needs. These providers are, in essence, just trying to be ethical in providing the best care for their patients but must act within a set of constraints that are not always consistent with providing optimal care.*

RANALD/LAW: *Years and years ago I worked for one academic year in what was then called the U.S. Department of Health, Education, and Welfare. Since then Education has split off into a separate department. I worked on grants—not writing them (it's illegal to write them while you're working for them) —but evaluating, and the word— even then the key word—was "outcomes." I think you were alluding to that in a sense. At some point, somebody—the persons who are receiving the money or the conduits for the money, since you mention here both the federal government and the state government, I guess state of Massachusetts—will want a formal report on the outcomes. This grant seems to be both theoretical and also providing care, multispecialty care—two very different things. Almost from the beginning one is going to have to conceptualize, I think, what the outcomes of this activity are going to be. In education it is often very difficult to show hard outcomes. In medical science I think it may be a little bit easier, but still outcomes. Who is going to be responsible for describing and recording the various outcomes, both theoretically and in terms of clinical care, and then other things, training for students and studying the factors that affect them? There really are four different sets of outcomes here. Ultimately, if this enterprise is successful in two of them, I suspect it will be highly successful as grant outcomes go. How to document them, that's what is not clear.*

BOCAGE/SOCIAL WORK: *I'm very concerned about our getting into this community and how we make ourselves known. This is not a homogeneous community. I think it sounds fairly heterogeneous, and it sounds like there are a lot of different stakeholders, so I don't think that everyone in the community is likely to share the same goals and values. I think it would be very important to begin perhaps with a community meeting where we invite members from the community to come and we make a presentation about our grant, letting them know some of what we're thinking and asking for their input, and then seeing what the reaction is and responding to that: what our assessment is of where the community and who the different stakeholders are.*

BARD/PSYCHOLOGY-PASTORAL CARE: *I agree with you. One danger that I can see, of course, is that how that meeting is structured will determine what people's expectations are. They can raise expectations that may not be met, so I think that how that meeting is constructed, how people develop their concepts, and what they understand is the purpose of the meeting needs to be thought through pretty carefully. This is a short-term project; at least there's a short-term expectation from this grant that ultimately, we hope, will have a long life. There should be clarification of what it can't be at this particular time, not necessarily knowing what it can be. There are certain things that it probably can't be in a short period of time. This would probably be the beginning of many opportunities for the community to get together and to look and see whether what is being created is actually serving the community in a meaningful way.*

BRUCE/LAW: *I also think that's a good idea, to hold a community meeting, although I agree that you have to structure it so the expectations are appropriate. This gets back to the issue of whether we're talking about control or advisory, which has to be quite clear when you're dealing with the community. I would also suggest that we ourselves do some brainstorming about what we know about the community because we here around the table might want to hear, be able to identify leaders in the community in the different components that we're trying to attract, and do some specific outreach to those people in addition to sort of just an open-door community meeting.*

SCIEGAJ/MANAGEMENT: *While I agree with what has been said by the last couple of speakers, my question is how we sell this to the dean or the vice president of the medical school that's overseeing the project. Because my experience with those kinds of bureaucracies is that they may not be favorably disposed to having a community meeting, to inviting the community and talking about a center that is still pretty amorphous.*

SAFRAN-NORTON/PHYSICAL THERAPY: *I wonder if we could break it down into smaller ideas or have focus groups on certain aspects of what we want to accomplish so that it's not just an open-ended community needs assessment, but we focus on smaller topics or smaller goals that we're trying to achieve. Then it might be more manageable and/ or it might be easier to promote. We would have more information to present and some more accurate facts. Another point I would like to make follows from Ellen Bruce's mention of funding. The grant proposal states that it is large, unrestricted funding from HealthCo, which is a company that markets medications and devices for older adults. I think it would be imperative to find out about the company stakeholders and their interests in funding the grant. Even though it states that it is unrestricted, there may be some concerns that we need to address, as Ralph Ranald had mentioned earlier.*

LOWENSTEIN/OCCUPATIONAL THERAPY: *I agree that we need to have community involvement, and focus groups are important. We also have 6 months to get this up and running, so I think we have to be cognizant of a very tight timeline because it can take a while to plan and get announcements out and those kinds of things.*

BHALOTRA/PUBLIC HEALTH: *I'm glad you brought up the 6-month timeline because I think that is, even with the best intentions, rather ambitious. I don't want to get us sidetracked, but I think perhaps we should be revisiting that timeline. It might be essential for us to spend a lot more time early on and then prevent a lot more damage down the line. I mean, that's what my topic's all about—prevention and promotion of health—so I would rather we did this very careful planning up front, involve the community in the best way that we possibly can. For example, John Capitman brought up the issue of power in the governing board. We need to build something into the plan that talks about board development. It's a small tactical point but one that gets overlooked very often. And then just one more point to follow up on the fact that we need measurable outcomes: We need to have an evaluation plan before this thing gets off the ground. That's hard to do, come up with measurable objectives for each of these goals that we have in mind.*

SATIN/PSYCHIATRY: *I appreciate a number of things that have been said. One is that we need to get some specific things accomplished—prevention, for instance. Another is that there is a timeline. Let me remind us that we ourselves in this meeting have a timeline. We've got to come out with some kind of plan within the next hour and a quarter, so we need to give ourselves some sense of direction as we need to give the project some sense of direction. One consideration is that we need to do planning, we need to do inclusion, we need to do evaluation, we need to do motivation of people; but this grant, like most, is going to demand an interim report within an absurdly short period of time, like a year. This means we've got to start writing it within 9 months, which means we have to have something done to write about. I have a feeling, both as a psychiatrist who thinks about human motivation and also as somebody interested in the disciplinary working relationships, that we need to get some direction, get some force working to get things done, and not evolve naturalistically. We have a complicated project here. Myrna Bocage, as a social worker, mentioned community organization and getting the community together to decide. Remember, the community, in terms of interest groups, involves not only the people who are living in the area, but it involves the medical center, it involves the Center for Medicare and Medicaid Services, it involves HealthCo, a for-profit organization, it involves the state and the city. If you talk about a community meeting, these are people who are going to be at the community meeting, negotiating with one another about their needs and their expectations. And some people are more equal than others. Some people have the purse strings. Some people are going to be talking to the funding agencies. And some people are going to be appealing through humanitarian need or through threat of withholding their agreement and their participation. You're going to have quite a melee going on. That can evolve over a long time, and it can end up with nothing, as has happened in other community projects. So I would think that there might be need for some structure. Somebody with some sense of direction needs to host and facilitate what is going on. And here's where we consider people who are able to do that and are able to have an overview of what needs to be done and the outcome. You're interested in prevention, I'm interested in mental health issues, and other people are interested in other things being a part of the project. So I think we ought to think about who needs to be the, how shall we say, the overseer, the facilitator for this, and what kind of person does that well. Is that a social worker who's used to running community meetings and getting consensus? Is that an administrator who knows when things have to be pulled together and what things have to be decided in order for the project to move ahead? Does that need to be somebody who is a natural-born community leader, comes out of the community, because such a person knows how to get people to work together? Who does this? What are the credentials for doing this? Is it disciplinary? Is it experience? Is it a democratic vote? How do you get somebody to get the thing organized and occupy a leadership role in this?*

BARD/PSYCHOLOGY-PASTORAL CARE: *David Satin, I appreciate the structures that you want to implement and I certainly would support that. I have an issue raised by Sarita Bhalotra, I think what many of us have talked about is the cautionary note that it's done properly the first time so that you don't have to reinvent it. On the other hand, I think that there's probably already an involved structure that's not represented here in our group now, and that is the medical center itself, which I think is very much interested in providing care, and certainly care for the elderly population. I can imagine that much of that care is time-bound. For example, as we're talking we're at the beginning of the flu season, and I can easily imagine that the medical center would like to create a flu clinic in the space that's available. It might have other agenda items that it wants to get to for the direct health care of the population. So I think what we need to do is probably to find an individual (this goes along with what you were saying, David Satin) who might begin to coordinate with the medical center to see what their timetable is in terms of immediate services, if they have any to provide to the community, and what that would take, and how that would or would not have implications for any programmatic development. So I would recommend that, before we depart today, we choose from among us one individual who makes that connection and then reports back to us.*

BRUCE/LAW: *I think part of what you're suggesting is also what Clare Safran-Norton was, at least in my interpretation, suggesting. It's that we break this down into pieces that we need to do. And if we think that one of the pieces that has to be done is just the setting up of this community base, the multispecialty clinic. So there is a constituency that we have to worry about in just setting it up, which is, are you going to get the different disciplines willing to go along with the model of care and work in the community? So maybe that's one discrete piece that is somewhat separate from the community piece of organizing a group from the community. They are really the patients, the other side, the other half. And figuring out how we can facilitate their gaining some voice, basically becoming a presence, to say what they need. Because right now my guess is that we don't have an organized group from the community to be able to express what they need, so they're not in a position to interact with this other provider group. They have to be in a position to interact. So maybe those would be two separate things we could talk about to come out of this meeting with a plan.*

BOCAGE/SOCIAL WORK: *Something that I'm struggling with right now is that it seems to me the heart of this is providing basic care to the community. And it seems to me before we can even begin to think about other kinds of structures it would make sense to have a better understanding of who and what we're dealing with. So I'm wondering if a place to start might be getting to know who the older people in the community are and what their particular needs might be because my guess is that there are going to be a lot of different kinds of needs. One of the things that come to mind is that it sounds like it's a very diverse community, so I expect that there are going to be some health disparities. I suspect that there are going to be some perceived and some real barriers to the utilization of the services that are provided. I'm concerned about where the clinic is located and the structure that it's located in and how that structure's going to be perceived by the people we want to use the services. There are a number of other issues, too, that I think we need to think about. It sounds like at least a sizeable number of the people aren't going to be covered by health insurance of any kind, and so financing services is another issue. So, to summarize, I think one place that we might start is getting a better sense of the community and what the needs are of the elderly in the community.*

FUNG/NUTRITION: *If it is possible to establish a physical location to provide clinical care, then the clinic itself can be a tool or channel in getting some ideas of community needs because the clinicians will be interacting with the people in the community.*

SCIEGAJ/MANAGEMENT: *I'm mindful that we have like an hour and five minutes to go. It seems to me one thing that we haven't finished discussing goes back to David Satin's point about leadership for this center to be successful. Coming out of a medical school, it seems to me that we need to have a physician to head the project, head the group, because there are two different constituencies that we're going to have to interface with. One is going to be the medical care establishment and the medical center itself and the other's going to be the community. And the medical person doesn't have to wear both hats, but it seems that, even though we want to talk about interdisciplinary, in order for this to be successful within the medical school, we'd need to have a physician at the top.*

KIRWIN/PHARMACY: *One thing that I would suggest we keep in mind when thinking about qualities of our leadership is that this is a novel model for this community, a demonstration project of sorts. The people leading the project need to have the vision to make this work, as well as strong interpersonal skills and experience interfacing with all these different stakeholders.*

BHALOTR/PUBLIC HEALTH: *With this interdisciplinary approach I thought we are trying to do something innovative and novel, and so falling back on the same things and the same methods we've done in the past isn't necessarily going to get us to achieve newer or different results. And so I agree, then, that it's not necessary to have a physician as the leader just because that's how we've always done it in the past. I had a vision of not retaining the model where we make plans and then we figure out ways to get different populations to accept those things that we've constructed. So when I look at this, this seems very much like a replication of what we've done before. Here's dentistry, here's medicine, here's surgery. It's really just following the same conceptual framework. And I'd rather turn it on its head and say, how do we really, truly come up with an interdisciplinary, integrated approach? And let's put the patient at the center of this, not our different departments. And one way, I think, to do it is to go and think about information systems and say each person has this unique identifier. And then we take this person and make sure that this person has a seamless transition through different departments to meet his or her needs, and take the focus away from our different departments to really make it patient-focused or customer-focused. One last thing that I'd like to add is one glaring omission: the fact that we're not looking at community resources. For example, there are senior wellness centers that we want to link up with. The flu clinic, for example, is more likely to be run by a senior center than the hospital. Also, for example, dealing with things like social isolation, which is a huge thing. There's nothing in here yet that says we have the system in place to deal with that particular aspect.*

SATIN/PSYCHIATRY: *I think that we have really four different projects with four different central foci. The patient is the focus for the clinical aspect; the student is the focus for the educational aspect; the community is the focus for the factors that affect health and functional status; and the planning group, the theoreticians, the academicians, are the central people for developing theories and planning and funding. It's not to disagree with you; it just means you replicate your model so that you keep your eye on each of these balls for the appropriate arena, and you get the appropriate person or group to provide the leadership because they know how to do it. And I agree that it should not necessarily be a physician, nor should it necessarily not be a physician. Lots of people have something to offer—social work has something to offer, occupational therapy has something to offer in terms of planning and organization, public health has something to offer, and so on. So look for the disciplinary opportunity and contribution but also the nondisciplinary. And don't overlook the commitment, the source of values contribution. What you want to accomplish, what are your priorities is also a credential that helps to shape your project. So an academician may have one set of priorities, a community person may have another set of priorities, a community politician who is climbing his or her way out of the community into the upper echelons may have another set of priorities. So those values are another set of credentials. How do you choose them? One off-the-cuff suggestion is that you get planning groups, minicommunities representing all the stakeholders, to decide who is the best kind of person to lead this particular project. Who has the training, who has the experience, who has the values, who has the commitment, the motivation to do it? And it will turn out to be a different person for each of the projects. And it will turn out to be a different mix of training, academic credentials, experience credentials, and ethnic credentials or whatever seems to be important. So here's a way of getting the right person for the right project and getting that person to facilitate accomplishment in that project and not waiting until something arises spontaneously out of the primordial ooze to get the job done.*

BARD/PSYCHOLOGY-PASTORAL CARE: *A short note, then I'll hand over. Sarita Bhalotra, you really touched on something that I very much resonate with. There's a danger here, if we use old concepts, that the novelty of what is created, that's owned by the community (which is really what I think you were advocating) needs to always be possible within the framework of what's created. Because it's so easy in creating the structure that the structure itself tends to take over. Now, I think that's what you were sort of saying. And it leaves aside the community or the members of the community that it's trying to serve. And they should really be the framers of this. And it should be an evolving reality. And probably, what I hear you saying as well, is that at least the best of concepts, maybe long-term, is that the community should be assuming a major leadership role in this, if I'm right in hearing you. And I think that's really important. Maybe we have to think of two ways of constructing this. Because of time we have to try to get something in place, but we can't have ownership of that. It has to be more fluid than that, so that at the same time we're helping them find leadership to create structures, we're at the same time investing ourselves in getting the community to invest itself in whatever's being created, so that it's owned by them, if I hear you correctly.*

BRANCH/PLANNING: *And, not to be cynical, but let us not forget that the medical center loses reimbursement for every accident, illness, trauma, or condition it prevents. We really do have the proverbial perverse incentives to deal with in this project.*

BHALOTRA/PUBLIC HEALTH: *Thank you so much, Terry Bard, for articulating this much better than I could. I bring these concepts from the whole concept of sustainable development, which is different from economic development, according to which we build the structure, we provide the resources, and then that will raise the level of health in this community that we're trying to serve. This is opposed to not just economic development but sustainable development that is more community-driven and maintained. Thank you.*

CAPITMAN/POLICY: *Although I really feel very excited about our discussion of shifting the pattern of ownership and moving to a model that has the patient at the center, the recipient of care at the center, I'm also aware of how we're funded for this effort by a for-profit organization concerned with maximization of utilization of its medications and other devices for older adults. Although our university medical center is nominally a not-for-profit organization, we function in the context of commodified medicine. I guess what comes up for me is to what extent we, as a planning group and as we expand this group, are going to examine our own values and our own goals in moving forward with this initiative. I, at least, would like to see this be a program that really addresses some of the fundamental challenges in the United States in the financing and delivery of health care for older people. And some of those fundamental challenges have to do with the gaps in the kinds of coverage there are. There isn't adequate coverage for preventive services. How can we put the client in the center if we have to get them once they're very sick or can't offer them chronic care services? There isn't adequate coverage for our services on a chronic basis. People need assistance to maintain themselves in their own homes. Those kinds of problems with the fundamental funding structure of health care should be at the basis of what we want to do. Also, within our* community and many communities are tremendous disparities in access to appropriate care and the quality of care based on race, ethnicity, gender, social class, and age, even among elders themselves. So, thinking about all that, I'd really like to go back to Dr. Bhalotra's comment as sort of a central organizing feature: Are we going to try to develop a system of care that maximizes utilization for the hospital, that maximizes the use of HealthCo's products, or are we going to try to do something that has as its goal really meeting the needs of the elders in this community, starting from realistic assessment of those needs?

RANALD/LAW: I have worked around hospitals and physicians, the military medical system, which I'm somewhat familiar with and which is the source of much of civilian medicine and not the other way around. The person in charge gets a better hearing and better support, I've found, if he or she is a physician. This is just an empirical statement based on one person's observation, a person who is not a physician, by the way, and so cannot be accused of self-interest in that respect. If the person in charge, whatever that happens to mean, the director, the coordinator of the program, is a physician, it is, in my opinion, a little easier to get cooperation from the various medical and medical-related disciplines than if the person is a nonphysician. I sense there was a difference of position around the table as to whether the director ought or ought not to be a physician. I would vote for that person being a physician, and preferably somebody who has relationships with the people who are going to provide the care or do the research or all of these four things—has a track record. That would be a primary credential in my opinion, at any rate.

SCIEGAJ/MANAGEMENT: To pick up really quick on something that John Capitman pointed out: We're getting money from HealthCo, Inc., within the medical center that is looking, in part, for referrals to them and to provide training for their students. And so there are economic considerations here, and if we turn it on its head and ignore the fact that we have these economic connections, we're going to have a short-lived center. And so, when I said that I thought the person ought to be a physician, it is because we need to have a strong connection with the medical center for political reasons, for survival reasons beyond the life of this grant. And it seems to me that you can have the interdisciplinary team, but also I think we need to recognize some of the political realities. Whether it's Harvard Medical School or the medical school at Fresno State University or the University of Iowa, there is, to put it in a very crass way, a caste system in medical schools that's operative.

BRUCE/LAW: I agree with the point that we have to look at this practically and try and set it up so there's a strength in this program that will continue. And a lot of the strength comes from where the money comes from and that part of the institution. And so the medical school is important, as is the whatever HealthCo is, where the money comes from. I don't take a position on whether it needs to be a doctor or not. I would say we need somebody who is an advocate within the medical school because that's a key component of it. So, whether it's a doctor or somebody else, we need an advocate there. Somebody with some kind of power within the medical school. But I think this is set up with a lot going against us, at least what has been articulated as an interest of this group—have it be a multidisciplinary, community-driven, patient-focused project and done with some results in less than a year. Those seem like enormous, absolutely enormous barriers against us on a couple of fronts. And the only way I can see of approaching it is to basically triage it and decide what it is that is most important for us to get out of it at the end of the year. And, given that, then focus on that and decide *what it is that you need to do. And if it's having the director, the choice of the director, I actually respectfully disagree with the proposal that we have multiple working groups focused on different things because it just seems way too time-consuming. Maybe we decide what is the real key to this, what's the innovative part of this that we want to make sure works. And then figure out how to make that happen and decide what's expendable in here.*

CAPITMAN/POLICY: *Building on that, one of the biggest problems in many hospitals is a high rate of readmission after brief stays. And so maybe we could think about using the new clinic to assist in solving one of the central challenges for the facility as a first step. This would be an approach that would resonate with many in the community. It would clearly resonate with the administrators in the hospital. It makes sense as a medical priority. I agree that we need to pick a challenge, a problem, a central area, and focus on that. And I think some of the issues around leadership and structure will sort themselves out as we make a little progress on a topic. What are people's reactions to that as a kind of first step?*

BRUCE/LAW: *I would say that. I like it, and I think if that is something that we decide to choose, then that's something tangible to build a community base around because then you can start saying, well, okay, what is it in the community that they're concerned with? You've identified something that is the hospital's concern; it is a financial concern. But then maybe the community has a different take on the same problem, such as African Americans aren't being followed up or we think we're being ignored— whatever it is. But it's something concrete to go to the community with to ask for their input.*

BARD/PSYCHOLOGY-PASTORAL CARE: *I think you're touching on a very important part, and that is a feature of this: There is a financial interest for success by the medical center. Unfortunately, there are competing pieces here, though: The medical center does gain income each time there's an admission and a discharge, but it also would probably do better if it were providing more curative care within the community. So we can think how to recognize how that interest could feed the medical center and how it can benefit the community in a different way by having supportive services and services that actually happen to contextualize a person's well-being. That would be something that they could buy into quite easily and might help to structure some of the community effort that you're talking about. So I think it's a very good place to begin. And it also begins with the pragmatic concern that's very real, and it's real in the community, and it's also real from the perspective of the funding source. And of course we're talking about devices—there's devices that get to be used in the community. And it actually may have potential for finding greater resources—financial resources—to service the community in the way that works best. And the medical center will do best if it serves all of the community—there's no question. If we can also address some of the inequities that we're talking about, so that it actually gets some of those rewards. And I think we can probably agree that we need a unique system that will allow that to happen.*

BHALOTRA/PUBLIC HEALTH: *Addressing your issue about the fact that, yes, every admission is a source of revenue. However, that's balanced against quality measures. A lot of payors will reimburse hospitals based upon the quality measures—readmission within 30 days, for example, is a quality measure for Medicare, and so on. So I think that administrators might look very seriously at trying to reduce those kinds of findings on their quality indicators. And I'm just picking up then on what was said starting with Ellen Bruce: I love this idea of starting with a small and manageable project on postdischarge care. We could come up with a handful of conditions that we'd say we will follow into the community, provide culturally competent follow-up care, and actually engage in the postevent prevention that I talk about in my chapter. So it's not just the nurse calling up to make sure that the person with congestive heart failure is taking his medication and not eating too much salt, but it's actually engaging very actively in the day-to-day—I don't want to say "management" because it's more about building patients' skills and self-efficacy—but encouraging them in more self-advocacy and in using their resources to optimize their health.*

SATIN/PSYCHIATRY: *I have two different issues to address: one in terms of how to organize the project. I think it's a great idea to pick a particular focus and get that done. But I suspect we do not having the option of jettisoning some of the goals of the project because that's what it's funded to do. We can't decide we're taking the money but we're not going to do half the job. We've got to come up with it. I think we probably can address all of these four issues in that one focus—you can talk about training in that focus, you can talk about community clinic service in that focus, you can talk about planning and funding in that focus, and you can talk about prevention and health maintenance and illness prevention. That's the hardest one to do if you're talking about posthospital discharge because you haven't prevented it if they've already been in the hospital and come out of it. However, you can prevent the recurrence of it. I think we may have to deal with the community in terms of whether they want to see health care focused in the hospital or they want to see health care focused at home or in community multiservice centers or in some other alternative setting. But you can work that out—that can be developed as part of a constructive dialogue.*

Let me go back to the other issue I wanted to address, which was from a psychiatric point of view. People's outcomes, people's actions are determined by people's expectations, people's attitudes. It doesn't come out of pure science. It doesn't come out of divine inspiration. It comes out of people's backgrounds and people's prejudices. And so, if we are tied too much to existing ideas, like from the medical center, the medical idea, we're not going to come out with a creative outcome. We have to be free enough to think about all the alternatives and, as I think it was Ellen Bruce who said, get the support, get the imprimatur of the medical center for this new idea without necessarily having a physician do it or having it done the same way as the medical center used to do it. The medical center has to see that this is useful to it because they got into this business because of increasing social and funding focus on the aging population. This is a new market—that's why they're there, and they have to make something from that market. But they don't have to do it the same way. It's going to be hard to get an established, powerful institution to change it's ideas, but to tell it, to convince it that there's a better way of getting your business done better may be helpful. So you need to have a person who does not come with an established set of attitudes, values, and ideologies. You have to get somebody who is able to bring the expertise that is useful and may come from a different source or a nontraditional background but come out with a product that is useful and get the stakeholders to agree that this is a good outcome and this is a good person to do it.

BARD/PSYCHOLOGY-PASTORAL CARE: *I agree with you. On the other hand, I wouldn't be so sour on the medical center. I'm impressed by the medical center's willingness to actually put in this grant submission. And it sounds like, from the description, that, in fact, the medical center may be stretching itself to look at new models of intervention within the community. So it may well be that the medical center is (and many that I've known and worked with actually are) thinking outside the box—they're thinking differently. And, in fact, they may be very eager partners in this enterprise, where, in fact, they're going to win. They're sitting around the table, anyhow. They're not going to leave the space. And if we can provide a better model that works in their best interest and serves the community, I think it works to everybody's advantage. So I guess sometimes our attitudes, as you were suggesting, also can taint the way we approach this. And I would suggest that we approach it with a more open mind and see if, in fact, their willingness is as great as ours is to create a new enterprise.*

BHALOTRA/PUBLIC HEALTH: *I do agree. I really do agree. And I think that underlying all our discussion about this is a really common feeling that we want to do something slightly different and, at the same time, getting all the stakeholders to have buy-in. We certainly can't alienate the medical center. We'll get nowhere if we do. And, having said that, I agree with Dave Satin that there's a whole new crop of physicians who've grown up with complementary and alternative forms of medicine that older physicians might never have accepted. Within our time we've seen things like aromatherapy in hospitals—who would have thought that? So I do agree that medical centers can participate. Perhaps they can't turn on a dime, but they do turn eventually, and we can't really leave them out of this equation. On the question of physicians, likewise physicians are not monolithic in nature. If we can find somebody who has credibility with multiple stakeholder groups and has built up trust and who is warm and sincere and if that person happens to be a physician, so much the better, given our constituencies.*

SATIN/PSYCHIATRY: *But if that person happens not to be a physician, that person should not be excluded.*

BHALOTRA/PUBLIC HEALTH: *Exactly right.*

SATIN/PSYCHIATRY: *I think that excluding nonphysicians would really be reinforcing a caste system.*

BRUCE/LAW: *I say we find out who wrote the grant, start there.*

SCIEGAJ/MANAGEMENT: *I guess the reason I had focused on the credential of the physician was primarily because of the economics, the sources of revenue. We need to have a strong sort of economic base. And, quite frankly, we're in cahoots with a for-profit entity. And regardless of the fact that this is an unrestricted grant, there is definitely an incentive behind giving us the money. And if we're going to have that kind of relationship, having someone who can talk that talk but also who can embrace the larger interdisciplinary nature of the center and the community constituencies is the kind of person who I think would be ideal.*

BARD/PSYCHOLOGY-PASTORAL CARE: *I'm getting a sense that there's a bit of consensus that's developing around our group this evening, and that is that we have a concept of an initial project that, John Capitman, you suggested and that is looking at outcomes and recidivism in the community. That we need to somehow develop an understanding of the medical center and its relationship to this project at the same time that we also need to have a better understanding of what is the nature of this care in the community. And it seems to me that we're beginning to develop what might be an agenda for our next meeting. Someone from the medical center ought to be contacted, perhaps the writer of the grant, to be present and participate. And perhaps someone from the Visiting Nurse Association in the community would know actually what's taking place within certain segments of the community and should be invited. And we should begin to focus on developing specifications for an administrator too. And develop some way to begin to work on this particular project and to measure it and to at least get its first demonstration outcome in place within the 6 months that the grant requires. At the same time we could then, once we focus on that, look at the other dimensions that this grant is supposed to include. I don't know what your thoughts are.*

SATIN/PSYCHIATRY: *Just a quick comment: If we don't want this to be born dead, we need to have other stakeholders part of the planning group, not just professionals. We need to have somebody from the Grey Action Coalition, somebody from the city health department. It need not be a large group, but it needs to be people who will not only contribute assent, they will contribute ideas. An interdisciplinary interaction means you get answers to questions you never thought to ask, so people will come up with issues that need to be addressed in terms of what needs to be done and who needs to do it. So I think they need to be a part of it. And we need, somewhere along the line, to have people who have the credentials, the training, the experience, and the commitment to do the job—to do the clinical work, the treatment; to do the training that's going to be a part of the project; to do the prevention—to have those people with those kinds of skills in on the planning. It may not be at the initial planning stage. It may be as it is developed later on into the more details, but don't forget the people with the skills that are necessary.*

KIRWIN/PHARMACY: *One last comment about other people that we might want to bring to the planning table: They are people who would have an interest both in assessing outcomes as well as setting up systems for training of all these various clinicians wherever they might be or however they might be involved. I think a motivated group of researcher-clinicians could do a lot for our program. And later on a motivated group of student clinicians may also be able to help to motivate the community, help raise awareness, and spread the message.*

SAFRAN-NORTON/PHYSICAL THERAPY: *I've been thinking about what David Satin said a while ago regarding this being an interdisciplinary project in nature, with four missions of the grant being interdisciplinary in themselves, and determining the importance of each. Ellen Bruce raised the issue as to whether it is practical to make all four missions equal. Is it possible in 6 months or 2 years from now to have goals for each mission? Is one mission more important than another? Picking one idea or one problem to solve may be one way to prioritize the four different missions. Can we actually create a program for research with students, with clinicians, and with patients all at the same time; or should we focus on the community and the patients in the next 6 months? Then the following year we address student issues. And then in 2 years we focus on research. Maybe in this meeting we should create an overall plan as to what it is we would like to accomplish, how to do it, and who is going participate. This way we break it down over a 2-year time frame to make it more realistic and practical.*

BHALOTRA/PUBLIC HEALTH: *I really do agree that a phase-in strategy will also protect us a little bit. And I also think that if we choose this circumscribed project as developed by Clare Safran-Norton and John Capitman and David Satin, I think we can address also those almost simultaneously. And if you give me a minute to explain how when I talk about postevent prevention, I agree it's not primary prevention in the true sense of the word, but what I'm trying to explain is that we can use all three levels of prevention concurrently after the event. So ask the person to stop smoking and exercise more, so that's the primary prevention. It's not going to prevent the primary myocardial infarction, but it's going to help him optimize his outcomes. And the same with secondary and tertiary prevention. And this, I think, will really lead us to identify a lot*

*of unmet needs, which again will be useful in terms of convincing the medical estab-
lishment because this is going to now bring revenue, for example, the new guidelines
for colon cancer screening. Let's just say that, OK, that's what we want in terms of
the prevention efforts that we're going to do with this community. That enormously
increases the revenue from colonoscopies and maybe polypectomies and so on, and
radiology. And so it becomes a win–win situation: We're improving the health status
and attracting more revenues.*

BRUCE/LAW: *I think I would support Clare Safran-Norton's faith. I'm not quite so sure
we can meet all the four goals at the same time, and I guess I'm going to make a plug
for the clinical. If we need to come out with outcomes for the goal, then I think that
I would pick the clinical one to be the first, as opposed to the research or the training
goals, because I think those are longer-term and they're going to take longer to show
up. I would support prioritizing where we focus. That is not to say that we don't have
it in our minds all along that we have to develop and research tools that are going to
come out of this. I'd also like to just raise another point that I think is part of the key to
this that needs some strategy on our part, and that is we talked about the community
care, part of it prevention. But how are we going to get the disciplines together or convince the medical school that they need to involve all the disciplines in this? It seems
to me that we haven't discussed this at all. And then we could very easily go to a "OK,
we'll go to two disciplines here." How are we going to say, well, it's not just the nurse
and the physical therapist that you put in there, but we also want to look at the social
setting we send this person home to. How are we going to involve the other disciplines
and convince the powers that be? I think we need to take a little time to discuss that.*

FUNG/NUTRITION: *How about quality of life as one of the goals? And maybe that can
expand into a research project as well. Though I have to admit that I am not familiar
with research in this area.*

BARD/PSYCHOLOGY-PASTORAL CARE: *I think that will occur quite naturally, probably
even at the next meeting when there's a more focused project that's evolved. I think that
I and certainly others will begin to look at some of our own personal disciplinary concerns as they relate to the population. So I think those would emerge quite naturally
and from the fact that all of us are involved, plus the additional people who we will
bring. I can't imagine us being silent about that as the project begins to be more robust.
We will all begin to have very particular concerns that we will bring to bear. So I guess
I'm a little less concerned about needing to model that at this moment, but I think it's
something that needs to be present at all future meetings once there's a specific focus.*

SATIN/PSYCHIATRY: *From experience I remember a paper I wrote titled "The Difficulties
of Interdisciplinary Education: Lessons from Three Failures and a Success." That's
an optimistic ratio. I think we're swimming upstream when we're looking for interdisciplinary education or clinical care. Most interdisciplinary training programs and
research projects end up seeing some disciplines making a lot more investment in the
project and others making a lot less, so I think eventually we're going to address that
issue. And I would suppose that somehow we'll have to convince the powers that be
that it is useful to be involved in this, it makes for good education, it makes for good
clinical care, it makes for good reimbursement, it makes for good recruitment for staff.
Somehow it's got to be successful in order to say that it's worthwhile investing in this
rather than whatever the alternative is. We may want to go crusading about it from the
beginning and alienating everybody, but we may have to make that case and push hard
for it even if diplomatically somewhere along the line, because it's not going to happen*

naturally, with all due respect. I don't think it's going to happen naturally unless there's a good reason for it to be done, unless it's on a pilot basis and not on a modal basis.

SAFRAN-NORTON/PHYSICAL THERAPY: *Well, after spending the last year reviewing the literature on this exact question for the chapter in this textbook, I have found that there is not a lot of good research on the difference between interdisciplinary and multidisciplinary team approaches. Most often, interdisciplinary is defined as multidisciplinary practice, which is different from our definition. In the current literature, outcomes are mostly based on mortality, and the outcome measures that have been used are not necessarily ones that would support our saying that an interdisciplinary model is better than a multidisciplinary model. I don't think that these are necessarily the right outcome measures for us to use. I think it's a great research question to consider—interdisciplinary versus multidisciplinary models of care—since most studies have published on multidisciplinary models. The examples that appear to be working quite well are in home care. Through my professional experience and from the literature I have read, home care appears to function in an interdisciplinary manner. So I think it would be easier to start an interdisciplinary team approach in a home-care setting. Many agencies are already using this model. They choose who to pick as the leader or who are the team members and how it all works. I believe this team approach and model of care is very different from that in a hospital setting.*

BHALOTRA/PUBLIC HEALTH: *I'm going to piggyback on what you were saying about the lack of literature on interdisciplinary work and the fact that most outcomes speak only about mortality and we probably will not see a difference in mortality within a year. I'm thinking that what we need to do, and this goes to the next phase of planning, is to come up with the process measures and then intermediate outcomes. The number of times primary prevention efforts were made and so on, not necessarily did this prevent colon cancer in the next 7 years, because we're not doing a long-term follow-up. I'm just affirming what you say, that it's going to be very difficult to come up with ultimate outcomes and that we might need to revert to just process measures and intermediate outcomes. Because it speaks to Ellen Bruce's point about being conscious about trying to do all four goals and maybe picking a couple and keeping the others in mind because I think we can probably incorporate some aspect of all four. For example, the fact that we are measuring process—that's part of the research goal. We may not be able to get into attitudinal factors, for example; that's a more ambitious thing to do.*

SATIN/PSYCHIATRY: *Have we answered your question about implementing the interdisciplinary aspect, Ellen Bruce?*

BRUCE/LAW: *Yes, because I interpreted that out of the three speakers that spoke after me, two of them agreed with me, even though the first one didn't. Out of the four that spoke after me, three agreed, so I don't know. Terry Bard has sort of, I guess. It's more of a question whether we convinced Terry of that.*

BARD/PSYCHOLOGY-PASTORAL CARE: *I don't disagree with what you're saying. I think it is a staged kind of approach, so I have no problems with that. I don't think that's a primary focus at the next meeting. I think it is something that's iterative, so I have no problem with that at all. I don't think that one can do it as robustly, however; we may have some sort of restrictions, and that is to get better clarification of what the expectations of the grant is, to see how much of that we must demonstrate within a short amount of time. If there's greater latitude, of course I think that prioritizing them and stratification is a much, much better way of approaching it. But we can be very inventive if we need to be to address at least the most up-front concerns that are necessary to maintain and renew the grant if we can. So I don't think I'm in any disagreement with you at all.*

SATIN/PSYCHIATRY: *Let me see if I've gotten some of the general principles that we've come up with. I think we've moved the process in the course of this meeting. In no particular order: One agreement is that all the interest groups need to be represented in the planning, and I would advocate in the actual organization and implementation. The second is that their interests need to be met, whether it's financial, a matter of recognition, a matter of health needs being met; that they have to see profit from this. The third that it has to be interdisciplinary, ways have to be found of contributions from each of the disciplines, and by disciplines I'm using small "d" relating to training, experience, and interest; that they have to have an opportunity to contribute what they have without offending any of the interest groups by having their people not recognized or some unacceptable people recognized; bringing them along so that they enrich what is done here, even if it's not done by their particular person or their tradition. And the fourth that comes to mind is that there has to be a phased approach, that we need to get all of this done. We don't need to get all of this done at the same time or in the first place. That we start with a project, such as posthospital discharge aftercare. That we incorporate all of the four goals that need to be involved, that they don't all have to be done at the same time, and that each of them can be phased in so that by the 1-year progress report we can say that we have done this and we have specific plans for doing that, and that by the end of the 2 years we can say that we have done this for 1 and a half years and we have done that for 6 months, and the other is still to be developed, but everything has proved that it is doable and that we know what it takes to at least get it started. Is that correct? Did I miss any points that need to be further developed?*

BARD/PSYCHOLOGY-PASTORAL CARE: *I think we need to set up right now the next meeting date and have something in place so we don't lose the steam that we have right now to move ahead. I propose that we meet 3 weeks from today.*

SATIN/PSYCHIATRY: *I agree that we need to have defined goals and milestones. By that time we will have a clearer idea about who participates in the next meeting and what it's agenda is. Maybe this group as a whole can be a kind of ad-hoc steering committee to get a more legitimate group going to develop an agenda. But we take the first step and we move on from here. Agreed?*

17

Interdisciplinary Health Management for Older Adults

Professional Education and Practice

EDITOR DAVID G. SATIN

PARTICIPANTS KIMBERLY ARMSTRONG, SOCIAL WORK; TERRY R. BARD, PSYCHOLOGY/PASTORAL CARE; KATHLEEN BOYLE, SOCIAL WORK; SHANNON BROVERMAN, ELDER CARE ADMINISTRATION; PEGGY BROWN, SOCIAL WORK; JEANETTE BURACK, OLDER ADULT; JOAN R. DREVINS, PHYSICAL THERAPY; PETER MARAMALDI, SOCIAL WORK/ PUBLIC HEALTH; JENNIFER PRITCHARD, NURSING/HEALTH CARE ADMINISTRATION; ERICA RAINE, SOCIAL WORK; JULIE SALINGER, SOCIAL WORK; DAVID G. SATIN, PSYCHIATRY; KIMBERLY SAUDER, GERONTOLOGY; MELANIE VAUGHN, PHYSICAL THERAPY

Learning About Interdisciplinary Gerontology

DAVID G. SATIN: *What do you know now that you didn't know before? What kind of thinking or what kind of ideas did this material stimulate?*

SHANNON BROVERMAN/ELDER CARE ADMINISTRATION: *I think that we learned about the meaning of interdisciplinary approach to care, which is a unique concept. It's not something that you have to learn through trial and error; you learn through role-plays and through in-depth group projects.*

JENNIFER PRICHARD/NURSING/HEALTH CARE ADMINISTRATION: *One of the things that I was really struck by was the number of creative individuals who are putting together very innovative programs to improve the quality of life for elders. I have a much greater appreciation of the multitude of initiatives currently in place and being developed. It is very concerning how truly underresourced we really are to care for our older adults in the future as this age group continues to grow. It will require continued ingenuity and creativity on the part of policy makers and providers to meet their needs.*

SATIN/PSYCHIATRY: *The two things that we had hoped to bring out were (1) an understanding of the health-care system and how it affected the health care that older adults get and how it affected professional practice. And the other was an interdisciplinary approach and how that applies. Did you learn about both of those things or one of those things, or did some things seem basic or irrelevant?*

JULIE SALINGER/SOCIAL WORK: *One of the things that I have a better grasp on—which I thought I understood but I probably didn't—is the following: When you enter situations where your role is to help people, which is what most of us are doing in one form or another, it is not necessarily sufficient to present your own expertise. It is also to learn from other disciplines: What do others know, and how can that information help you do your job better? In theory, I may have thought that I was doing just that; in reality, I don't think I had the appreciation of other disciplines that I have now. At this point I believe I can go into a patient review meeting and say, for example, "What did you see when you were working with this person in physical therapy? What did you see that might be useful to me?" Additionally, I can share what I have seen that may be useful to others. I don't think I really thought about client or patient care like that. I think you enter a situation thinking that you're the social worker or you're this or you're that and that's what you're there for. And then you lose half of what you could be gaining from others.*

SATIN/PSYCHIATRY: *What do you mean you lose half? What half do you lose?*

SALINGER/SOCIAL WORK: *The half that you lose is what you learn form other disciplines and the potential to increase your effectiveness as well as theirs. Assuming that clients are the center of discussion, our role should be to gather as much information about them as possible. As professionals we need to be attuned to what others may know and use that information.*

JOAN DREVINS/PHYSICAL THERAPY: *I'm looking at you and nodding my head because I totally agree with you. I've been a physical therapist for a number of years, but I think I learned a lot more about everybody's discipline because everybody was open in sharing that. Oftentimes when we are in the work setting we're all focused on having to present what we know about the patient, not about the process, and without as much openness to really listen to what other people say. So I think I hear what you're saying and I do agree with it because I have actually learned that too.*

TERRY BARD/PSYCHOLOGY/PASTORAL CARE: *I think I have learned from all of you—I do every year in many ways—but what I just heard that I want to support is the growth experience. A lot of people who are seasoned professionals and have experience, even they know how difficult it is to create a relatively structuralistic orientation to a program so that people have to struggle with defining what they need to get out of it, how best to navigate what actually works in a team. And I think that openness to the process is important to finally understand the difficulty in not knowing a lot about each other's disciplines in order to provide more of an even template. Templates, even though they are uncomfortable, provide opportunities. When you have to struggle more, you have to listen more, you have to listen to other people differently and what they're saying. Out of discomfort comes a new reality of working together. I've really gained a new appreciation of that, even though some of you still don't like that model.*

PEGGY BROWN/SOCIAL WORK: *This may seem like a little thing, but I learned the difference between "multidisciplinary" and "interdisciplinary," where with the interdisciplinary you really are entering into each other's disciplines and crossing over some of those boundaries, as opposed to just staying within your discipline and offering what you have and listening to what the other person has. You really do become much more enmeshed. And I do find that I think a little bit, maybe, like a pharmacist and I think a little bit like a physical therapist, and it has changed how I look at medical care.*

MELANIE VAUGHN/PHYSICAL THERAPY: *I was thinking along the same lines as Peggy. I now have a better understanding of what "interdisciplinary" means. I thought that*

I knew prior to joining this education program, but it was more of the multidisciplinary approach that I know of. I was challenged in this program to see the value of all disciplines and not claim that one is more important than another. I gained a new appreciation for the value of working together and learning from each other's disciplines. It is neat to see how our disciplines do overlap and support each other.

ERICA RAINE/SOCIAL WORK: *As one of the seasoned students, this class was an eye-opener for me. I realize I'm sort of stuck in my own little world. I am used to working with experienced professionals in health care on multidisciplinary teams and, at times, interdisciplinary teams. Working on teams and with colleagues in other disciplines is the norm for social workers. I loved the opportunity to interact with new professionals. For example, I learned from our pharmacist about how the pharmacy field is changing with pharmacists having more clinical contact with patients and partnering with physicians. I learned that pharmacy and physical therapy programs are moving away from granting master's level degrees and going directly to doctorates, which may give them more influence on treatment plans and the future of health care.*

I think Keith, a pharmacy student, and Kay, a physical therapy student (on our project team), were surprised about how interested the social workers were in their disciplines. When you are a social worker in geriatrics, you really need to know about medications and their interactions. You need to understand what the physical therapist is doing to help clients/patients function in their environments. So often social workers meet with clients/patients and learn that they don't understand their medical problems, their treatment, or their medications. The more we know, the better we can support and empower clients/patients to ask questions and get answers and participate in their treatment plans. Ideally, patients should feel part of the treatment team.

JEANETTE BURACK/OLDER ADULT: *Some elderly people frequently visit every conceivable aspect of medicine and therapeutic professionals. This education that I've been partaking of has made me hungry to see changes from my aspect as the patient. And I must confess that I keep looking because I spend a lot of time being treated. It hasn't happened yet, from my vantage point. Interdisciplinary is something I haven't seen as a patient.*

Multidisciplinary, yes! But they are all tied into the computer for their information. Working together as an interdisciplinary group leaves much to be desired from the patient's point of view. But the left hand sometimes doesn't know in time what the right hand is doing. And I have to confess to you that it is a long row for you guys to hoe because until such time as it becomes a procedure—interdisciplinary care becomes a standard operating procedure so that it will be fluid and affect the outcome of the patient's care—it is going to be a struggle, and you people are my hope. I say this each year that I am blessed with being here. There's so much out there that needs you. So when you are involved in interdisciplinary care—or hoping to be involved—remember Jeanette because I have hopes for all of you. I really do!

PRICHARD/NURSING AND HEALTHCARE ADMINISTRATION: *I do feel that the interdisciplinary team brings a richness to patient care because you have so many perspectives on patient care. It is almost like seeing something in three dimensions versus two dimensions in other kinds of health care with a multidisciplinary team. There is just such a richness that you can treat the patient in a more holistic fashion, I think, and really have a greater chance of meeting the needs—all the needs of the patient—or at least addressing them. So I think that's a wonderful, wonderful outcome of the interdisciplinary team.*

SATIN/PSYCHIATRY: *Some people have said how much they benefit from understanding other disciplines and from learning from other disciplines and from sharing the task with other disciplines. One of the objections to interdisciplinary work is this crossing of boundaries because some people have said, "At the least this waters down the education of the individual disciplines. If you are spending this much time learning pharmacy, then you are not spending this much time learning social work. If you are spending time in an interdisciplinary class, then you are not spending time in a pharmacology class or in a nursing practice class or in a management class. So it is taking away from the time that is already too packed in the discipline." The other objection is that you are losing your disciplinary identity. That if you learn from pharmacy or physical therapy or biology or something else, then are you still a good nurse or social worker or other primary discipline? You are something else—you're a hybrid. And you're not clear enough about what your role is and what your contribution is. So it is seen as a waste of time and undermining. What would you say to those objections to your learning outside of your discipline?*

BROVERMAN/ELDER CARE ADMINISTRATION: *We had an exercise where we learned about each other's discipline, and that really helped us to gain a different appreciation for the disciplines of our classmates. As part of our presentation we were asked to share some of the key components of each of our educations. As someone who had one elective to take out of her whole curriculum, I chose this class and I am thrilled that I did because I really think that I got the most enriched learning experience that I could. Instead of taking a class solely about one discipline of studies, such as management, I was able to learn about an approach to care services that is multidimensional. This education really challenged me to think creatively "outside the box" and beyond my role definition and allowed me to learn about the possibility of expanding my developing new career in elder-care administration beyond the prescribed role definition.*

KATHLEEN BOYLE/SOCIAL WORK: *When I listen to your question, the thing that comes to my mind—and I'm sure it's why you posed the question—is: who are we talking about? Who are we worried about here? Are we worried about ourselves as social workers or physical therapists or doctors? Or are we worried about the patient? What's the goal? So if you assume that the goal is to give better care to the patient and not to sort of create our little boundaries for ourselves so that we can feel more like what we were trained to be or whatever, I think it is really hard to argue against interdisciplinary work. I know if I walk in to see somebody that I work with and I can understand better about what kinds of questions to ask about the medications they are taking or what sort of physical therapy they are doing and why and so on—I mean, those things are going to be much better for the patient. Does it water down my being a social worker? I wouldn't say so. I would just say it augments it more than waters it down. But I think it's a question of patient-centered versus professional-centered, and so I think that's the key.*

RAINE/SOCIAL WORK: *I would agree with that, and I think that is a good way of putting it. The goal is to provide care to patients. I think interdisciplinary care has the best chance to provide coordinated care. My experience is that patients expect their providers to communicate with each other. When they don't communicate patients are disappointed and confused and lose confidence in their health-care providers, and that extends to all their providers.*

There is a place for individual disciplinary identity. Developing that identity is important while you are learning your field but less in the actual care of patients. I don't think you compromise your professional identity by working on an interdisciplinary team or having the experience of studying an area of mutual interest with other health-care students. I'd like to make a strong case for a place for training health-care professionals to work with each other. Perhaps it is at the postgraduate internship level. Terry Bard pointed out that Hebrew SeniorLife brings together doctors, nutritionists, and physical therapists at a postgraduate level; but those fellowships are not widely available to all health-care professionals in geriatrics. For example, social workers are not eligible for training fellowships at Hebrew SeniorLife despite the strong psychosocial orientation in the long-term care units. Despite the role social workers play in geriatrics, I'm not sure that other health-care professionals understand what we do. In my experience as a clinician and a supervisor, whenever social workers join health-care teams there is a long educational process before the full range of social work is accepted and valued by nurses and physicians. I was startled when one of our project team members said that he did not feel there was a "strong psychosocial presence." We had two social workers on our project team! Our project included a lot about social justice and public policy.

SALINGER/SOCIAL WORK: *But don't you think that their statement is a misconception of what social work is anyway? One of the important lessons of this education is to accept the fact that we don't always fully understand the focus of other professions. Often, we have preconceived notions that turn out to be wrong.*

RAINE/SOCIAL WORK: *Right.*

SALINGER/SOCIAL WORK: *In this situation we see another discipline asserting that psychosocial assessments define social work professionals. We know our profession is much more complicated than that. We have to be careful not to make assumptions about what other professions do.*

RAINE/SOCIAL WORK: *I find even well-educated people don't understand the value of social work skills in health care. Martin Solomon talked about his frustration with advocating for his patient to have her medication provided under Medicare D. If Dr. Solomon had social workers as part of the team in his office, they would have developed the network to resolve the problem. Dr. Solomon's dedication to his patient is laudatory, but what a waste of his medical skills and energy! Maybe private medical practices need to include social workers. Sometimes even the most educated and experienced people think that social workers just take away people's children or administer welfare policies.*

SALINGER/SOCIAL WORK: *Or therapists.*

RAINE/SOCIAL WORK: *Or therapists.*

SALINGER/SOCIAL WORK: *There is a great deal in between welfare work and psychotherapy.*

PETER MARAMALDI/SOCIAL WORK/PUBLIC HEALTH: *In response to Erica's comment about post-master's training. I know some of you are members of the Gerontological Society of America. That is a truly interdisciplinary organization. If you attend their annual meeting, if you read their journals, if you go to any of the offshoots like the Association for Gerontology in Higher Education, all those meetings, if you even look at the abstracts, most of the presentations, papers, and studies are truly interdisciplinary. So there are venues to participate in.*

SATIN/PSYCHIATRY: *It's been a very interesting and very rewarding educational program. It's a learning experience for everybody, including the faculty. That's how we can stand participating in this program for 30 years and not get bored because it's different each time and you're learning something different each time and you are seeing people learn from one another. I have learned from dentistry the importance of dry mouth for oral health and speech and nutrition and the effect of psychiatric medication on the mouth. I have learned from occupational therapy the importance of functioning in daily life for people's ability to overcome illness and disability and depression. I have learned from pharmacy the way medications are absorbed and distributed and deactivated and excreted and the way they work on different organs. I have learned from pastoral care the importance of religion as a support and an answer to existential questions. I have learned from social work the dignity and equality of patients as people. So it's an extraordinarily rewarding, remarkable educational program that we appreciate.*

Interdisciplinary Gerontology Education Compared with the Usual Disciplinary Education

BARD/PSYCHOLOGY/PASTORAL CARE: *I have a question as we are talking about this dimension and the capacity or the benefit of having some interdisciplinary, integrated care. One of the observations that we often make, and one that David Satin usually notices directly in our first class and also noted again in our last class, is that if you look around you are sitting in a relatively small class among a very large cohort of fellow workers or other students in your schools who have not elected to take this class. Is there something different about you, about us that this class speaks to that doesn't speak to others? Therefore, even though we are saying we should make this part of the curriculum and in practice and in professional development, is that really possible, or is there something almost hardwired in those of us who sit around here, that this is the orientation that we have toward our world and that what we come here is to discipline it, to amplify it, and to play out an undercurrent that is part of us? I don't know. I have that question that I want to ask you because I think those are real questions. Not everybody is breaking down the doors to take what you took.*

KIMBERLY ARMSTRONG/SOCIAL WORK: *I think that it is in part the way I'm wired that I chose this education. I wonder about the value system of the interdisciplinary approach because there aren't any medical students in this education. That being said, I wonder about the value the medical system attaches to interdisciplinary teams. It seems that a medical person is key on the interdisciplinary team. If they are not a part of this education are they really committed to this idea? And what does that mean for the future of interdisciplinary teams? To complicate matters, I wonder about the value system in medicine with managed care, with reimbursements, and all the struggles talked about by the two interdisciplinary teams we heard from. Can interdisciplinary teams make it? I think this education has helped me as a social worker become a better social worker. I now have a greater understanding of resources for my clients and my patients, but I am uncertain of the future of interdisciplinary teams within the current medical system.*

BARD/PSYCHOLOGY/PASTORAL CARE: *I think that is certainly an accurate criticism. We can't choose who participates in terms of discipline. We can try as much as possible to enrich the mix. We have had medical students in the past. I think proportionately you'll find that medical students are represented over the course of years, probably very much the same that you are in your discipline. There are fewer doctors trained than there are social workers in this country. I am not going to defend those who are not here, but*

I think there needs to be more promotion. There needs to be more awareness of what it is all about. And they are taught differently. But I'm not so sure I would indict them quite so much because those medical students who have taken this course have made considerable inroads into how they manage their care. And you've had a number of people come as guest lecturers who are physicians, who clearly understand what's going on. Some have even taken the lead to make this happen in your work setting. So I guess, just to try to put it in a broader spectrum. I don't know if I would "go there" quite yet.

MARAMALDI/SOCIAL WORK/PUBLIC HEALTH: *And anecdotally, Terry, if I could, the one medical student who started this course and left this course, I happened just to see her just before class and she said, "Are you here for that gerontology class?" And I said, "Yes." And she said, "I would love to have taken it, but there were many pressures on the curriculum this year and so there were demands for time." And so there are reasons for things; it is very, very difficult.*

BARD/PSYCHOLOGY/PASTORAL CARE: *Earlier today I spoke with one of the medical school academic leaders. At this point you can count on one hand the number of courses in geriatrics in medical school. So it's not been a focus. And we are, of course, considering two different dimensions of health and geriatric care: We are looking at macrocosmic and microcosmic dimensions of health care and caring for the older person. At the same time we're considering ways in which one can create interdisciplinary teams that really cross all age boundaries and look at how we work together.*

SATIN/PSYCHIATRY: *To answer this, to put more perspective on this question, over the years the largest number of students in this course have come from social work, occupational therapy, and public health. The largest numbers of students in this course are female. There have been medical students in the course but very sporadically and maybe one at a time. In one year there were four or five medical students because another elective course had been canceled, and these guys were sitting around wondering what to do with their time and picked this and stuck it out. This year we had eight medical students inquire about the course. Three elected to take the course: one never showed up, one wanted to come every once in a while, and one came for one or two sessions and then was "too busy."*

BARD/PSYCHOLOGY/PASTORAL CARE: *She had a conflict in her curriculum.*

SATIN/PSYCHIATRY: *That still amounts to being too busy. I don't know whether it is a comment on her priorities or those of her curriculum.*

BARD/PSYCHOLOGY/PASTORAL CARE: *I don't think she has any latitude, David, in the first year.*

SATIN/PSYCHIATRY: *That's significant. That is significant.*

BARD/PSYCHOLOGY/PASTORAL CARE: *A structural issue.*

SATIN/PSYCHIATRY: *How come social work has time in its curriculum? Occupational therapy has time in its curriculum. Public health has time in its curriculum. Medicine does not. Physical therapy and occupational therapy at two institutions do not have time in their curriculum for this. Why physical therapy at a third university does have time in its curriculum for this I don't know, but I suspect it's a matter of values and educational philosophy, rather than time or geography.*

Most medical education programs focus on the basic sciences, clinical sciences, and clinical practice of medicine. They see many new discoveries that change medicine greatly and have to be taught in a limited amount of time (it's already 7 to 13 years, not counting undergraduate premedical education). And it is assumed that they teach physicians to be researchers and educators as well as clinicians. And it is an article of faith that physicians are leaders of the teams in which they work. Medical education includes other disciplines mainly in support or supplementary roles in multidisciplinary teams. Many of you must have had the experience of physicians being available for team meetings, planning projects, and teaching only when they are not called away by more important responsibilities. This education program starts with the very different premise that all disciplines are equally valuable and needed, and all are responsible to the strength, success, and enrichment of the team for the benefit of the task. I think this causes "cognitive dissonance" for medical students and postgraduate medical trainees—it sounds reasonable, but it doesn't fit with their disciplinary socialization. That's why medical students have had a hard time deciding to "find time" for this education rather than the easier task of seeing the importance of genetics, epidemiology, or even health policy. And medical students who do take the course tend to have a hard time fitting themselves into the role of team member. I have great compassion for those who do complete the course and try to find some place for this perspective and skill in medical education. Perhaps those who want to apply it to medical practice may have an easier time finding members of other disciplines and task settings where this approach is well received and useful. But that is not likely to be in an academic medical setting. Are we then left with the hard question as to whether interdisciplinary education is compatible with medical education?

I wish people who are in social work would tell us how this compares with their other social work courses, people in nursing how it compares with nursing; and we don't have the people in medicine, but the medical courses don't have time for this and are focusing on physical examination, on biology, on stuff like that. What's the comparison of values that translate into education and, later, professional practice? I think this all is relevant to the comparison of this course with the other education that you get in your professional training.

BROVERMAN/ELDER CARE ADMINISTRATION: *This experience has been unlike any other I have had in the coursework at my disciplinary education program. I think that it's partly related to a structural setup of my program because not all the classes meet every week; some of them meet every other week, and some meet online. I feel that because I had the opportunity to participate in an education which is more the traditional model as opposed to the modern method of hybrid and online learning, I really got a different breadth of experience than I would have in online and the hybrid courses. I feel that I really grew into this program and have been challenged to learn as an individual as well as within our small group. Initially, I was hesitant to participate in the group discussions as I am not accustomed to having an open discussion forum; rather, I am used to having to raise my hand to participate. But after a while I became more familiar with the format and more engaged in our group discussions. I have learned from the other participants through our lectures and other learning formats, as well as from members of my small group. In both settings I feel I have grown as during the program I became more comfortable with my own contributions and voicing my opinions in the meetings. I also took on more of a leadership role within my small group, whereas in the beginning I did not feel confident working with a group of "strangers" from outside my education program and discipline. In addition, we grew in understanding the purpose of the small group presentations, implementing the concept of collaborating as an interdisciplinary team rather than solely demonstrating our knowledge of the content. After many weeks we finally clarified our understanding of this material as demonstrated in our presentation to the whole group. I've been honored to have this educa-*

tion. *Perhaps the traditional form of education where we meet every week really has its value and advantage as opposed to the more modern conveniences of online, etc.*

SALINGER/SOCIAL WORK: *I'm going to go in the opposite direction. It became clear to me and to some of my fellow social work students early on that the interdisciplinary focus of this program was, in many ways, similar to how a social work school curriculum teaches us to view our profession. In the first semester of our MSW program, we are presented with a picture of patients/clients at the center of a large circle. Like spokes in a wheel, the multitude of areas that influence people's lives (school, family, religion, community, etc.) create a multidimensional understanding of people's lives. Similarly, this program also sees patients in the center of the circle, with each of our professions becoming the spokes in the wheel. But the program also adds another important dimension to that picture by proposing that the spokes do not stay separate as on a wheel but instead intertwine with one another.*

BURACK/OLDER ADULT: *My theory is that the reason that the doctors or medical students are not present in this education is that they haven't gotten the context of what we represent. They are the distributors of treatments, but they send the patient to seek out the disciplines. They do not interact with the multiple disciplines as a group. The patient is the one who is sent out into the field for herself or himself. And I'm talking about an elderly geriatric patient who needs to have interdisciplinary help, who has to go to an "ist." Do you know what "ists" are? I've been to every "ist" because I have been sent by my primary-care doctors, of whom I have had a variety, to occupational therapists and physical therapists, and all of the "ists." But I'm the one who has to go and make appointments and find out from all of these specialists. And there is no melting pot other than the computer. I don't mean to be facetious about this computer, but the computer has the disciplines all inside of it but nobody to work out the problems for the patient. You hit the nail right on the head from my vantage point: Social workers are the practitioners of interdisciplinary care. Because from my own experience with social work after surgery or after therapy in nursing homes, it's the social worker who saw to it that I had the proper medications, who saw to it that I had help at home having been discharged to go home and live alone, who saw to all of the patients' needs which the doctors do not do. The doctors are busy; they're trained to do wonderful work, but I don't think they can be persuaded to address the quality of what we experience. And therefore the nut that you're going to have to crack professionally in the future is going to be a very difficult one but so important because I speak for the elderly—I'm 83 years old and I have been through hell and I am so enthused about what this education represents. And I just hope from year to year that we will have more people who'll be blessed. You used the word "blessed," and I appreciate your sentiments about participating in this education. It is such an unusual opportunity that if we spread the gospel and send the word around that there exists an education that could be an open door for the future of geriatric patients. Or even nongeriatric patients—interdisciplinary work doesn't necessarily mean you have to be old to have it. It's important, it's important to have a network but to focus on the patient and not on the computer. It has to be a personal effort.*

RAINE/SOCIAL WORK: *To respond to the educational question "How come social work students made time or the social work curriculum provided time for social work students to participate in this program?" I think communication and collaboration is a core value of social work. My MSW program at the University of Michigan emphasized this from the first day. Despite the values of social work and the fact that social workers* are very active in health care and geriatrics and we often practice in multidisciplinary or interdisciplinary team settings, there is not much course work on these topics in the social work curriculum. Social work students recognize that this class is a golden opportunity for them.

I was disappointed at the paucity of medical and nursing students in this program. It seems as if it is a question of scheduling or maybe a question of core values. Or maybe it is taken for granted that health-care professionals will learn to work effectively together through clinical experiences. Maybe there needs to be a meeting of all the health profession training programs in the area to talk about the importance and the opportunities for students to learn together so that they will communicate and collaborate to provide better care. What I am hearing from Mrs. Burack is that, with more specialization and new technology, doctors may be communicating to each other about patients; but the synthesis is missing, and patients are left to figure out how it all fits together on their own. If there were more effective interdisciplinary teaming, older adult patients might not feel this way. Those who don't participate in this education are missing the opportunity not only to study with each other but to hear from older adults such as Mrs. Burack and our older adult panelists.

DREVINS/PHYSICAL THERAPY: I just wanted to talk a little bit about the physical therapy background. When I received my physical therapy training—and at that point it was a bachelor's degree—I think in all my 4 years of education, I didn't really have any interdisciplinary courses. My freshman year you took courses with all kinds of different students, but once you get into your professional training it is very specific to that profession. For us it was just physical therapy students. As it turns out, there was so much crammed into the curriculum that now the entry level is at the doctorate level. The students who are now in physical therapy programs again might take their chemistry class, their biology class, some of their basics with other students; but at that point all the students don't have their disciplines set because they are entering totally different degree programs. This type of education is very different because of the mix of disciplines. It's the first interdisciplinary class I've ever been involved with. I've been teaching for 15 years, and all I teach is physical therapy students, so it is very interesting to see this perspective. So I just wanted to clarify what the physical therapy background is and how different this approach is. When David Satin asked why other students don't participate, it really depends on what year you are targeting them. Many of the students are out in the clinical areas; they are doing their clinical rotations, and they are in the hospital settings and in the private practices working until five, five-thirty, six o'clock at night, so they couldn't build in a night education experience and it's not the right timing for them.

I can clarify what we do in our hospital facility. I get calls from the hospitalists all the time—physicians who work primarily in the hospital setting—they call and they say, "Set me up with an occupational therapist. I want to shadow an OT. I want to shadow a physical therapist. I want to see what they're doing." We have these regular programs go on. Okay, it's 4 hours out of their day maybe once, but at least they're asking for it. So I do think that that's a push for interdisciplinary understanding. And in the outpatient setting, the same thing: The orthopedic residents are shadowing our outpatient physical therapists to find out what they're doing because they realize there's a knowledge deficit and they have to learn it. They also learn to respect the different disciplines, so I think that's another piece. So some things that we're doing in this educational approach is cotreatment in the clinical setting. And you get more respect cotreating; a patient may require both occupational therapy and physical therapy or *speech therapy, and we'll do that together because maybe in order for a patient to have their speech therapy they have to be sitting upright but they can't support themselves sitting unassisted so a physical therapist will go in and work on that while the speech therapist is doing treatments. And we get respect—mutual respect—for the different disciplines. I think it just makes you a better clinician by being more exposed to these other areas. I think you're very narrow if all you do is interact with your own discipline or profession. It makes you a better clinician all around to be exposed to other disciplines.*

KIMBERLY SAUDER/GERONTOLOGY: *Coming out of a PhD research program, this is a very different educational experience. And I found it really refreshing because I used to be a social worker, and when I first went into the PhD program I had a bit of a transition shock, if you know what I mean. I knew I was stepping away from direct care, but I still wasn't totally prepared for the disconnect between academia and research and the frontline staff and direct care. And I am just really struggling with where I fit in. I don't want necessarily to be a social worker for the rest of my life, but—goodness!— I don't want to sit and, you know, just punch numbers and get completely sucked into the world of academia and then completely forget my days as a social worker. What I appreciate about this educational approach is that it felt very clinical to me. And whenever I would say that, one of the physical therapists on my team would say, "I don't understand why you're saying that because this education is so not clinical." But for me it was. Because I'm sitting here surrounded by social workers and nurses and physical therapists and, you know, it's like being back in my social work days again and talking about the patient and talking about what's best for the patient. How can we come together and put a plan together? And it was just a good reminder to me that, yes, that is really what is most important. And so, as a researcher, as a gerontologist, being challenged to think when you do research and when you try to change policy or make policy proposals or things, to keep that at the foundation, as the goal, I just found very different and important. I wish that there would be more students in the research domain who would be interested to come into the more clinical domain and learn about it because this is really where the rubber hits the road. As researchers, if you don't have an understanding of what the problems are or how the system is failing or you know who is falling through the cracks and how are the older adults really feeling when they're dealing with this health-care system—how are we as researchers supposed to know what can we do to help bring change at the bigger picture?*

PRICHARD, NURSING/HEALTHCARE ADMINISTRATION: *Speaking about my basic preparation at a baccalaureate level 20 years ago, we really focused on a multidisciplinary approach, not so much an interdisciplinary approach. But in retrospect we really crossed one another's roles. For example, if physical therapy was on at night, the PT would teach us how to do whatever we needed to do. Speech therapy would teach swallowing. We would do all of that. So there's always been a lot of give and take; that's been part of our basic education. Now I'm in health-care administration. At my school there is another interdisciplinary course that's being taught. I haven't been mixing with my own usual crowd of students, and I did have the opportunity about a month ago and was anxious to compare notes. I still haven't got a full perspective, but I'm so glad that I took this educational approach because it's given us an opportunity to apply some of the techniques of an interdisciplinary team and to experience the development of an interdisciplinary team. I have learned so much about elder care that's going to change my practice. I've been encouraged by the fact that they included this in the health-care administration program because they really need to have an appreciation of the value of an interdisciplinary team. Health-care administrators are in a key position to really make that happen. And to address the issue around medical students, it is concerning that more medical students are not involved in this kind of a program because, in the end, we often look to the medical folks to lead the team and they're usually the most ill-prepared because they haven't gotten the experience. Maybe they don't need to be the team leaders, but they can certainly interface better if they have an appreciation of what the interdisciplinary team can offer and the value to the patient.*

DREVINS/PHYSICAL THERAPY: *I'm just looking at you again when you talk about how nurses do things to help out physical therapists or other disciplines. That's absolutely right. And I think in many hospitals the nurse is sort of the hub. But it doesn't make you a physical therapist, nor would you pretend to be one. And that goes back to the question as to whether we lose our identities. We don't. Just because we carry out a part of another disciplinary role doesn't mean we pretend to take over that whole role. For instance, in acute care if I do something that nursing traditionally would do, it doesn't make me a nurse. So, again, it's being respectful of other people's professions and also doing what the patient needs at that point in time. I think it's a good point that you raised.*

Interdisciplinary Gerontology Applied to Professional Practice

SAUDER/GERONTOLOGY: *Coming back to the question about the medical system or the medical students, where are they? One of the things that I've been struck by, especially in this last module when we've had the example of teams coming in, is that the system, I think, is really the problem. And I think these teams that came in were really commendable because they were really making a lot of effort to work around a system that really is not supporting this concept of interdisciplinary teamwork. And I think if you look at the medical programs and that Terry Bard said there are very few classes that are geriatric, you know the medical education system is training people to work within this medical care system. In order to function and to survive, you need to learn to work within the system that we have. It would be great if doctors would intuitively just step up and put together more interdisciplinary teams and see the vision, but I think everybody is trying to do their best within the system that we have. I think the challenge is more changing the system and trying to impact policies or changing how the health-care system in general is structured and trying to get the word out that an interdisciplinary approach to care is much better than the structure that we have now. I think if it doesn't change at the systemic level it's going to be really hard to get the individual players to do it. You have teams here and there and you have people making a difference, but I think there needs to be also the energy put in at the big level—the glue that binds the system together.*

BARD/PSYCHOLOGY/PASTORAL CARE: *I think that you touched on a very sensitive issue for me. I know that some of us, reiterated many times by Martin Solomon from his long experience in acute care, had this fantasy wish, even a prediction, that a change in the health-care system is not going to happen. Rather, we are watching what we call a system—which is really a nonsystem system of systems—ultimately just totally collapse and implode. It's a fantasy wish, because once it implodes and doesn't exist, maybe we can start building what should be there. But that's unlikely to happen, and that's the frustration too, because if it could implode I think a number of us would work very hard to hasten that. But since that's unlikely to happen, the question is how do we go about strategically identifying and making the health-care system work in a way that is not just helpful to individual patients (which is the focus for all of us) but also helpful to communities and to large populations? It's interesting that one or two of you have said that we've learned that this dysfunctional system exists in a context of so many surplus resources. Some of you then went on to say, "But what happens in rural America, what are their resources?" I have spent a good deal of time in rural areas in the Midwest, Arkansas, and I have a small place in New Hampshire, and I have found that communities themselves actually take on the role of interdisciplinary care without the benefit of specialists in various disciplines. And somehow they survive better than we because in these rural communities people realize their connection with one another more than they do in urban communities, where people are much more autonomous. So I don't know what the answer is, but I share your concern and your observation. Maybe we should all move to small towns. Maybe that's the answer.*

BURACK/OLDER ADULT: *The Mt. Auburn Hospital Multiple Sclerosis Comprehensive Care Center team recently exemplifies a potential that could conceivably blossom out. You see, they have the advantage of meeting at the same time, at the same place, together—all the disciplines. And their focus is on a group of patients that they all share and they're all concerned about, and they work together. From my vantage point, it's the only one I've seen that has been successful. Because it's compact, and they have the time to work together in a small group. We're talking about big hospitals, and I can't see how it will ever happen there.*

BROWN/SOCIAL WORK: *The unique thing about that Mt. Auburn program is that they have a doctor who's very committed to interdisciplinary teaming. I would wonder that when that doctor retires . . .*

BURACK/OLDER ADULT: *If she ever croaks, that's the end of that program—I'm telling you right now.*

BROWN/SOCIAL WORK: *That's a critical piece there to get that program . . .*

BURACK/OLDER ADULT: *That's a separate problem.*

SATIN/PSYCHIATRY: *They don't have the time, they make the time.*

BURACK/OLDER ADULT: *Exactly!*

SATIN/PSYCHIATRY: *At great personal sacrifice.*

BURACK/OLDER ADULT: *Absolutely. But it works!*

MARAMALDI/SOCIAL WORK/PUBLIC HEALTH: *Before we leave that, I think a lot of it depends on your clinical experience. You see this in the leadership of the team, and it lends itself to the question of professional practice. As you ascend into positions of leadership, you will have the ability to really instill interdisciplinary collaboration. I'll just talk about some of the hospitals at which I have worked. You'll see interdisciplinary teams that go so far as to include support staff—the receptionist, the telephone operator. It's not uncommon now to see the senior oncologist walk out to the reception desk and ask the receptionist a question about the patient before going in to see the patient. Unheard of! In the same hospital, the same clinic area, a different team leader wouldn't even acknowledge the existence of the receptionist—today, right now. Things are changing, there's a shift, and we're all in positions to influence that. And a lot of it has to do with competency.*

BROVERMAN/ELDER CARE ADMINISTRATION: *One of the things that I have gained from this education is a greater understanding of being a creative problem solver and thinking outside of the box. In my future role as an elder-care administrator in whatever setting that may be, I will have a lot of respect for everyone involved in the care process. As people said before, whether that's the front desk receptionist or the trained professionals, I think that now I have a broader understanding and appreciation for everyone involved in caring for the patient/client/elder.*

PRICHARD, NURSING/HEALTHCARE ADMINISTRATION: *I work currently as the coordinator of a diabetes program, and we're in the process of revamping our whole program and developing a business plan. We are required under the American Diabetes Association guidelines to have a multidisciplinary approach to patient care, and I'm hoping that will include an interdisciplinary approach. So I'm in the process now of bringing the team together and, I hope, can begin to share some of my little kernels of knowledge and continue my education in this field and hopefully spread the word, not only of interdisciplinary teams but the care of elders. And I hope to be more sensitive in terms of our curriculum development and our educational tools to the unique needs of this patient population. This is often not just about giving knowledge, but it's about changing behavior and really looking at the patient and what their unique needs might be and what the team can offer. So this education has acted as a stimulus to continue my education in both those areas—the care of the elder and also interdisciplinary teaming as a goal.*

SATIN/PSYCHIATRY: *Isn't there anybody here who will say this is utopian, this is impractical, it isn't going to work in the outside world? "This is a nice restful interlude, but now we have to go back to business."*

BOYLE/SOCIAL WORK: *OK, I'll say it. I don't think it's utopian; I think it's a lofty goal to strive for, worthwhile, meaningful. I think it requires a lot of scratching and fighting because there is, as you said, that sense on the part of some people that they're sacrificing their disciplines or it is slipping away from them, they're giving it away, or they're becoming less focused themselves. But also I think it's money. Money, money, money, money. I don't think it's practical, but I think it's worth pursuing. And my own experience is one of being part of an interdisciplinary team for 7 years, so this is a refresher course for me. And it comes at a good time because this is the end of my 2-year Master of Social Work program. And I have realized in the course of the last 2 years that I have been functioning in two settings, serving the elderly population as a solo practitioner, as a social worker. And I love social work and I love social workers and I'm proud to be part of the profession. But it's lonely when you're serving an elderly population. They have a lot of needs, and you're going through the door as an individual, not with a team, as you are in hospice. You're not going through with a nurse in the background or the doctor, with a physical therapist, with a pastoral care person, with a home health aide. You're going through by yourself. And I'm going to see people in their homes, out in the community, where their lives are rocking and rolling. They are trying to maintain their equilibrium, but it is very difficult for them as they age, as they have more and more challenges. And I have felt very sad to be doing this on my own. I feel that I'm at risk of prying because in some cases I'm going through the door and seeing what their lives are like. I'm the only one going through the door in the week, other than the person who hands the "Meals on Wheels" food through the door. And I come back looking around at my fellow social workers in the agency in which I'm interning and they're all kind of feeling the same way. But there's no time to sit and* talk, even with my fellow social workers. And there is no one to share the physical strain, and there's no one to share those spiritual challenges with. You know, I can't be it all, I can't do it all. So I'm lonely, I'm isolated, I'm stuck. I'm not serving this population as well as I could if I weren't alone. So I'd like to go out and look for a job making home visits to people but as part of an interdisciplinary team. But is there a mechanism to pay for that? So I think that each of us was drawn to this education maybe for the interdisciplinary piece or, as you pointed out, the three different components. I was drawn to it because of all three coming together. And I feel as though, for an elderly population, it's a very important point of view to hold as a goal, to share that point of view and to be in it together because it helps you stay in it longer, you serve better, you share the weight. The intensity of all of those needs that people have as they are proud and independent and they don't want to give up their homes. And yet they don't want to go to another doctor's appointment on the elderly transportation system, and I can drive them to just so many appointments. So I'd like to think that this idea of mine would exist out there as something to look for. I hope to find it. If any of you hear about it, please send me an e-mail.

BARD, PSYCHOLOGY/PASTORAL CARE: We tend to look at the situations we find around us as opportunities to act in an interdisciplinary way, contributing our disciplinary thoughts. But one of the dreams of mine—I think it is shared by many, if not all, of my faculty colleagues—is that your vision doesn't have to be so focused on the orbit in which you are serving right now. We live in many worlds at the same time: We live in our family worlds, we live in our professional worlds, and we do live in the larger world. Maybe some of you (and this is my fantasy maybe because I've taken some of it on; I know some of us as well have done so) is that this system of health care that we are living in today is broken. There is not a person I know who doesn't acknowledge its brokenness. No one is saving it. There are lots of visions. There is not a lot of will from the government. Some states have taken a step. But there is nothing except ourselves to prevent us from taking a much broader role, from becoming people who advocate with lobbyists. For people who join efforts to make change at the macro level (which we addressed at the beginning of the education program) as well as at the micro. We don't necessarily have the vision of how this should take shape, but we know where it is failing. And we also know how the pieces work best together: That's what we're trying to represent in this education. In that respect we can become advocates. So I would suggest that we advocate at every level. When the opportunity or the inspiration arises don't hide from it. If you need to speak you don't have to speak out just at home or just in the office where there is a bunch of people who don't have time to process what they're struggling with. We can also yell on a bigger stage and make a difference because I think this is where the leadership will come from. You and people like you around the country who are getting inspired and have a vision that's different from what currently exists. Otherwise, all we do is exert our efforts managing what comes our way, what is currently "on our plate." It is hard to picture ourselves as shapers as well as managing as best we can what our plate gives us (though we manage pretty well). But I think that we can become shapers as well. That's my advertisement and my wish for the future for all of us.

PRICHARD/NURSING/HEALTHCARE ADMINISTRATION: Just to comment on what you were saying earlier about feeling lonely, I absolutely share that feeling working where I'm working. I just had an incident last week, and I called Erica Raine because I needed a social worker because I felt so overwhelmed by this situation, and it happens over and over and over again. That's why I'm angry, that's why I want to develop a team *that is more integrated—because the patients are becoming more complex and we're living with chronic disease. We absolutely need this interdisciplinary approach to help and support one another because the weight is very heavy. So I absolutely share your sentiments—absolutely! So it's lonely from the nursing perspective as well.*

SAUDER, GERONTOLOGY: *To add to that, I really appreciated listening to the functioning interdisciplinary teams. You could see how they really did support each other. There was definite camaraderie among them. As a former social worker and dealing with the stress of really complex situations and just not knowing which way to turn and feeling like your hands are tied, the times when I am able to talk with the people that I worked with really help support me. Then you feel like, "OK we can get through this. We can work it through." It's another component of interdisciplinary teams that is really invaluable, which was very well demonstrated, I think, by the teams we saw functioning in the real world today.*

BROVERMAN/ELDER CARE ADMINISTRATION: *One of the things that other folks have commented on is being part of the team and feeling a sense of belonging and feeling some camaraderie with other people. That was demonstrated throughout this educational experience. We all got to know each other and what disciplines we represent. It would be grand to have these teams in every setting, but as other people have said, the reality is that it may not be possible. I think we need to use our skills to create a kind of team, even if it be with one other person who can provide support, to help manage the difficulties we encounter in working with older adults and the health-care system. We are dealing with a very challenging, vulnerable population that has multiple needs. Sometimes we need to get support for ourselves in order to support the clients that we're trying to help. That can only be done by having an outlet such as a team mechanism. I do agree that the two teams we met demonstrated that they had a formal structure but also that they had informal structures so that they could vent about what they were feeling. I think that is so, so important. Coming from a practice setting that lacks support and structure, I can testify that it is very frustrating. We've had a lot of mechanisms taken away from us. We don't have a venue to have supervision, to talk about what our thoughts or feelings are, and try to work to improve things. I think it would be important to have a list of people who are in the same profession, maybe work together on a similar case, and then expand in the interdisciplinary realm.*

BURACK/OLDER ADULT: *Has it ever occurred to any of you that in the community called "geriatrics" there might exist people who are not in need of your services but can be helpful in providing services to their peers? It could be possible to tap into this resource.*

MARAMALDI/SOCIAL WORK/PUBLIC HEALTH: *The Atlantic Philanthropies has a civic engagement initiative nationwide that is trying to tap into older people who have professional life experience that can be given back to communities.*

BURACK/OLDER ADULT: *I mean multiply me by thousands . . .*

MARAMALDI/SOCIAL WORK/PUBLIC HEALTH: *Right.*

BARD/PSYCHOLOGY/PASTORAL CARE: *Remember the elderly panel that came and represented that kind of constructive involvement. They were involved in helping their peers in a variety of ways. They worked very hard with people their age, and they were devoting their time and their energy and their expertise and their experience. So even in our midst there are many ways to do that. In many of the communities their various offices on aging may have a younger person who is managing the desk, but the people* who are really working there are the volunteers who are elder people in the population of that town who are helping to care for the other people and looking after their needs. So I think you are absolutely right. I think it is actually something that is not advertised well, it is not integrated well, it is sort of a separate service that people are providing rather than figuring out how this really fits with such formal agencies as the Visiting Nurse Association or how does this really fit with the people who are making funding decisions. No one has really ever integrated that with other services as far as I know. But all the tools are right there. Maybe one of the things that someone here who is going to be working in a community leadership role can say is, "Let's go to this office and see how do these pieces articulate with one another?" Because we all know that in most towns and cities the offices don't talk to each other.

VAUGHN/PHYSICAL THERAPY: *Thinking about the older adults who do not necessarily need services but could help provide them reminds me that we can positively influence others by just being us—people—independent of our disciplines. Everyone can be supportive of others in various ways. I am personally challenged to start thinking of simple ways in which I can further serve the older adults in my own family, whether by being a physical therapist or not. I agree that it would be very effective to advocate and encourage elders to be the volunteers and active servers in their own communities. People can be very influential without being health-care professionals.*

BURACK/OLDER ADULT: *The senior centers that exist in the communities, the couple that I'm familiar with, attract senior citizens who are bored, lonely, intellectually almost deprived, and seek entertainment, common ground with their peers. They're the ones to start with: Give them some respect, give them a challenge, and give them something to think about instead of playing bingo and doing inane stuff. And make them look within themselves and realize that there is a worth there.*

RAINE/SOCIAL WORK: *How will this education apply to my future work? I have an internship with the Boston Partnership for Older Adults. I've served on their mental health committee for a long time. I choose to work there as I study cancer, which I didn't know much about. I'm choosing to look at different things outside my experience, so I got interested in business. The gentleman from Hebrew SeniorLife surprised me greatly when he said that they were supporters of the elder-friendly business districts. Nobody at the Boston Partnership knew that. I work with a group in an elder-friendly business district. That is an effort to bring a group of elders together to have them do surveys and focus groups and discover how elders use their business district, the idea being that if elders are going shopping in the business district, it will improve the quality of life for everybody. In one neighborhood of the city there are 10,000 elderly people who are potential customers in their shopping area. What I've used this educational program for is to make this elder-friendly business project really interdisciplinary by bringing the sources together to work together and training them that they each have something to bring—as a community organizer and those kinds of things. And that's a direction in which I'm going to continue. I really haven't thought of doing it in quite that way until I had this education experience. I told them I was having this education experience and I had to do it, so they were willing to go along. The other thing is that I incorporated the stuff that I was learning in this program. I teach bench building to 6th-graders, and I incorporated a lot of what I was doing in this program to help them build stronger teams and better relationships. What I really want to do is to get involved much more in public education and advocacy. I've been a clinician for 30 years, and that's my plan. And this was the first start. So I really appreciate everything I learned from everybody here. You've all inspired me—each and every single one of you—to do more writing, for example. I got up the courage to e-mail the gentleman who wrote the article in the New Yorker because I had some questions for him. And that's a lot of what I've been doing, is getting the courage to do some of things. Well why not? So I just wanted to say that it's led me to expand my thinking. Partly it's the interdisciplinary approach but also how to bring people together and empower older adults. They are going to be certifying businesses as elder-friendly businesses, and then they will be promoted as such. It's going to eventually list the 19 neighborhoods in the city. Right now, it's just one of them.*

MARAMALDI/SOCIAL WORK/PUBLIC HEALTH: *One of the interesting things about these civic engagement initiatives and civic enterprises locally is that, rather than looking at how seniors participate, they are looking at how seniors will contribute to those businesses. Someone who's a retired chief executive or chief financial officer can consult with private business and bring tremendous skill. You've all heard the famous line of the human relations director who went to volunteer at a hospital and she was quoted coming out the door saying, "Candy striper, my ass!" She never set foot back in the hospital. The mantra here is that people are retiring more than ever before with tremendous skills. It's important to anticipate the curve.*

BROVERMAN/ELDER CARE ADMINISTRATION: *I think that one of the things to add to what other people have said is that our group presentation was about NORCs, naturally occurring retirement communities. One of the things that our group learned from our presentation is the importance of involving the seniors in the process of care and not making the choices for them. So I think that one of the things that I will take away is involving the persons we're talking about, if at all possible, instead of making decisions for them. That's why we chose to use the format that we did, to involve the seniors within our town to see what their needs are. Certainly, we could come in with a business plan about formulating a NORC and tell you all the things we're going to do for you, but it might not meet any of your needs and it might just be fruitless. So one of the things that I take away is involving everyone in the whole process of their care and including the patient if they have the capacity to do so.*

MARAMALDI/SOCIAL WORK/PUBLIC HEALTH: *Hear, hear!*

SATIN/PSYCHIATRY: *I can think of three levels of involvement. One is personal: The way you deal with your colleagues, the way Ms. Raine is encouraging the people in her workplace to work with one another, the way you were going to make contact with other people who work with the same patients and talk with them and make it a communication circle with them. The second level is to create a team: to create an agency or a program that does this interdisciplinarily. The two interdisciplinary teams we learned about were not appointed by somebody, were not invited by somebody. Somebody there decided that this would be a good thing to do and found a way of doing it and found people who wanted to do it with them. The neurologist, Lynn Buchwald, had this idea of what is good multiple sclerosis care and found people who are willing to do it, more or less on their own time, to get together. The Urban Medical Group was started by somebody who decided that poor people in an urban setting needed good medical care and there was no reason why it couldn't be paid for through Medicaid. He was not entirely right; it's been limping along for a lot of years powered by people who want to do that. This education approach was started by students who said, "Why can't we meet students from other disciplines. Why can't we learn about older people as a whole rather than be stuck in our own small pigeon holes?" And faculty members who were willing to say, "Why not? That's a good point." And got together and did it. And continue to do it, not with the suggestion and encouragement of the institutions in which they exist but on their sufferance. It found a place in between the other courses and the other schools, a place where people could come together, a time when people could get together, people who are willing to do this and a place which was willing to give it free heat and light and equipment. The third level is to do something with the system as a whole. Do something with the society as a whole. One example is the Massachusetts Association of Older Americans or the Gray Panthers, groups which got together to say, "We want to advocate for older adult services." If I understand it correctly, the Massachusetts Association of Older Americans was started by a union organizer who retired from union organizing, so he organized old people and developed it as an effective advocacy, lobbying group. Another example is a student in this program who graduated from the program and was invited to join the core faculty and was on the core faculty for several years and then (she was a nurse) got herself (on the second try) elected as president of the American Nurses Association with the idea that nurses should suggest and lead the way in certain kinds of care, adequate care, including for older people. I don't know but I suspect that Howard Dean stopped being an internist and started being a governor and wanted to be president because he had something in his mind about what health care, among other things, should be and thought that these would be positions from which he could do this. So that things can be done on that level also. I think people find their levels. What level are you comfortable on? What level do you think you could make most of an impact on? And you work on that level or you could say, "That was a nice dream, now let's get down to reality and do what the system allows us to do."*

BARD/PSYCHOLOGY/PASTORAL CARE: *Or you can grow into your level.*

BURACK/OLDER ADULT: *You just said the magic word—do what the system allows us to do. That's the rotten bottom line of the whole thing—the system. I don't like the system.*

BARD/PSYCHOLOGY/PASTORAL CARE: *You sound like a '60s radical. We certainly want to wish those who participated in this educational program well. There is not a formal alumni association, although some of you are proposing to do something about that.*

BURACK/OLDER ADULT: *I think they should have class reunions with other classes and see how to build on what they learned here.*

BARD/PSYCHOLOGY/PASTORAL CARE: *Those who participated in this program get back to us sometimes after an absence of 5 or 6 years, and then all of a sudden we hear from them out of the blue and it's really interesting to see what they're doing as life went on, and they said, "Gee, you know I'm just doing something that I learned back here or experienced there."*

MARAMALDI/SOCIAL WORK/PUBLIC HEALTH: *I really challenge you to create the things you think need to be done.*

PRITCHARD/NURSING/HEALTH CARE ADMINISTRATION: *I really enjoyed the program as well and so much so that I approached David Satin about the idea of developing a newsletter so that we can try to maintain some kind of communication.*

RAINE/SOCIAL WORK: *I, too, liked the program and became very interested in interdisciplinary teaming. It would be interesting to see what we do with this education, what career paths people take, how do they implement some of the things that we've learned. A newsletter would help explore this.*

ARMSTRONG/SOCIAL WORK: *How about some sort of a website?*

BOYLE/SOCIAL WORK: *That we'll set up where people can just put their thoughts in and like a blog . . . whatever those things are.*

BURACK/OLDER ADULT: *Don't forget, there's also a telephone.*

PRITCHARD/NURSING/HEALTH CARE ADMINISTRATION: *That's true, but providing people access to a website allows individuals to communicate when they have the opportunity regardless of the time of day. However, it may eliminate those without computer access.*

MARAMALDI/SOCIAL WORK/PUBLIC HEALTH: *Actually if you're interested, there's a way to do this for free—with social networking sites that restrict access. Some are free, you restrict. So you have a social network, but it's a venue, it's a platform to do what you're saying about having a website. You can do blogs, you can post photographs, you can put in whatever.*

BARD/PSYCHOLOGY/PASTORAL CARE: *I sort of hear you suggesting that this is not simply for the group this year . . .*

SAUDER/GERONTOLOGY: *Right—exactly!*

BARD/PSYCHOLOGY/PASTORAL CARE: *. . . but for all people who have participated in this experience. It can have a life of its own.*

BROVERMAN/ELDER CARE ADMINISTRATION: *Right.*

DREVINS/PHYSICAL THERAPY: *I was thinking this would be a great opportunity to not only keep connected but also offer some ongoing education, some highlights of some kind—so it would serve two needs.*

MARAMALDI/SOCIAL WORK/PUBLIC HEALTH: *Links to important articles.*

BROWN/SOCIAL WORK: *We'll have Erica and anybody else write articles, anybody who wants to submit them.*

PRITCHARD/NURSING/HEALTH CARE ADMINISTRATION: *So, Dr. Maramaldi, may I contact you then with some ideas?*

MARAMALDI/SOCIAL WORK/PUBLIC HEALTH: *Sure, sure.*

BURACK/OLDER ADULT: *In the interest of the class, we talked earlier about doctors. We have seeds planted in Sweden through a program participant last year. We have a seed planted in Korea about interdisciplinary care for the elderly from a participant the year before. And who knows, someday those plants will rise and become our heritage.*

SAUDER/GERONTOLOGY: *That's great!*

PRITCHARD/NURSING/HEALTH CARE ADMINISTRATION: *So I welcome everyone's ideas and anybody who'd like to help me with this initiative. I certainly would be most appreciative if you want to e-mail me, we could plan to get together and have a little strategic meeting to further explore and investigate what resources are available. That would be great.*

SATIN/PSYCHIATRY: *We will help as much as we can.*

PRITCHARD/NURSING/HEALTH CARE ADMINISTRATION: *Great. Thank you!*

BURACK/OLDER ADULT: *Bear in mind that you're working with people who are at the mercy of natural attrition. You know you can get all worked about with something and then, all of a sudden, you're dead and gone. But I'm going to hang around for a while.*

SATIN/PSYCHIATRY: *It seems that this group is developing an interdisciplinary action team. Apparently, this educational approach can be applied in the real world!*

Index

AAA (Area Agencies on Aging), 201
Access Project, 122
Access to care, 149–161
    for children, 119
    cultural issues, 155–157, 154f, 155f
    definition of, 51–52, 62
    demographic changes and, 150–152,
        150f, 151f
    equitable/fair, 108–109, 111
    financial/economic issues, 155–159
    health law and, 136–137
    language barriers and, 153–154
    medical profession changes and, 160–161
    racial/ethnic health care disparities,
        114–115
Activities of daily living (ADLs)
    improvements
        interdisciplinary practice model and, 214
        occupational therapy for MS patients
            and, 255–257
    limitations, prevalence of, 81–82, 81t
    outcomes measurement, in interdisciplinary
        practice model, 217–218
Acute care
    access to. See Access

preventative. See Preventive care
ADA (Americans with Disabilities Act), 73,
    136–137
Adjusted average per capita cost, 62
ADLs. See Activities of daily living
Administration, health care
    education/training for, 328–329
Administration, interdisciplinary model
    and, 15–17
Adult day services (ADS), 199–200
Advocacy
    for community-based care, 200–201
    by health care professional, 142–143
    at Mt. Auburn Hospital Multiple
        Sclerosis Comprehensive
        Care Center, 248–249
    responsibility for, 26–28, 30, 31
African-Americans. See Race
Aging
    impact on health, 21–26
    models of, 87–88
    natural history of
        description of, 87–88
        needs of older adults and,
            91–92

Aging (*Cont.*)
  normal, 88, 89*t*
  personal reflections on, 21–26
  physiological changes, 88, 89*t*
  successful, 87, 88, 89*t*
  usual, 87
Allostatic load, 87–88
American Association of Homes and Services
    for the Aging, 163
American Medical Association (AMA), 40, 41
Americans with Disabilities Act (ADA), 73,
    136–137
Ancient Greece, 39
Area Agencies on Aging (AAA), 201
Armstrong, Kimberly, 323–324
Arthritis self-management program, 94
Asian-Americans. *See* Ethnicity
Assignment, 62
Assisted living, 195
Assisted suicide, 137–139
Assistive technology, 199
Attitude, interdisciplinary model and, 15–16
Attorneys. *See* Lawyers
Autonomy, 67–77
  conflict with beneficence, 70–71
  contextual model of, 69–70, 69*t*
  definition of, 67–68
  dimensions of, 68
  hindrances, 70, 70*t*
  ideal, 68
  motivation for, 6
  OACTRPP and, 76–77
  Older Adult Care, Training, Research,
      and Planning Program and, 76–77
  supportive factors, 70, 70*t*
Autonomy in Long-Term Care Initiative, 68

Balanced Budget Act of 1997, 92, 191
Bard, Terry R.
  on applying interdisciplinary gerontology
      to pastoral care, 329, 332–337
  on interdisciplinary gerontology education,
      323, 324
  views on interdisciplinary care, 302, 303,
      306–319
Beneficence
  conflict with autonomy, 70–71
  definition of, 71
Beneficiary. *See* Medicare, beneficiaries
Bhalotra, Sarita, 302, 303, 305, 308–316
Blue Cross Blue Shield, Medicare extension
    plans, 28
Bocage, Myrna D., 301, 304, 307

Boston Partnership for Older Adults, 167
Boyle, Kathleen, 321, 331–332, 336
Bragdon v. Abbott, 137
Branch, Laurence G., 302, 304, 309
Broverman, Shannon
  on applying interdisciplinary gerontology
      to professional practice, 331, 333,
      335, 337
  on interdisciplinary gerontology, 318, 321,
      325–326
Brown, Peggy, 319, 330, 337
Bruce, Ellen, 302, 303, 305, 307, 310–316
Burack, Jeanette, 20–23, 27, 320
  on improving health care system, 29, 30
  on interdisciplinary care education, 326–327
  on interdisciplinary gerontology practice
      applications, 330, 333, 334, 336, 337
  on intergenerational relationships, 33, 34
  views on health care for older adults, 20–23,
      27, 320

Cancer mortality, racial/ethnic health care
    disparities, 115
Capitation rate, 62
Capitman, John A., 302, 303, 309–310, 311
Caregivers
  cancer. *See also* Prince, Joanne
      Yacker, Charlotte, 20, 26
  personal reflections of, 21–26
  strains on, 151
Case coordinator, role of, 260
Case studies
  for class discussion, 99–102
  of interdisciplinary practice model,
      217–219
  OACTRPP, 35–37
Cash and Counseling Demonstration and
    Evaluation Program, 74–76
Catastrophic care, 55
CCRC (continuing care retirement
    communities), 163–164, 170, 195–197
CDSM (Chronic Disease Self-Management),
    94
Centenarians, 80
Center for Medicare and Medicaid Services
    (CMS), 42, 43, 46, 53
Choices for Independence, 76, 201
Chronic conditions
  by gender, 82, 82*f*
  health care expenditures on, 84*t*
  prepathogenesis period, 88
  prevalence of, 81, 81*t*
  protections against, 88–89

self-management, 93–95
    Wagner's Chronic Care Model, 93
Chronic Disease Self-Management
    (CDSM), 94
Chronic illness breakthrough collaboratives, 94
Civil Rights Act of 1964, 136–137
*The Clinical Care of the Aged Person: An
    Interdisciplinary Perspective,* 3
Clinical training sites, development of, 13
CMS (Center for Medicare and Medicaid
    Services), 42, 43, 46, 53
Cognitive function improvements,
    interdisciplinary practice model and,
    211–212
Coinsurance, 62
Collaboration, motivation for, 6
Collaborative care, 93
Collopy, Bart, 68
Common law, access to care and, 136
Commonwealth v. Hunt, 39–40
Communication, within interdisciplinary team,
    233–235, 245–246
Community-based care, 190–204
    advocacy for, 200–201
    coordination of, 200–201
    definition of, 189–190
    forms of, 190
        comprehensive health approaches,
            190–192
        HMOs. *See* Health Maintenance
            Organizations
        housing approaches, 193–197
        social health maintenance organizations,
            192–193
    future considerations, 202–203
    interdisciplinary approach and, 203
    justice in. *See* Justice, in community care
    long-term, 112–114, 120–121
    nonhousing options, 197–200
        in-home services, 197–199
        out-of-home services, 199–200
    OACTRPP and, 203–204
Community Partnerships for Older
    Adults, 122
Competence
    primary, 6, 6*t*
    secondary, 7, 7*t*
    tertiary, 7, 7*t*
Competency, 141–142
Competitive market-based perspective
    long-term care and, 112–114
    racial/ethnic disparities and, 114
    in solving prescription drug cost problems,
        109–112

Confidentiality, 139–140
Congregate older adults housing, 194, 195
Congress "contract with America," 73
Consumer-directed long-term care, 67–77,
    71–72
    barriers to, 72
    efficacy of, 75–76
    reimbursement mechanisms, 72–73
    trend toward, 72–75
Consumer direction, OACTRPP and, 76–77
Continuing care retirement communities
    (CCRC), 163–164, 170, 196–198
Coordination, of community-based care
    services, 199, 201–202
Costs, health care
    for chronic conditions, 84*t*
    for older adults, 157
    health care policy and, 52
    indirect, 82
    for interdisciplinary practice model,
        216–217
    rise in, 42
Cost sharing, 62
Coté, Janet, 19, 22
    on improving health care system, 29
    on intergenerational relationships, 32
Cross-training, of interdisciplinary team, 232
*Cruzan v. Director, Missouri Department of
    Health,* 138, 141
Cultural humility, 118, 122–123
Culturally competent care, need for, 115–116
Curriculum, interdisciplinary
    content of, 13
    development of, 11–12
    implementation barriers, 12
    planning, 11–12

Death, leading causes of, 84*t*
Death with Dignity Law, 139
Decision making
    within interdisciplinary team, 235
    sharing policy decision making with
        patients, 122
Deductible, 62
Deficit Reduction Act of 2005, 134, 192–193
Department of Health and Human Services,
    Independence Plus Initiative, 76
Diabetes self-management program, 94
Diagnosis code, 62
Diagnosis-related groups (DRGs), 41–42,
    62–63
Dignity, community-based care services
    and, 202

Disability/disabilities
  Americans with Disabilities Act and,
    136–137
  description of, 113
  health-promotion efforts and, 91–92
  inconsistent responses to, 112
  prevalence of, 81, 81*t*
  rates, for older adults population,
    173–174, 174*f*
Disciplines
  differences among, 5–6
  examples of, 5
  expertise overlap, 6–7, 15
  health care, training, clinical role and team
    role of, 224–230
  identity, power and security of, 6
  infrastructure of, 16
  knowledge of, 223–237
  organization of, 16
  overlap of, 254–255
  practice models. *See* Interdisciplinary
    practice model
  multidisciplinary practice, 208
  subdivision of, 6
  working relationships of. *See* Working
    relationships, interdisciplinary
Discrimination, federal legislation and,
  136–137
Disease, chronic. *See* Chronic conditions
Doctors. *See* Physicians
Drevins, Joan, 319, 327–328, 329
DRGs (diagnosis-related groups), 41–42,
  62–63
Dual eligibles, 63
Duggan, Jane, 261–262, 268–269
Durable medical equipment, 63

Education, professional
  disciplinary *vs.* interdisciplinary gerontology,
    322–328
  interdisciplinary
    clinical training sites, 13
    developmental barriers, professional
      and disciplinary, 13
    faculty and, 12
    resources for, 13–14
    timing of, 12
  for interdisciplinary team, 215
  for nurse/nurse-practitioners, 224
  for occupational therapists, 226
  for pharmacists, 226
  for physical therapists, 227

  for physicians, 228
  for registered dietitians, 225
  for social workers, 229
Educational status, of older adults population,
  172, 172*f*
Elder autonomy. *See* Autonomy
Elder care administration, interdisciplinary
  gerontology applications, 331, 333,
  335, 337
Elder-care policies
  epidemiological transition and, 106–107
  fairness and, 108–112
  goals, 123
  inequalities in
    description of, 119–123
    solution proposals, 119–123
  just/fair, implications for, 121–123
  local decision-making, patient-professional
    engagement in, 123
  OACTRPP and, 123–125
  racial/ethnic health care disparities and,
    114–118
  reforms, 121
  U.S. health inequalities and, 107–108
Elderly. *See* Older adults
Elites, 278
Emergency Medical Treatment and Active
  Labor Act (EMTALA), 136
Employment benefits, for military
  servicemen, 40
End-of-life cases
  assisted suicide, 137–139
  informed consent doctrine and, 137–138
Ethnicity
  chronic conditions and, 153–154, 154*f*
  discrimination, federal prohibitions
    against, 136
  diversity of older adults population and,
    172, 173*f*
  elder care and, 107
  health care disparities. *See* Racial/ethnic
    health care disparities
  health insurance and, 155*f*
  physician visits and, 155*f*
Excess charges, 63
Exclusions, 63
Exercise, importance of, 90, 92
Expenditures, health care
  average per capital, 82
  on chronic conditions, 84*t*
  on institutional long-term care, 174, 175*f*
  out-of-pocket, 108
Extended families, 33–34

Faculty, interdisciplinary education and, 12
Fairness, in elder care policies, 123
Fallon, Terry
    on insurance coverage for hospice care, 264
    interdisciplinary team planning for hospice
        care, 259–260
    need for hospice care, 258–259
    role of nurse in hospice care, 261, 264, 265,
        269–270
    on volunteer staff, 263
Families
    caregiving, 197
    strains on, 151
    support from, 153–154
Family/team conferences, 247
Federal General Revenues, 63
Fee-for-service payment, 48, 63, 203
Fee schedule, 63
Financial support, for interdisciplinary
    education, 13
Financing, health care
    financing, OACTRPP and, 59, 61–62
Financing of health care, policy implications,
    95–97
First-dollar coverage, 63
Food and Drug Administration, 158
"Friendly Visitor" program, 199
Functional limitations, prevalence of,
    81–82, 81t
Funding, for community-based care services,
    202–203
Fung, Teresa T., 302, 307, 315

Gender
    differences in chronic conditions, 82, 82f
    elder care and, 107
Generic drugs, 63
Geriatric assessment programs, 95
Geriatric care textbook, need for, 3–4
Geriatric Interdisciplinary Team Training
    (Siegler, Hyer, Fulmer and Mezey),
    13–14
Geriatric Interdisciplinary Team Training
    programs (GITT), 215
Gerontology, interdisciplinary, 318–323
Global Burden of Disease Study, 107
Governance, social policy and, 273–276, 274f
Government, homeostasis. See Homeostasis
Grandparents
    raising grandchildren, 34
    relationship with grandchildren, 33–34
Great Depression, 40

Harlem Hospital Patient Navigation
    Program, 117
Harvard Cooperative Program on Aging, 167
Health
    effect of lifestyle behaviors on, 90–91
    ill, causation in older adults, 88–92
    impact of aging on, 21–26
Health care
    access to. See Access
    continuum for seniors, 163–164, 164f
    costs. See Costs, health care
    disciplines. See Disciplines
    in emergency rooms, 136
    needs of older adults, alignment with
        policy, 109
    primary, coordinated with preventive
        care, 120
    racial/ethnic disparities. See Racial/ethnic
        health care disparities
    spending. See Expenditures, health care
Health care policy. See Policy
Health care professionals. See specific types
        of health care professionals
    as advocate, 142–143
    cultural humility of, 118
    humility, 122–123
    implementation of preventive care for
        elders, 96–97
    interdisciplinary practice model benefits
        for, 214–215
    reimbursement for, 159
    sharing policy decision making with patients.
        See Decision making
Health care proxy, 142
Health care settings, for low-income
    elders, 120
Health care system
    autonomy and, 70, 70t
    components of, 38
    early beginnings of, 39–41
    improving, suggestions for, 29–31
    interdisciplinary practice model benefits
        for, 214–215
    older adults and, 26–29
    reforms, 41–42
    structure, OACTRPP and, 59, 61–62
Health Disparities Collaboratives, 117
Health insurance. See Insurance
Health Insurance Portability and
    Accountability Act (HIPAA),
    63–64, 140
Health law, 130–145
    access to care and, 136–137

Health law (*Cont.*)
  assisted suicide, 138–139
  competency issues, 141–142
  interdisciplinary care and, 302, 305,
      311–312, 316, 317
  lawyers and, 130–131, 144–145
  Medicaid. *See* Medicaid
  Medicare. *See* Medicare
  patient confidentiality, 139–140
  patient self-determination, 137–139
  private insurance and, 135–136
  role of professional as advocate, 142–143
Health Maintenance Organization Act, 41
Health maintenance organizations (HMOs),
      41, 192
  definition of, 64
  personal experiences with, 26, 27
  premiums, 28
  social, 95
  vs. PACE, 192
Health management, professional practice
      and, 56–57
Health outcomes, cross-national, 107
*Health Professions Education: A Bridge
      to Quality,* 236
Health status outcomes, 90
Hebrew Rehabilitation Center for Aged
  cost-per-day *vs.* Medicaid gross daily rate,
      168–169, 169*f*, 170
  geriatric research and, 167
  history of, 167, 168
  long-term acute-care unit, 181
  operating environment, 168–170
  post-acute care unit, 181
  program sponsorships, 167–168
  redefinition of mission, 180, 180*f*
  SeniorLife Facilities, 168, 185–188,
      186*f*, 187*f*
  simplicity within the three circles,
      178–179, 179*f*
  strategic plan
      development of, 176–181, 177*f*
      implementation of, 182–188, 184*f*,
          186*f*, 187*f*
HIPAA (Health Insurance Portability and
      Accountability Act), 63–64, 140
Hispanic patients. *See also* Race
  chronic conditions of, 153–154, 154*f*
  language barrier to health care, 153, 154
HIV (human immunodeficiency virus), 91, 137
HMOs. *See* Health maintenance organizations
Homebound older adults, illustration of,
      152–155
Home care agencies, 152

Home health aide, role of, 260, 261
Home health care services, 164, 197–198
Homemaker assistance services, 198–199
Home nursing care services,
      hospital-based, 152
Homeostasis
  power/privilege and, 277–278
  social practice, policy and, 276–277, 277*f*
  through human service economics, 279–280
  via policies and industry of care, 278–279
Hospice care
  health aid role in, 260, 261, 267, 268, 270
  insurance coverage for, 264
  medical order for, 264
Hospitalization, length of stay, interdisciplinary
      model and, 210–211
Housing approaches, for community-based
      care, 193–197
  assisted living, 195
  congregate older adults housing, 194
  continuing care retirement communities,
      195–197
  motivation for, 194
  naturally occurring retirement communities,
      195–197
Human immunodeficiency virus (HIV),
      91, 137
Human service economics, 279–280
Humility, professional and cultural, 122–123

IADLS (instrumental activities of daily living),
      212, 253–255
Illness, causation in older adults, 88–92
Incentives
  to address racial/ethnic health disparities,
      118
  for practice settings, 121–122
Independent Choices Program, 75
Independence Plus Initiative, 76
Industrialization, 39–40
Informed consent doctrine, 137–138
Institute for Aging Research, 167
Institute of Medicine, *Health Professions
      Education: A Bridge to Quality,* 236
Institutional reorganization, benefits of, 16
Institutional support, for interdisciplinary
      education, 12–13
Instrumental activities of daily living (IADLs),
      212, 253–255
Insurance
  coverage for hospice care, 264
  employment-based support, 39–40
  health care, racial/ethnic disparities and, 116

inadequate, 107–108
industry-wide cost cutting measures, 157
national, 40–41
premiums, 27
private, health law and, 135–136
private vs. Medicare, 53
race/ethnicity, 155f
Insurance companies, 29–30
Integration, of community-based care services,
    202
Interdisciplinary gerontology
    applied to professional practice, 329–337
    education, vs. disciplinary education,
        323–329
    program, 30
Interdisciplinary practice model, 9t, 159,
        208–209. See also Interdisciplinary teams
    administration and, 15–17
    benefits of, 210–214
        health care system-related, 213–214
        patient-related, 210–212
        provider-related, 212–213
    challenges for, 214–217
    community-based care services and, 203
    conceptual schema for, 7
    conference on, 302–317
    contributions to professional thinking, 16
    costs of, 216–217
    delivery of, policy implications for, 95–97
    effect on health management policy and
        practice, 16–17
    governance structure, 303
    levels of prevention and, 17
    OACTRPP and, 219–220
    policy and, 15–17, 119–123
    relevance for elder care, 209
    resources for, 16, 216–217
    settings for, 209
    successful, 223–224
    supportive attitudes for, 16
    task performance and, 17
Interdisciplinary teams
    administrative structure and, 230–231
    advantages of, 207
    communication, interpersonal, 233–235
    conflicts in, 214–215, 233–235
    decision making, 235
    development, function/maintenance, 223–237
    functioning. See Mt. Auburn Hospital
        Multiple Sclerosis Comprehensive Care
        Center; Sawtelle Hospice House
    goals of, 231–232
    leadership, 208–209, 232–233, 245–246
    members. See also specific team members

training, clinical role and team role of,
        224–230
    membership, 231
    for multiple sclerosis, specific roles of
        members, 249–258
    OACTRPP and, 236–237
    organizational support for, 230
    other roles in, 235–236
    planning, for hospice care, 259–260
    policy/administration and, 15–17
    power structure of, 232–233
    structure of, 214
    teaching, 11–14
    teamwork
        blurring of professional role in, 12
        teaching, 11–14
        value of, 207
        vs. multidisciplinary teamwork, 12
    training programs, 232
        implementation, 14
Intergenerational relationships, 31–34
International Classification of Disease, ninth
        edition, Clinical Modification
        (ICD-9-CM), 62
Interpersonal issues, within interdisciplinary
        team, 233–235
Interpretive services, 154
"Invisible hand" concept, 278–279

Jack Satter House congregate housing facility,
        169–170, 182
John A. Hartford Foundation, 14
Justice, in community care, 106–125
    fairness of elder care policies and, 108–112
    long-term care and, 112–114
    OACTRPP and, 123–125
    socioeconomic inequalities and, 107–108

Kaiser Family Foundation survey, 56–57
Kassenbaum-Kennedy law, 63–64
Key, Joan, 263
Kindbettfieber, 284–285
Kirwin, Jennifer L., 301, 308, 314
Kumph, Pat, 259, 261, 263, 264, 265–270

Labor unions, 39–40
Language
    barriers, access to health care and, 153, 154
    complexity, policy and, 282–283
    policy change and, 289
Larson, Leonard W., 79

Last dollar coverage, 64
Lawyers
 health law and, 130–131
 role in OACTRPP, 144–145
 views on interdisciplinary care, 301
Learning exercises, 57, 59
Legislation, 32, 157
Legislative process, 30
Length of hospital stay, interdisciplinary model
  and, 210–211
Life expectancy, 80, 150, 151f, 171–172
Lifestyle behavior
 changes, disability rates for older adults
  population and, 173–174, 174f
 changes in, 96–97
 effect on health, 90–91
Limiting charge, 64
Long-term care, 163–188. *See also* Hebrew
  Rehabilitation Center for Aged
 case-managed community-oriented,
  120–121
 changes in, 165–166
 congregate housing facility, 169–170
 consumer-directed. *See* Consumer-directed
  long-term care
 institutional, spending on, 174, 175f
 justice in, 112–114
 life expectancy increase and, 171–172
 Medicaid spending, 174, 175f
 OACTRPP and, 186–188
 options for, 163–166, 164f
 public television documentary on, 166–167
 system, autonomy and, 70, 70t
 waiting lists for, 169
 Wellspring Model, 175–176
Lorig's Chronic Disease Self-Management
  (CDSM) program, 94
Lowenstein, Nancy, 301, 305

Malpractice insurance premiums, 29
Managed care programs, personal reflections
  on, 28–29
Maramaldi, Peter, 322
 on applying interdisciplinary gerontology
  to professional practice, 330–331, 333,
  335, 336, 337
 on interdisciplinary gerontology education,
  324
Married couples, Medicaid eligibility for
  institutionalized spouse, 134–135
McGuire, Kay
 on health care for older adults, 19, 21–23,
  25, 28–29
 on improving health care system, 29, 30, 31

on intergenerational relationships, 32, 33, 34
Medicaid
 adult day services, 201–202
 definition of, 64
 description of, 133
 eligibility rules, 133–135
 gross daily rate vs. long term cost per day
  170–171, 171f, 174
 home health services, 199–200
 Patient Self-Determination Act, 142
 physically and mentally disabled patients
  and, 137
 purpose of, 41, 49–50
 reformulation of, 74
 spend-down method and, 134
 waivers
  applications, Independence Plus Initiative
   and, 76
  1915C Home and Community, 72–73
  1115 Research and Demonstration, 73
Medicaid Community Attendant Services and
  Supports Act (MiCASSA), 73–74
Medical director, role on multiple sclerosis
  interdisciplinary team, 251–253
Medical information privacy, 139–140
Medically necessary services, 64, 132
Medicare, 131–133
 advantages/strengths of, 52–54, 56t
 appeal process, 132
 Balanced Budget Act of 1997, 191
 beneficiaries, 109
  definition of, 62
  flu shot recipients, 86f
  with functional limitations and poor
   health, 83f
  in Medicare Advantage plans, 132
  with self-reported conditions, 82f
 coverage, 92
  denial of, 132–133
  for hospice care, 266
 definition/description of, 43, 64, 132
 diagnosis-related groups, 41–42
 disadvantages/limitations of, 54–55, 56t
 effect on health care for older adults, 49–51
 electronic claims, 56–57
 eligibility for, 132
 emergency room care, 136
 enrollees, functional status of, 83f
 enrollment, 52
 financial solvency of, 54
 health care providers and, 50
 health maintenance organizations and, 192
 home care benefits, 50
 home health services, 198–199
 inconsistent responses to disablement, 112

medical benefits, 92–93
medically necessary services and, 64, 132
out-of-pocket expenses and, 108
Part A, 43, 44t, 46–47, 49, 50, 54, 55
Part B, 42, 43–44, 45t–46t, 46–47, 50, 55
Part C or Medicare + Choice, 43, 47–48, 53
Part D. *See* Medicare Prescription Drug
   Improvement and Modernization Act
passage of, 41, 49
Patient Self-Determination Act, 142
payment schedules, 53
preventive geriatrics program and, 96
preventive health services, 42
purpose of, 109
reforms, 51
reimbursed clinical preventive services,
   utilization of, 85t–86t, 93
reimbursements, 120, 304
spending, 57, 58t, 60f
Medicare Advantage, 42
Medicare approved amount, definition of, 64
Medicare Modernization Act of 2003, 42, 48,
   92–93, 192
Medicare Prescription Drug Improvement and
   Modernization Act (Medicare Part D)
administrative complications, 133
ban on national prescription drug
   formulary, 110
coverage, 48–49, 93
doughnut hole, 157
prescription coverage, 108
provisions of, 42, 133
Medicare Summary Notice (MSN), 56, 64
Medications. *See* Prescription drugs
Medigap policies, 42, 46–47, 135–136
Mental disabilities, Americans with Disabilities
   Act and, 136–137
Military servicemen, employment benefits
   for, 40
Minimum Data Set, 167
Models of care, Wagner's Chronic Care
   Model, 93
Moore, Deborah, 261, 267, 268, 271
Mortality
cancer, racial/ethnic health care
   disparities, 114
rates, interdisciplinary practice model
   and, 211
MSN (Medicare Summary Notice), 56, 64
Mt. Auburn Hospital Multiple Sclerosis
   Comprehensive Care Center
advocacy, 248–249
concerns/needs of health care
   providers, 241
evaluation and screening, 244–249

interdisciplinary team
   communications, 247
   leadership of, 246–247
   size, 244
   specific roles of members, 251–260
outcomes, anticipated, 247–48
problems/obstructions for, 242–243
rationale for, 240–241
recruitment issues, 243–244
Multicultural Coalition on Aging, 167–168
Multidisciplinary model, 7, 8t
   teamwork, *vs.* interdisciplinary
      teamwork, 12
Multidisciplinary practice model, 208
Multiple sclerosis, 242
   interdisciplinary approach for.
      See Mt. Auburn Hospital
      Multiple Sclerosis Comprehensive
      Care Center

National Council on Disability, 75
National Health Program, 40–41
Naturally occurring retirement communities
   (NORC), 194–196
Network, 65
Neurologist, role on multiple sclerosis
   interdisciplinary team, 250–252
New Deal, 40
New Freedom Initiative, 76
1915C Home and Community Medicaid
   waiver, 72–73
Nonhousing options, for community-based
   care, 197–200
Nonparticipating physician, 65
NORC (naturally occurring retirement
   communities), 194–196
Nurse coordinator, role on multiple
   sclerosis interdisciplinary team,
   251–253
Nurse practitioners, 224–225
Nurses
   clinical and team roles, 224–225
   role in hospice care, 264, 266
   training, 224–225
Nursing home care
   alternatives, 165–168, 164f
   description of, 166–167
   human service economics and, 279
   Medicaid eligibility levels and, 134
   Medicare and, 55
   residency ratios, 157
Nutritionists
   clinical and team roles, 225–226
   training, 225–226

views on interdisciplinary care, 302,
307, 315

OAA (Older Americans Act), 108–109, 201
OACTRPP. *See* Older Adult Care, Training,
Research, and Planning Program
Obesity, 91
Occupational therapists
clinical and team role, 228
role on multiple sclerosis interdisciplinary
team, 255–257
views on interdisciplinary care, 302, 306
Older Adult Care, Training, Research, and
Planning Program (OACTRPP)
administration of, 36
catchment area, mixed ethnic character of,
124–125
community-based care and, 202–203
in community setting, 219
consumer direction and, 76–77
disciplines, 36–37
elder autonomy and, 76–77
elder care policies and, 123–125
evaluation, 36
funding for, 36
health care funding/resources and, 160–161
health care structure/funding and, 59, 61–62
lawyer's role in, 144–145
lobbying for, 36
long-term care and, 189
in medical center, 219–220
missions, 35–36
monitoring, 36
primary prevention and, 97–99
residential population, 36
Older adults
control over health and health care, 26–29
demographics, 80–81
functional decline, causation of, 88–92
health and, 21–26
health care system and, 26–29
health law. *See* Health law
illness and, 21–26
on intergenerational relationships, 31–34
needs of, based on natural history of aging,
91–92
Older adults population
community-based care for.
See Community-based care
definition of, 158
disability rates for, 173–174, 174*f*
diversity of, 172, 173*f*
educational status of, 172, 172*f*

epidemiology of, 81–82, 84
GI Generation or Greatest Generation, 174
growth of, 156, 156*f*
New Dealers, 174
population demographics, 171, 171*f*
poverty rate and, 172, 173*f*
racial/social diversity of, 81
Silent Generation, 174
Older Americans Act (OAA), 108–109, 201
"Oldest old," 80
Omnibus Budget Reconciliation Act
of 1993, 51
1115 Research and Demonstration Medicaid
waiver, 73
Orchard Cove continuing care retirement
community, 170
Oregon, assisted suicide and, 139
Organization of care, racial/ethnic health
disparities and, 117
Outcomes measurement, in interdisciplinary
practice model, 215–216, 305
Out-of-pocket health care expenditures, 108
Overweight, 91

PACE. *See* Program of All-Inclusive Care for
the Elderly
Pandisciplinary model, 10, 10*t*, 10*f*
Parents, responsibilities of, 34
Pastoral care
interdisciplinary care and, 303, 304, 306
interdisciplinary practice and, 303, 304,
306–307, 309, 312, 313–314, 315,
316–317
intergenerational gerontology applied to,
332, 333–334, 336, 337
Paternalism, definition of, 71
Patient confidentiality, 139–140
Patient-provider partnerships, 93
Patient Self-Determination Act, 142
Peer review organization (PRO), 132
PEPP (post-event prevention program), 98–99
Personal care assistance services, 198–199
Personal needs allowance, 134
Personal representative, 140
Pharmacists
training, clinical and team roles, 226–227
views on interdisciplinary care, 300,
308, 314
Physiatrist, role on multiple sclerosis
interdisciplinary team, 257
Physical disabilities, Americans with
Disabilities Act and, 136–137
Physical function improvements,

interdisciplinary practice model and,
    211–212
Physical therapists, 227–228
    education/training of, 327–328, 329
    interdisciplinary care and, 301–302, 303
    role on multiple sclerosis interdisciplinary
        team, 255–257
    views on interdisciplinary care, 301–302,
        303, 305, 314, 316
Physicians
    clinical/team role of, 233
    cultural humility of, 118
    difficulty in finding, 156–157
    education/training, 228
    insurance and, 29–30
    nonparticipating, 65
    unequal care for racial/ethnic groups,
        116–117
    visits to, race/ethnicity and, 155f
Policy
    change, strategies for, 285–295
        action and, 291–292
        dialogue, role of, 288
        external power, removal of, 292–293
        group work in, 288–289
        internal power, removal of, 293–294
        language and, 289
        questioning, 286–287
        research for, 290–291
        using different focus/perception,
            285–286, 286f
    cornerstones of, 51–52
    disconnect between public and
        decision-maker views, 110
    for elder care. See Elder care policies
    governance and, 273–276, 274f
    health care delivery and, 95–97
    health care financing and, 95–97
    homeostasis and, 276–278, 277f
    institutional/social knowledge, history of,
        274–276, 275f
    interdisciplinary care issues and, 302, 303,
        309–310, 311
    interdisciplinary model and, 15–17
    invisibility, 280–281
    language complexity and, 282–283
    making, local, patient-professional
        engagement in, 122
    problems, complexity in numbers, 281, 281f
    security/solidary goals for, 110–111
    social context, 274
Post event prevention program (PEPP), 98–99
Poverty rate, older adults population and,
    172, 173f

Practice, health management, interdisciplinary
    model and, 16–17
Practice settings, incentives for, 121–122
Preferred provider organization (PPO), 65, 192
Prescription drugs
    affordability of, 157
    costs, 30, 42
        Medicare coverage for, 109
        private sector health plans and, 109–110
    generic, 63
    for hospice care, 266
    Medicare benefits, 55
    national formulary for, 110
    spending on, 158
Preventive care
    activities of, 89–90
    case studies, for class discussion, 99–102
    coordinated with primary care, 120
    misconceptions about older adults and,
        95–96
    OACTRPP and, 97–99
    racial/ethnic disparities and, 116–117
    U.S. Preventive Services Task Force
        (USPSTF)-recommended services,
        85t–86t
Prichard, Jennifer
    on applying interdisciplinary gerontology to
        professional practice, 329, 333, 337
    views on interdisciplinary care, 318, 320,
        328–329
Prince, Joanne
    on cancer caregiving, 19, 21–29
    on improving health care system, 29, 30–31
Private insurance, health law and, 135–136
Private sector health plans, prescription drug
    costs and, 109–110
PRO (peer review organization), 132
Professional humility, 122–123
Professional training, as barrier to
    consumer-directed long-term care, 72
Program of All-Inclusive Care for the Elderly
    (PACE), 95, 190–191
    health care system benefits from, 213–214
    length of hospital stay and, 210–211
    professional-paraprofessional teamwork
        and, 213
Property tax, 30–31
Prostate cancer survivor. See Taylor, Albert
Provider, 65
Psychiatrist, views at interdisciplinary care, 302
Psychiatry, in interdisciplinary team
    approach, 302
Psychology
    interdisciplinary care and, 302, 303, 304

Psychology (*Cont.*)
interdisciplinary practice and, 302, 303, 306–307, 309, 311, 312–314, 315, 316–317
intergenerational gerontology applied to, 329, 332, 333–334, 336, 337
Public health
applying interdisciplinary gerontology to professional practice of, 330, 332–333, 335, 336, 337
interdisciplinary care and, 302, 303
perspective on interdisciplinary care, 302, 303, 305, 309–317

In re Quackenbush, 141
Quality assurance, as barrier to consumer-directed long-term care, 72
Quality of care
health care providers and, 143
questions on, 52
racial/ethnic health care disparities, 114–115
Quality of life
community based care services and, 201
improvement of, 79–80
improvements, interdisciplinary practice model and, 212

Race
chronic conditions and, 153–154, 154*f*
discrimination, federal prohibitions against, 136
diversity of older adults population and, 172, 173*f*
doctor visits and, 155*f*
elder care and, 107
older adults population diversity and, 81
health care disparities. *See* Racial/ethnic health care disparities
health insurance and, 155*f*
Medicare beneficiaries, flu shot recipients, 86*f*
Racial/ethnic health care disparities
in cancer mortality, 115
competitive market-based perspective and, 115
in elder care policies, 114–118, 124–125
racism and, 114–115
solution proposals
cultural humility, 118
incentives, 118
Raine, Erica
on applying interdisciplinary gerontology to professional practice, 334–335, 337
views on interdisciplinary care, 320, 321–322, 326–327

Ranald, Ralph, 301, 304, 310
Reauthorization of the Older Americans Act (2006), 76
Registered dietitians (RDs), 225–226
Rehabilitation, physiatrist role on multiple sclerosis interdisciplinary team, 257
Rehabilitation care, 180
Research, for policy change, 290–291
Respite care, 199–200
Retiree health benefits, employee-based, health law and, 135–136
Retirement, 39, 156
Retirement Research Foundation, Autonomy in Long-Term Care Initiative, 73
Retirement Research Foundation, Chicago, 68–69
Right to health care, 111
Risk adjustment, 65
Robert Wood Johnson Foundation, 74–75, 122

Safran-Norton, Clare, 301–302, 303, 305, 314, 316
Salinger, Julie, 319, 322, 326
Satin, David G., 318
at interdisciplinary care conference, 302, 305–306, 308–309, 312–317
on interdisciplinary gerontology applied to professional practice, 330, 331, 335–336, 337
on interdisciplinary gerontology education, 324–325
Sauder, Kimberly, 328, 329, 333, 337
Sawtelle Hospice House, 258–271
advantages of hospice care, 264
interdisciplinary team roles
administrator's views on, 259, 261, 263, 264, 265–271
chaplain, 262–265, 268–269, 270
home health aide, 260–261, 268
nurse, 260–261, 264, 266, 270–271
planning for, 259–260
social worker, 266, 267, 268
volunteers, 263–264, 267
medication issues, 268
need for, 258–259
privacy issues, 267
room/board fees, 265
Schools, promotion of intergenerational relationships, 32
Sciegaj, Mark, 301, 303, 305, 307, 310, 313
SCO (Senior Care Options), 191–192
Security/solidarity value frame
long-term care and, 113–114

racial/ethnic health disparities and, 116
Self-Determination Program, 74
Self-directed care, 143
Self management, of chronic disease, 93–95
Self management education, 93
Semmelweis, Ignaz Philipp, 284–285
Senior Care Options (SCO), 191–192
Senior centers, 200
Senior Wellness Project, 94
Sherwood, Dr. Silvia, 169
SHMOs (social health maintenance
    organizations), 95, 192–193
"Simplicity within the three circles," 178, 179f
Smith, Adam, 278–279
Smoking, 90, 91
Social health maintenance organizations
    (SHMOs), 95, 192–193
Social policy. See Policy
Social problems
    complexity in numbers, 281, 281f
    disregard for, 284
    ignorance of, 283
    invisibility
        conquering, 284–285
        consciousness and, 283
Social Security, 31, 32, 157
Social Security Act, 40
    amendments, 41
    Title XVIII, 92
Social Security Act of 1965, 92
Social security administration, 65
Social workers, 229–230
    applying interdisciplinary gerontology to
        professional practice, 335–336, 337
    hospice care role, 266
    interdisciplinary care, 302, 305
    role on multiple sclerosis interdisciplinary
        team, 258
    views on interdisciplinary care, 302, 305, 308
Socioeconomic class
    industry of care and, 278–279
    power/privilege and, 277–278
Socioeconomic inequalities, elder care and,
    107–108
Spend-down method, Medicaid and, 134
"Spheres of competence," 7
Staffing, of community-based care services, 202
State government, structure of, 273, 274f
Substance use, 91
Suicide, assisted, 138–139
Summers, Renée
    on health care for older adults, 18, 19, 22,
        24, 25, 28
    on improving health care system, 29–30, 31

on intergenerational relationships, 31, 32, 33, 34
Support, for older adults, 151–152
Supportive health services, definition of, 106

Taylor, Albert
    on health care for older adults, 18–19, 22,
        24–28
    on improving health care system, 29, 30, 31
    on intergenerational relationships, 32–33
Teaching, teamwork, 11–14
Title XVIII, 92
Training, of interdisciplinary team, 232
Transfer of assets, Medicaid and, 134
Treatment refusal, 138
Treatment termination, 138

Unidisciplinary model, 6t, 7
Uninsured population, 28
United States Preventive Services Task
    Force (USPSTF), preventive services
    recommendations, 85t–86t, 87
Universal health care, 29
Usual and customary rates, 65

Vacco v. Quill, 138
Vaughn, Melanie, 319–320, 334
Villermé, Louis René, 275
Visiting Nurses Association, 152
Volunteer assistance programs, 199
Volunteers, on hospice care team, 263
von Bismarck, Chancellor Otto, 39

Wagner Bill of 1939, 40
Wagner's Chronic Care Model, 93
War Risk Insurance Act of 1917, 40
Washington v. Glucksberg, 138–139
Wellspring Model, 175–176
Widowhood, 81
Workforce participation, of older adults, 158
Working relationship, defining/distinguishing
    factors in, 10
Working relationships, interdisciplinary, 3–4.
    See also Interdisciplinary teams
    conceptual schema for, 7, 7t, 9t, 6f–10f
    history/theory of, 5–11, 7t, 6f–10f
    tension in, 6

Yacker, Charlotte, 20, 26
Young adults, 30, 31, 32–33